Slow Kill

EVERY MEAL MATTERS

Dr Rodney Lopez
MBBS (University of Sydney), GradCertNutriMed (RMIT)

Self-Published: Print-On-Demand

Printed in Australia

Educational intent

This publication is to be strictly regarded as an educational tool only. It is not meant to encourage self-diagnosis or self-management of any medical condition through dietary, exercise or nutraceutical means in isolation of qualified professional medical advice.

Medical advice is vital

Dietary information in any publication can only be general in its scope. To apply any information to an individual, will take knowledge of that individual's current medical situation, family history, medical treatment, dietary sensitivities or dietary allergies, exercise abilities and limitations. It is thus vital that any information in this book is only ever acted upon after discussion with your treating medical practitioner or specialist. Exercise should never be undertaken without medical clearance by your practitioner/s and only after you have had a functional assessment by an Exercise Physiologist (EP) who is trained to look at any medical or physical limitation you may have and design an exercise program around this to minimise the risk of injury.

Accuracy of information

All care has been taken to provide a true and accurate account of the information at the time of publication. However, changes in research understanding may occur, and new findings and insights may or may not impact on the accuracy of the information provided. This information may change at any moment, and the author is not liable for this accuracy as we live in a dynamic scientific world that constantly challenges conventional wisdom through new technology and research lenses. The author intends to make regular changes, and the print-on-demand structure enables this to happen with reasonable ease to ensure currency of information. However, any user needs to interpret the information provided in this context of shifting understanding and ensure the veracity of this information through self-directed research.

Book Layout ©2017. Cover designed by Dr Rodney Lopez

Ordering Information: http://www.a8h.com.au or http://www.nutridesk.com.au
Print-on-Demand publication

Slow Kill/ Dr Rodney Lopez. —2nd Edition.

ISBN: 978-1-7643837-1-4

Contents

I dedicate this book to my extended family, to my daughters Courtney and Caitlin
and a great little man called Jamison

Contributors

I would like to thank my brother Don Lopez for his proofreading efforts. I would also like to thank the following professionals greatly. Through their highly trained, highly educated and expert eyes, they have provided me with valuable feedback on this books early draft. The Exercise Physiologists (EP's) kindly provided feedback on the exercise chapter, and for this, I am very grateful.

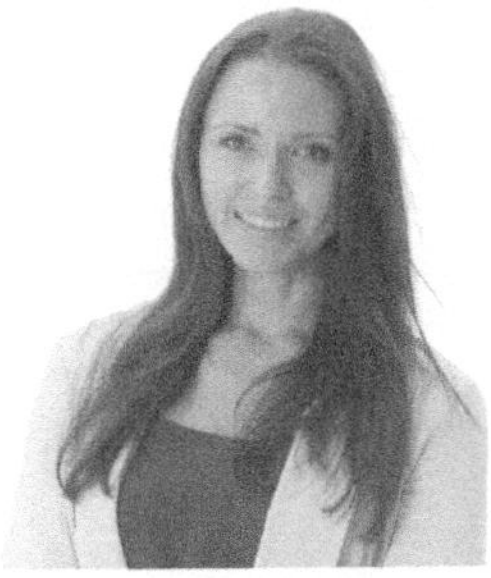	**Lisa King APD BNutrDiet (Hons), Dip Nut, Cert III/IV Fitness** Accredited Practicing Dietitian (APD) **Lisa** has over 10 years of experience in the health and fitness industry, with qualifications in Dietetics, Nutrition and Fitness. Lisa graduated with Class 1 Honours in Dietetics and a Deans Merit Award for Academic Excellence. Lisa works in Clinical Dietetics and Private Practice in Sydney, and has a special interest in gastrointestinal health, behaviour change, the microbiome, nutrigenomics and nutrition research.
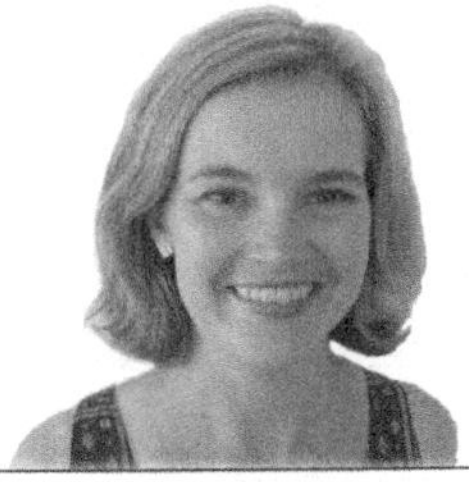	**Olwen Chell APD BSc.Diet Postgrad Dipl Diet (Hons)** Accredited Practicing Dietitian (APD) **Olwen** is an experienced dietitian with 12 years of dietetic experience and is a Class-1 Honours graduate in dietetics who has practised in South Africa, New Zealand and Australia. Olwen is a master trainer in the Stanford Model of care, which is a community-led six-week programme for clients with chronic disease covering a variety of topics.
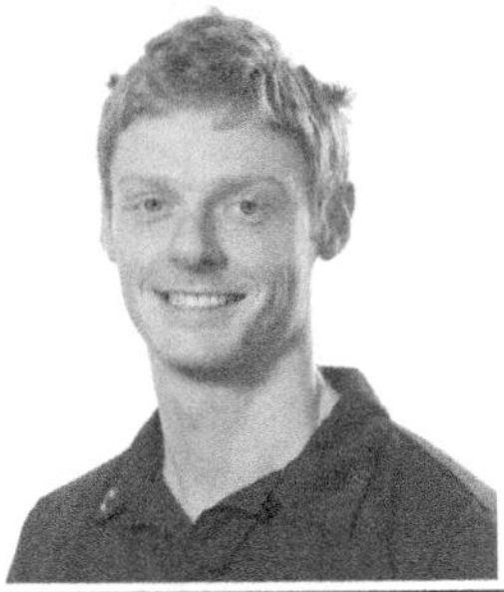	**Luke Dorizas – BSc (Health and Ex) UNSW ESSAM AEP ASCA** Accredited Exercise Physiologist (AEP) Level 1 Strength and Conditioning Coach **Luke** is an experienced Accredited Exercise Physiologist based in Sydney. He has worked with the UNSW Exercise Physiology Department as well as in various private practice settings in Sydney. He specialises in individualised exercise programs for chronic disease, weight loss and sports conditioning
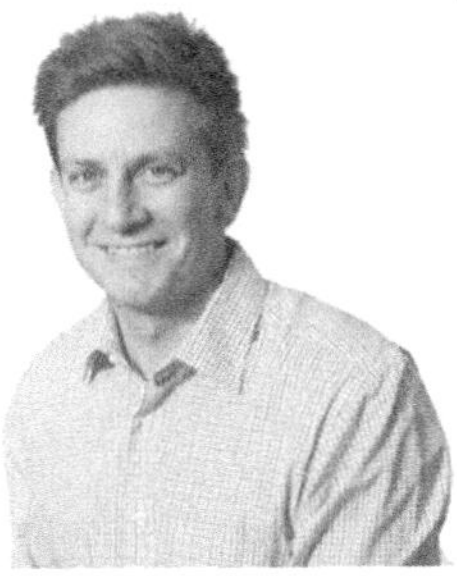	**Brendan Cummins - BExSc&Rehab(Hons) (University of Wollongong)** Accredited Exercise Physiologist (AEP) **Brendan** has been in the industry for more than 14 years and currently runs an Exercise Physiology business based in Sydney, predominantly servicing those who require management of chronic and complex health conditions, injury prevention/rehabilitation and improving health outlook. He is a member of the Australasian Society of Lifestyle Medicine and has presented seminars in various forms to health professionals, corporate, and community audiences.

Life is a tragedy of nutrition

—ARNOLD EHRET

Introduction

Just imagine your favourite meal with the aroma of this wonderful food choice wafting upwards to your olfactory consciousness and the sublime sensations of taste and texture in your mouth as you savour every mouthful. This degustation delight savoury or dessert is no doubt occurring in the presence of enjoyable company with either friends or family, making this meal even more delightful. This lovely sensory experience is however very short-lived. It is enjoyed fleetingly and essentially over minutes, but the effects of this one meal on your blood glucose and blood fat levels will linger in your bloodstream for 6 hours or more.

In fact, there are many changes in your blood after eating that goes beyond just elevated glucose or fat levels, and collectively these changes are termed **postprandial dysmetabolism**. These are the destructive postprandial (after-eating) effects that persist in your blood and body long after that oh so brief, and yet enjoyable eating experience is forgotten. But this is an ongoing process as you need to eat to live and so the next meal is not too far away on the horizon when the process continues, meal-after-meal over your lifetime.

It is highly unlikely that anyone apart from the boffins of nutrition will acknowledge that food can be so damaging and ultimately deadly over a lifetime of consumption, but this is an undeniable fact of life!

We eat to live but the very thing that keeps us alive, food, damages us! Food is nothing more than an amalgam of dietary chemicals that will need to be broken down into energy or where the nutrient components are used to build cell architecture, functionality, receptors, neurotransmitters and cell signalling molecules.

In the process of creating energy from food or using food components to build cellular structures, free radicals (atoms, molecules or ions with unpaired electrons) and reactive oxygen species (ROS) are released causing damaging effects on cell components and proteins and subsequent inflammation throughout your body. However, this is not the only way that food harms you as you will soon find out. This cellular and organ damage is not noticeable or even felt after just one meal although some meals in the wrong individual can kill during or soon after eating and I will show you how and this has nothing to do with an allergy.

This food-related damage is cumulative over your lifetime. It ages you incrementally and increases your risk of obesity, heart disease, vascular damage, diabetes, dementia and a range of cancers. Unhealthy diets can lead to telomere shortening. Telomeres are the 'shoelaces' at the ends of chromosomes that will ultimately shorten and limit cell division. Telomeres are an excellent marker of health and reflect the damaging effects of bad diets or destructive environmental factors through telomere shortening. Telomeres will be discussed further in this book.

There needs to be a change not only in mindset but knowledge as well about the dangers of food no matter how healthy you perceive that food to be.

ALL food ultimately damages you. Your meal composition is a critical factor in determining the extent of food-related damage caused by every meal you consume!

This book provides you with that detailed understanding of the damaging effects of food and how to avoid this ongoing and cumulative damage over your lifespan. This insidious process is the 'Slow-Kill' that I am talking about in this book. Control how rapidly you age by controlling your meal composition.

Decades of medical and nutritional knowledge enables me to see clearly how these food-related effects lead to chronic illness and premature death which, to a large extent, are eminently preventable.

Truth is emerging through all that dietary 'noise' out there.

The key to a long healthspan and looking far younger than your years is to understand **how** food damages your body meal-by-meal. The composition of each meal and the quantity of food eaten in the context of your genetics, your age, microbiome and lifestyle will determine how strong an impact every meal consumed will have on your body. It is important to know, that your genes are malleable and that you can control gene expression through epigenetic mechanisms. **Epigenetic changes are the result of some possible molecular signals that enable you to turn your genes 'on' or 'off'**. These epigenetic mechanisms are powerfully controlled by food and exercise, and by your environment and lifestyle.

Telomeres are a part of this epigenome, and as such, we can modify telomere length. Use these personally modifiable factors to your advantage! This book has valuable insights for anyone struggling with a serious illness.

So you think you are all human?

You are a walking, talking mass of human cells and microorganisms. You are a part of what is called the holobiome where you live synergistically with a host of microscopic creatures and their collective genomes. You cannot survive in the real world without them.

What you eat profoundly affects your gut microbiome and what is emerging from a scientific perspective, is the understanding of how important your human microbiome is to your overall health, immune system, healthspan and lifespan.

Each meal can alter the gut microbiome! As a holobiont, you as the host live in synergistic harmony with a range of microbiota that also lives in or on you hopefully in symbiotic harmony. It is vital to understand that you are not simply human but a human-microorganism hybrid where these microbial cells outnumber our human cells by a few orders of magnitude and that their genomes outnumber your human genes by a possible 100 to 1. It is staggering to think that for every human gene there are 100 microbial genes in your body.

Meal composition needs to embrace this understanding and that these organisms, particularly the bowel microorganisms depend on your dietary choices to survive and thrive. You are eating not only for yourself but your gut microbiome as well.

Your gut microbiome can change after each meal, and your overall diet will determine the type of organisms that will reside in your bowel. These organisms are also thought to drive your food choices not for your benefit, but for their survival through a range of gut-body signalling processes that are yet to be determined.

What a scary thought that your bugs are manipulating you. This book will let you show them who's the boss! Importantly, your gut microbiome powerfully determines your metabolic response to a particular meal. Two people may consume a meal similar in every respect, and yet your blood glucose may soar to very high levels, and the other person's blood glucose response may be far lower and less damaging with that identical meal.

I hope this book inspires you to take action to increase your healthspan, look young, lean and fit through your lifetime and to stay strong for as long as you can.

Dr Rodney Lopez MBBS (Sydney University) GradCertNutriMed (RMIT)

CHAPTER 1

The triage theory of nutrition

Individuals who only eat out of habit, preference or taste without giving any consideration at all to meal composition, face a bleak future regarding their health. Let's face it, how many individuals know the exact composition of the meals they eat regarding nutritional adequacy?

There are many nutritional elements that need to be in place that are critical to your short and long-term health outcomes, and these should never be left to chance. From consuming all your essential amino acids to having enough energy to drive cellular processes to the myriad number of vitamins, minerals, essential fatty acids, fibre, choline and trace elements you need daily to keep you alive and to keep your cellular processes ticking along. You also need all the phytochemicals necessary for hormesis and health, and yet all of these essential elements are often never considered in the context of meal adequacy.

Professor Bruce Ames, a clever professor of Biochemistry and Molecular Biology Emeritus at the University of California Berkley, has come up with a very clever theory, known as the 'Triage Theory of Nutrition'. This theory states that when there is a shortage of nutrients consumed by an individual, the body will allocate these nutrients to specific organs with the aim of short-term survival at the expense of long-term health and longevity. Prof Ames stated in an interview that:

"There's a known triage between organs. If you're short of iron, you take it out of the liver before you take it out of the heart because if you take it out of the heart, you're dead. And one of the things that's long-term is DNA damage, which doesn't show up as cancer for 20 years — so to hell with it if you're starving." (Downey, Edmonds 2001)

So *'to hell with it if you're starving'* simply means that your body is concerned with the 'here and now' not the distant future possibility of cancer. With starvation pressures, you are in fact facing an existential threat right here and right now and thus your body needs to take preemptive action to sustain life currently.

So this was a forceful and beautifully put statement on the importance of shuffling around micronutrients to keep an individual alive if there is a shortage of nutrient resources (famine pressures). Micronutrient deficiencies put you at risk of DNA damage and cancer long-term. Micronutrient deficiencies are absolutely commonplace in Western populations where bucketloads of calorie-rich and micronutrient-poor foods are consumed throughout the day!

The micronutrient shuffle

So what happens when you do not have enough of a particular nutrient? It is estimated that there are 37.2 trillion cells in the body (Bianconi, Piovesan et al. 2013). Each of these 37.2 trillion cells needs to have an optimal supply of nutrients to function efficiently and effectively. If you have a low-level intake of let's say, the nine essential amino acids, then any cell lacking these particular amino acids cannot produce (synthesise) proteins because even one amino acid substituted for another can change the character of a particular protein in many ways and make it non-functional. Anything classified as 'essential' in the body means that the body cannot produce it and thus requires this nutrient component from food.

There are 14 essential minerals, 13 universally recognised vitamins, six macro-minerals (Sodium, Calcium, Magnesium, Potassium, Chloride and Phosphorus), nine trace minerals (Chromium, Copper, Iodine, Iron, Fluorine, Manganese, Molybdenum, Selenium, Zinc) and two essential fatty acids (Linoleic Acid and Alpha Linolenic Acid). This was stated in the Merck Manual, the professional version of which is available online.

To this list is added the essential vitamin choline as de novo (new) synthesis of this important compound in humans is not sufficient to meet metabolic needs. So you see that your body needs a very large number of essential nutrients in the diet to simply survive. Some vitamins like Vitamin-A are produced in the body provided that enough Provitamin-A carotenoids are also consumed, and Vitamin-D can be produced in the skin provided enough ultraviolet-B radiation (UVB) is available for this conversion to occur. Your bowel organisms can produce enough Vitamin-K2 provided enough Vitamin-K1 is regularly consumed from dark green leafy vegetables.

Very low intakes of vegetables and fruits predispose populations to insufficient or deficient levels of micronutrients and vitamin precursors. Western populations are found time and again in nutritional surveys to consume far fewer portions of vegetables and fruits recommended for good health.

Glucose is not essential

One thing that is not essential is glucose. We do not need carbohydrates to provide us with glucose hence 'carbs' are not essential because your body can convert numerous glucogenic amino acids to glucose via a process called gluconeogenesis in the liver and your body can use triglycerides which are 3 fatty acids attached to a glycerol backbone. The three fatty acids can be stripped from this glucose precursor backbone allowing glycerol to undergo conversion to glucose in the liver through gluconeogenesis. More on carbohydrates later on. This process of stripping fatty acids from the glycerol backbone is key to fat loss provided you understand the mechanism and the biological imperative behind this.

You will be provided with tremendous insights into fat loss to enable you to lose weight or maintain weight to stay healthy throughout your life.

Let's look at how the triage theory works

The best way to think of this theory is to consider just one very important molecule. This one molecule could be any of the essential micronutrients we need for our bodies to function at its best. If we only have one (1) vital molecule available for the body to use, the body then has to decide which organ system will get this important molecule.

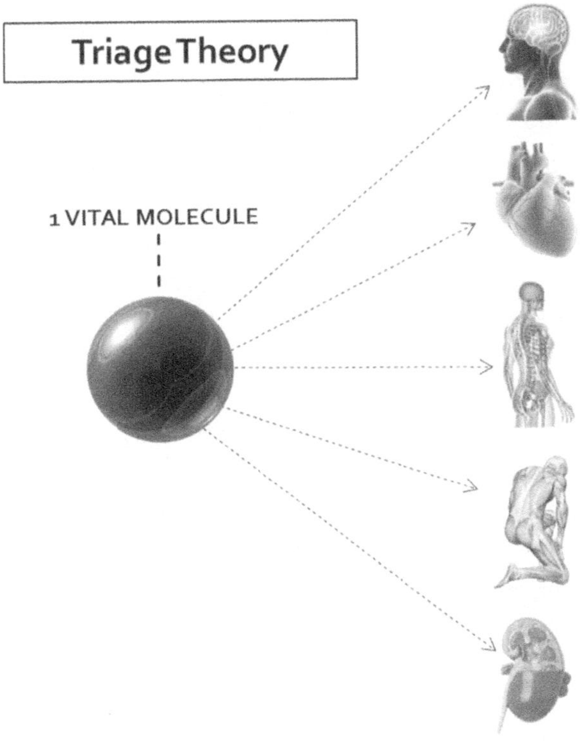

What do you think would be the body's considerations in deciding which organ this one vital nutrient will go towards? The answer is simple; this molecule will go to the most important organ that is critical for short-term survival. Organs like the heart, kidneys and brain are vital for immediate survival and if they stop functioning so do you! Anatomical systems like the bones or muscles are not so immediately vital. These organ systems can undergo slow deterioration over decades, and you will still survive although in a much-weakened state and undoubtedly suffer numerous chronic illnesses as a result. You will age poorly.

Organ systems chronically starved of nutrients due to the consumption of nutrient-poor meals day-in and day-out will shrink and become dysfunctional eventually. You lose lean muscle mass (sarcopenia), and your bones become brittle (osteoporotic) because limited nutrients are shunted (triaged) to organs needed for immediate survival. Nutrient-poor meals lead to long-term disastrous effects on the body.

This triage mechanism juggling act is a daily phenomenon. Robbing Peter to pay Paul is a precarious act that will eventually unravel with your long-term health ultimately paying the price. Medicine almost invariably focuses on immediate causes of ill health as this fits in with the interventionist model we are all taught in medical school. Less appreciated is the slow and inexorable damage done by poor diets over the long term. The sooner society adapts to this understanding, the better off we will all be.

How accurate is this theory?

As per usual, science will test this theory relentlessly for the next few decades until someone calls an end to the research and declares the theory a fact. However, an important paper on Vitamin-K by Ames and McCann established the accuracy of this concept (McCann and Ames 2009). Intuitively this makes sense that malnutrition will cause a deterioration of organ systems. Do we know this? Absolutely! Starvation and malnutrition are still rife on the planet, and the consequences are well known to everyone.

In Western societies, acute malnutrition is not the issue. Acute malnutrition or starvation becomes blatantly obvious fairly early on in the process so that 'Blind Freddy' can pick this up and deal with the issue in that interventionist medical way that is the hallmark of Western medicine. The irony is that in Western populations, it is a slow deterioration in health and vitality due to diet-related mechanisms of damage as outlined in this book. The micronutrient deficiencies associated with the **Standard American Diet (SAD)** adopted currently in developed and developing countries are killing millions of people every year. A slow kill indeed! SAD can also stand for the **Standard Australian Diet**.

Thus, being overfed and yet undernourished is truly a sad fact in Western societies, which is seeing the relentless march of chronic diseases that may manifest in your early 40's or just beyond.

Intrauterine undernutrition and adult health.

How well-nourished you were as a baby developing in your mother's womb is an indicator of future adult health. Intrauterine (in the womb) programming can determine adult disease. Why this happens is very interesting. We know that in a developing foetus, different organ systems will undergo rapid development at critical times in the growth of that foetus. So each tissue will have a 'critical period' or 'window' of development while in the mother's womb.

Foetal undernutrition can occur at these critical periods in organ development, and this undernutrition will have immediate and long-term health effects for the individual. Foetal undernutrition (or overnutrition) will also affect generations to follow due to epigenetic programming in the foetus which will be passed on to the following two to three generations through the germ cell line (ovarian eggs and spermatozoa). These germ cells are themselves, affected by poor nutrition. Undernutrition and a shortage of foetal nutritional resources is the triage theory in action within the mother's womb.

We only need to consider mothers who eat a typical SAD Western diet who are 'overfed, yet undernourished', to understand how this would affect the countless millions of babies being born today.

Around 50% of pregnant women in Australia are overweight or obese, and you can easily guess what constitutes a good diet for these women. In other tragic circumstances where a mother may be alcoholic or drug dependent, one can only imagine how malnourished that individual would be, let alone the toxic effects of the alcohol or recreational drug being used on the developing foetus, placing the mother and developing foetus at huge risk. All of this once again will have generational consequences.

The nutrition and environmental exposures of the mother (diet, hormones, toxins etc.) seal the fate of *three generations (mother, foetus, the children of the foetus) through* **epigenetic mechanisms**. The father seals the fate of two generations and all because the epigenetic markers once thought to have been wiped clean at conception are still present thus exerting their DNA on/off commands for genetic expression in the foetus and subsequent generations.

To make matters even worse, with poor nutrient intakes during foetal development, the triage system for nutrient allocation favours the foetus by diverting essential nutrient resources away from the mother's organs and tissues to the developing baby.

The Barker Hypothesis

The following findings show you how important your mother's diet is to your health as an adult. Research has shown that undernutrition in the first trimester of pregnancy, causing low birth weight with a reduced weight at one year of age, increased the risk of high blood pressure and stroke as an adult (Barker, 1995).

An undernourished developing foetus in the second trimester that was born underweight, but who had a normal weight at one year of age, had an increased risk of cardiovascular disease and type-2 diabetes mellitus (T2DM).

Of interest, a foetus undernourished in the third trimester with a normal birth weight but reduced weight at one year of age, suffered from increased blood pressure, high LDL and increased fibrinogen that could lead to thrombotic (clot-based) stroke as an adult (Barker, 1995).

So you can see that nutritional event or events before birth can have a profound impact on adult health outcomes. However, most people think that only lifestyle modification in our adult lives matter. Our health destinies have been programmed long before we were born and perhaps the most effective way to determine your health outcome is to look at your mother's lifestyle and diet while you were developing in her uterus if this is at all possible and to check if your birth weight was normal or low. I will discuss later in the book how cardiovascular disease is a childhood disease!

Public health measures should be concentrating on optimising nutrient intake from pre-conception onwards and governments should consider subsidising maternal nutrition especially in lower socioeconomic groups. A simple measure such as this would save society a tremendous amount of money ultimately because, we will move away from the interventionist medical action to a preventative strategy, and this will undoubtedly decrease hypertension, cardiovascular disease and cancers.

In all probability ensuring optimal brain maturation through an optimal intake of nutrients including Choline may prevent mental illness all because we would ensure optimal development of the brain in utero throughout its critical period of neurogenesis and foetal brain maturation.

Iodine deficiency in women preconception and through pregnancy is extremely common where 60% of women in this group in Australia, had evidence of mild to moderate iodine deficiency (Li, Ma et al. 2001). The significance of this is that a moderate iodine deficiency may result in the child being born with around 15 IQ points below their peers. This will place them at the bottom rung intellectually in a world that rewards those with high intelligence. This common micronutrient deficiency has far-reaching effects on the country as a whole, and yet this issue is not addressed with the public health intensity one would expect. A 'clever country', I do not think so!

All the research points to neurodevelopmental delay when the mother and foetus are exposed to thyroid insufficiency. We do not have the technology yet to see clearly how this impacts on the developing brain at the molecular level and how an iodine deficiency can have a profound impact on the brain at the Micro-Anatomical level. But the subtle and long-term effects on receptors, synapses, signalling molecules or neurotransmitters can easily be anticipated. We do not need to see or measure anything to know this must be happening.

That these molecular and microanatomical changes occur is beyond doubt. Unless doctors can quantify these changes through blood tests, markers or imaging, these subtleties are downplayed or ignored to the detriment of everyone in the country let alone the individual who has to live with the often irreversible consequence of a micronutrient deficiency that may have been prevented for a few cents per day. I discuss this further in the chapter on micronutrients and also the emerging knowledge about an essential micronutrient called Choline that may have a profound impact on preventing common mental health problems in society.

Ah, perhaps this is all too logical and idyllic. Cynically I would state that the waste in medical expenditure needs to reach a crisis point where countries are forced onto their 'knees' and financially crippled before real reform will take place. So where does this leave you? Hopefully, your mother had the most optimal of nutrient intakes while you were developing in her uterus, but to ensure your health outcomes are good in adult life, you need to look at your food intake, meal-by-meal to offset any disadvantage you may have had during foetal development.

If you are a woman intending to fall pregnant or you are pregnant, the most precious gift you can give your child and future generations is to ensure your nutrition pre and post-conception is as perfect as you can get it and that you keep your weight near to ideal as you can. Every woman needs to ensure nutrient adequacy before, during and after delivery when breastfeeding will place significant demands on nutrient needs. Supplementation cannot take the place of a good, nutrient-dense, phytochemical-dense and protein adequate diet. This is not to say that supplementation is not important in this circumstance.

Do not become a statistic from easily preventable factors

It is important to understand how micronutrient inadequacies may impact your life. In the chapter on micronutrients, I will outline the importance of a handful of these essential dietary elements and how they have an impact on each other and how multiple biochemical pathways are affected all because of suboptimal intakes of various nutrients.

This small selection of micronutrients discussed is important to you because they are common in society and will at least give you an insight into the complexities involved in micronutrient interactions. I am hoping, reading this important chapter will prove to you beyond doubt how important meal planning is to your current and future health and ensure you do not suffer from an insufficiency or deficiency of any essential nutrient.

Do not become a statistic - Avoid an inadequacy of any nutrient

Supplementation should be a part of your nutritional toolkit to ensure your body has all the resources at hand to function. Chronic ill health and DNA damage are well established, research-backed findings due to micronutrient inadequacy. Supplementation can fill in the 'gaps' to ensure adequacy of compounds critical for health. Your need for nutrient resources can skyrocket if you are acutely ill, taking medications, suffering from a chronic disease or due to a jump in the level of exercise intensity.

Food in the 21st Century is becoming famously inadequate for a multitude of reasons that I will make blatantly clear in this book. Try to have the most optimal of diets as you can but an optimal diet in this day and age is a mythical 'beast' riddled with shortcomings.

Those resistant to this concept of supplementation in dietetics and medicine will be the first ones to fall among their peers from a variety of diseases and cancers and all because of rigidity and ignorance in the face of overwhelming evidence. Medicine is riddled with stories of doubt when faced with ground-breaking findings and treatments where pioneers and Mavericks were challenged from Lister to Pasteur. I am hoping to take away any doubt in the chapters that follow.

CHAPTER 2

Micronutrients in health and disease

You now have a working idea of how the body manages a scarcity of nutrients. Please keep in mind the triage theory of nutrition when reading this chapter on micronutrients. As I have stated, previously, it always has amazed and saddened me that practitioners or researchers in the disciplines of nutrition or medicine seem to focus on the overt, observable and manifest effects of deficiencies on medical problems, but cellular dysfunctions almost invariably begin with even mild insufficiencies in Western populations. These wealthy populations do not have to contend with immediate starvation pressures. These insufficiencies won't show up as a clinical problem or in blood tests for quite a while. These are the **long-latency micronutrient deficiency diseases**. In other words, these slow to manifest deficiency states, damage you gradually and silently over your lifetime, hence the title of this book.

Although some vitamins are produced in the human body, many like Vitamin-C cannot be created by humans, and so we need to acquire this from food. **None of the minerals, on the other hand, can be synthesised in the human body**. It is important to know that the mineral elements used to create life only occurred in the cosmos from dying stars through a cascade of solar fusion products beginning with helium which fuses to form carbon and oxygen with the fusion process continuing to form magnesium and then onward to other elements to the very last element, iron. Iron just doesn't fuse, and so this is the last element formed in a dying star before a tremendously powerful explosion occurs called a supernova.

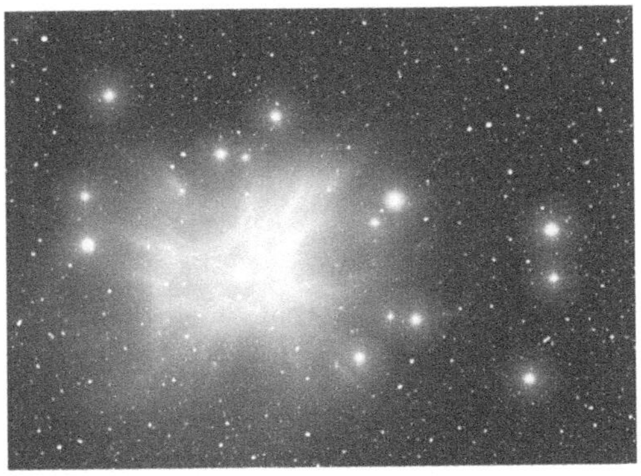

Supernova explosions scatter these elements into the cosmos enabling the genesis of life on this planet and in all probability, on many planets scattered throughout the universe yet to be discovered.

Complex interactions of micronutrients in the absorption phase may compound insufficiencies and amplify their effects on an individual's future health. These effects are often poorly understood or taken into consideration in research or clinical practice. I will describe nutrients that are inextricably linked and the synergies of which will determine nutritional deficiency outcomes. This will provide an important understanding of how micronutrient deficiencies or insufficiencies can have a profound impact on your healthspan and perhaps lifespan. Consider your diet and meal composition strategies when you read this.

Iodine deficiency

Iodine is a thyroid critical trace element and was one of the first to be discovered as being essential. 70-80% of all iodine is concentrated in the thyroid. The female breasts avidly take up iodine and concentrate this mineral for the benefit of a newborn baby.

Many people are iodine deficient and do not know it. 60% of pregnant women may be iodine deficient (Li, Ma et al. 2001). Iodine deficiency places foetal brain development at great risk with the child being born with a much lower IQ than their peers which may put them at the bottom of their class forever as I have indicated in the chapter on the Triage Theory of nutrition. Iodine deficient changes in the affected brain are irreversible! How sad is it that a child's intellect can be so profoundly affected by a micronutrient deficiency when this is so easily prevented and so cheap to do so.

A huge number of pregnant women are falling pregnant oblivious to the fact they are deficient in an element that is so easy to acquire and relatively very inexpensive. When we compare the cost of intellectual disability and all that extra care and attention this will entail, it will be staggering. Imagine the added financial cost and emotional concern by parents trying to overcome a hardwired problem in the brain that just cannot be reversed with the medical interventions that currently exist. This situation is analogous to what parents of autistic children try to do for their affected child in a remedial sense that can be costly not just in a financial sense but also in the price paid emotionally.

If we think of that tremendous need for extra support in the future with special courses and educational care and what about the consequences of an intellectual impairment in a digital, cyber world where intelligence counts, how irresponsible is it to allow this to happen without a strong public health message to would-be mothers. Let's not forget the fathers who are just as likely to be affected, and this will impact on their health and quality of sperm.

I have mentioned that a moderate iodine deficiency so common in pre-pregnancy and pregnant women can result in a child being born with 15 IQ points below their peers (Thyroid Foundation Ltd). Such an IQ level is the bottom of the class kind of lower intelligence in a competitive world where intelligence counts. It is interesting that Australia is regarded as suffering from a 'mild' iodine deficiency (Gallego, Goodall et al. 2010). It is as if 'mild' doesn't matter because you cannot quantitate (yet) the great impact a 'mild' deficiency can cause at the molecular level. Professor Creswell Eastman knows only too well how a mild deficiency can have an impact on the health of an individual. He stated this in the paper he co-authored;

"...we know that even mild maternal iodine deficiency can result in a decrease in cognitive capacity and subtle psychomotor defects in the population." (Li, Ma et al. 2001)

You often find 'gurus' underplaying deficiency states and over exaggerating the possible adverse effects of incredibly low-risk supplementation by stating 'mild' doesn't matter and that one should go and eat that mythical 'optimal diet' to overcome these deficiencies. There are no optimal diets in the real world! We can see how amazingly effective these 'gurus' are in preventing disease when 60 -70% of people are overweight or obese in the population, where 50% of pregnant women are overweight or obese and where at least 60% are iodine deficient in pre-pregnancy and pregnancy.

In this instance, it shows the absolute silliness of asking the vast majority of people who have no idea of what an optimal diet is to go and eat one! Labelling things as 'mild' smacks of political sensitivities because labelling anything as concerning means that you need to do something about it and this will cost money.

Thyroid hormones (T3 & T4)

There are four (4) elemental iodine units that are attached to the non-essential amino acid Tyrosine. This four iodine unit complex forms the inactive Thyroxine molecule or T4. The T4 molecule has to be stripped of one iodine unit (deiodination) to form Triiodothyronine (T3) which is the active form of thyroid hormone, and it is this form that is responsible for the regulation of your metabolism. T3 will determine how efficiently you will use food for energy or whether you will store food as fat. A lack of iodine and hence T3 will result in a sluggish metabolism causing you to put on weight, and this condition is called hypothyroidism. The iodine units are designated 'I' in the graphic.

So with a lack of iodine, you will impair thyroid hormone production, but there is a catch, for you to convert T4 to T3, you need an adequate supply of selenium. Selenium is incorporated into a molecule called **selenocysteine** and enzymes that incorporate selenocysteine to enable their metabolic activity are called **selenoenzymes**. The selenocysteine, in turn, depends on a steady supply of the sulphur containing amino acid – **cysteine** (See NAC in Appendix 7).

So even if you had enough iodine in your diet, a lack of selenium would ensure that you cannot create the active form of the thyroid hormone, T3. A dietary lack of cysteine and selenium will magnify the problem immensely putting your thyroid at risk.

Many in Western countries are at significant risk for thyroid disease. These are commonplace deficiencies in populations. It is a known problem that iodine is deficient in Australian soils. Iodine in soil diminishes the further inland you go from coastal areas (Fuge 1996). It is also a known fact that most foods are low in iodine content. Irrigation and fertilisers decrease iodine in food even further (Capra, 2006).

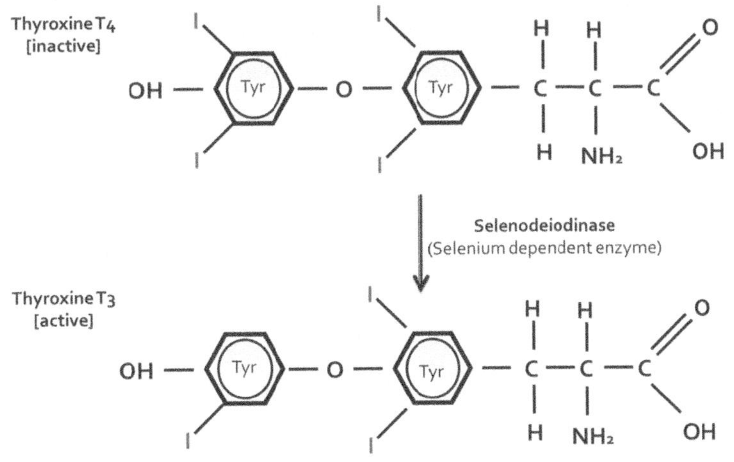

Goitrogens include the sulphur-containing thioamides found in brassica vegetables such as broccoli, cabbage, Brussel sprouts. These can interfere with the synthesis of thyroid hormones. Likewise, the cyanoglucoside goitrogens found in sweet potato and maize can interfere with thyroid hormone formation.

Mineral synergy and interdependence illustrate the complex nature of nutrition. Try not to avoid Brassica vegetables as these have important compounds that assist with the biotransformation of hormones and cancer-forming compounds through upregulation of Phase-1 and Phase-II liver detoxification enzymes. What you can do is to ensure you aim for nutrient density and food variety in the meals you choose as this can override any excesses or negatives in food composition. Eating the same foods every day may result in toxicities and deficiencies that you have never considered.

Hashimoto's Disease: A common autoimmune condition

Hashimoto's Disease is a common autoimmune disease affecting up to 10 percent of females and 2 percent of men (Nordio & Pajalich, 2013). The autoimmune process destroys the thyroid through the body's immune system (antibodies) attacking the gland. This autoimmune attack will make the person ultimately hypothyroid and dependent upon taking Thyroxine a T4 thyroid hormone medication for the rest of their lives. Unless treated, hypothyroidism will cause many metabolic effects from an increase in blood cholesterol and thus cardiovascular risk, to hair loss, weight gain, loss of the outer third of their eyebrows, to a sluggish metabolism, swollen ankles and sensitivity to cold weather.

Even a mild deficiency in selenium may trigger Hashimoto's Disease

A gold standard, double-blind, placebo-controlled trial, has shed some light on the causation of Hashimoto's disease. It is stated that even mild selenium deficiency may impair glutathione peroxidase (GPx) an enzyme extremely important to dampen down oxidative stress in the thyroid gland. Remember, all organs are a hive of activity, producing energy or synthesising proteins or hormones and a myriad number of other structural or signalling molecules including intrinsic antioxidant enzymes like GPx to help neutralise (quench) the free radicals generated by all this high-level metabolic activity.

Without enough selenium, the production of glutathione peroxidase a selenium-containing enzyme is diminished allowing unchecked free radicals to damage cells within an organ or gland. If you take Thyroxine (T4), you still have to convert this to T3 the active form which you have seen from the T4 →T3 conversion graphic, requires a selenium-dependent enzyme called Selenodeiodinase.

Where do you get your required selenium? Do you even consider this in your daily dietary intake? What about iodine? Where do you get this element? Do you consume the RDI (Recommended Dietary Intake also known as RDA in the USA), for iodine on a daily basis?

As the thyroid falters, a signalling hormone from the pituitary called TSH sends out a message to your thyroid gland to demand more T3 from T4, and as the thyroid continues to fail, higher and higher TSH is released as if to demand that the thyroid does something urgently to supply the T3 needed by the body.

What I posit is that with rising TSH levels and the fact that the thyroid gland cannot produce T4 and then T3 due to iodine or selenium deficiency or both, the TSH acts like a powerful stressor on the thyroid gland causing apoptosis (cell death) with the consequent release of cellular proteins that stimulate the immune system, increasing the risk of autoimmunity.

Ensuring an optimal intake of iodine and selenium may just halt this process and prevent Hashimoto's Disease if autoantibodies are discovered early in the disease and supplementation implemented. A pregnant woman deficient in iodine is put in harm's way because Mother Nature will ensure the foetus gets all the iodine it needs, at the expense of the mother as discussed under the Triage Theory of Nutrition. If the mother is also selenium deficient and lacks sulphur containing compounds, like cysteine required for the synthesis of glutathione an important intrinsic antioxidant, it may then trigger Hashimoto's or other thyroid disorders in pregnancy which are not uncommon. Plasma or urine selenium can be measured, and urine iodine can also e be determined easily in a random urine specimen done on the spot in a GP's office. These test should be carried out in pregnant women who are showing signs of thyroid gland disease.

A simple intervention of ensuring adequate micronutrient intakes may be all it takes. It is interesting that one study looked at supplementing with both selenium and **myoinositol**, a compound that can be created from glucose in the body. This intervention helped to significantly decrease thyroid antibody levels in those with early Hashimoto's Disease (Nordio and Pajalich 2013). A logical step for individuals who have thyroid autoantibodies present in their blood is to start a program of selenium supplementation and iodine if deficient. Just one Brazil nut per day would provide a full day's worth of selenium provided it was an **Amazonian** Brazil nut. To prevent Hashimoto's Disease, including myoinositol with the selenium +/- Iodine, is now an evidence-based way to avert Hashimoto's Disease especially in the early stages of antibody production.

Whey protein is rich in the sulphur containing amino acid cysteine necessary for glutathione production, and organic kelp is rich in iodine and many other minerals and trace elements. Simple prenatal supplementation may prevent iodine deficiency in pregnancy. Such supplementation is a safe, evidence-based approach using the gold standard of research, i.e. the double-blind, placebo-controlled trial. It will take a long time for this knowledge to filter through to clinical practice. These simple and very safe approaches to nutrient sufficiency in pregnancy should be broadcast loudly in the name of public health.

Subtle micronutrient deficiencies in a mother may have powerful adverse effects on the developing foetus resulting in long-term epigenetically determined medical problems for that baby as it develops into adulthood. These impacts were discussed under the Triage Theory of Nutrition and the Barker Hypothesis.

Hashimoto's Disease: Do you need to worry?

The prevalence of Hashimoto's Thyroiditis (HT) is high with up to 12% of the adult population suffering from this condition. One of the largest national health surveys, the National Health and Nutrition Examination Survey (NHANES) III in the United States of America, showed that 18% of the population had elevated thyroid antibodies without previously known thyroid disease regardless of age or gender (Zaletel & Gaberscek, 2011). Statistically, this includes almost 1 in 5 people. You have seen how micronutrient deficiencies may cause the thyroid to malfunction and self-destroy as explained above. Unfortunately, this can happen with even mild deficiency! If you consume a predominantly Western diet, the risk of iodine and selenium insufficiency is high due to calorie-rich, nutrient-poor dietary choices.

The second nutrient I would like to discuss is Vitamin-A

From the outset, I would like to establish the importance of Vitamin-A to your health. In a paper titled, 'The effect of vitamin A on epithelial integrity', the authors stated:

*"No nutritional deficiency is more synergistic with infection than vitamin A" (*McCullough, Northrop-Clewes, & Thurnham, 1999)

Not only is this vitamin critical for the immune system to function, but it is also absolutely vital for the integrity of the epithelial cell linings of your genitourinary tract (bladder, urethra, vagina), respiratory tract (lungs, sinuses, nose, trachea, throat), skin and salivary glands. Many children suffer from recurrent colds, and middle ear infections and many adults suffer from frequent acute or chronic nasal or sinus infections, from urinary tract infections or cold after cold due to respiratory viruses. Ensuring Vitamin-A adequacy may just treat the foundational cause of these problems rather than taking antibiotics time and again. Vitamin-A supplementation would be a rare recommendation in general practice.

Vitamin-A insufficiency is readily understandable when we consider that the dietary intake of provitamin-A carotenoids is so very low in many Western populations. Over 90% of people do not eat the required amounts of fruit and vegetables. Low intakes of coloured fruit and vegetables severely limit the intake of provitamin A carotenoids which are the orange, red pigments in fruit and vegetables that can indeed be converted into Vitamin-A, but even this may be limited in many people who are low or non-responders.

Individuals who are non-responders, may not absorb or convert the provitamin-A carotenoids to retinol (Vitamin-A) (Lin, Dueker et al. 2000). Genetic influences are involved, but one factor that is vitally important and yet commonly ignored is how you consume these carotenoids in your meal. Vitamins A/D/E/K are all fat-soluble vitamins, and so are the provitamin-A carotenoids. If there isn't enough fat or oil in the meal, you simply won't absorb the carotenoids and hence won't be able to form the essential Vitamin-A needed to protect the epithelial linings discussed above or support your immune system. When did you last eat a salad with some oil on it or as vinaigrette? A lost tradition in societies!

In generations past, people would eat a salad and pour vinaigrette made with one of many oils, vinegar and perhaps herbs and spices. The oil in the vinaigrette would ensure that the carotenoids in the vegetables or fruit consumed would be absorbed adequately which in turn would ensure Vitamin-A sufficiency in most people. A small amount of oil like a teaspoonful of good oil should always be put into a vegetable and fruit blend or poured onto a salad. However, this knowledge and practice seem to have been lost in modern societies, and individuals, in reality, consume a markedly low intake of fruits and vegetables avoiding anything green and anything that looks like a vegetable. Poor fruit and vegetable intake puts any individual who has an aversion to fruit and vegetables, at great risk of harm from micronutrient, fibre and phytochemical deficiencies.

Children under five years are at great risk because of their legendary aversion to, and hence avoidance of vegetables. Children love white foods like potato, bread, pasta and dairy and this puts them at risk for many nutrient deficiencies. Perhaps parents just do not provide vegetables and fruit to their babies and toddlers because of their aversions or preferences. Is it any wonder then that so many children are constantly fighting off infections and getting secondary complications like tonsillitis or middle ear infections?

Vitamin-A deficiency is also one of the most common global deficiencies and a leading cause of blindness on the planet. Iron, Iodine, Folate, Zinc and Vitamin-A are the most widespread micronutrient deficiencies (Bailey, West Jr, & Black, 2015). It is estimated, that more than 50% of the world's population is deficient in iron, 50% are deficient in zinc, 25% are deficient in iodine and 20% deficient in selenium (Graham 2008). Many important agricultural soils of the world are also deficient in Molybdenum and Boron.

Vitamin-A and your thyroid

Just to reinforce the complexity and interconnectedness of these micronutrient deficiencies once again, if you have a low Vitamin-A intake, this can lead to a goitre which is an enlargement of the thyroid gland. Goitre development is a defensive mechanism to compensate for iodine deficiency, and so a Vitamin-A deficiency in association with a low iodine intake could result in large swellings in your neck called goitres.

Vitamin-A deficiency will, unfortunately, result in decreased thyroid iodine uptake and will also decrease thyroglobulin production. Thyroglobulin is the precursor for the thyroid hormones T4 & T3. Zinc is just as critical for your immune system and is synergistic with Vitamin-A in ensuring a robust and effective immune system. So a deficiency in zinc along with a low Vitamin-A level will dramatically compound any dysfunction in the immune system. Lacking any micronutrient is never a wise thing!

Vitamin-A is also vital for incorporating iron into cells. A deficiency of Vitamin-A, iron and protein (protein-energy malnutrition or PEM), often coexists in developing countries that are highly dependent on cereal grains for energy and protein. Remember, these are also common deficiencies in Western populations. Once again each deficiency magnifies the effects of the other. When does a medical practitioner ever consider the addition of Vitamin-A when they try to rectify an iron deficiency anaemia? When do they consider Vitamin-A deficiencies when they have a patient that presents to them time and again for recurrent upper respiratory infections or frequent urinary tract infections? The answer is almost never apart from that rare breed of medical practitioner that understands that the human body is simply a highly complex amalgam of 37.2 trillion cells in the body, where all these cells are entirely interconnected and dependent upon an optimal supply of all the essential micronutrients to function efficiently and synergistically.

How many antibiotic scripts could be prevented through judicious supplementation of Vitamin-A? However, what you will often hear time and again is how dangerous an excessive dose of fat-soluble vitamins can be. Potential overdose is such an irrational argument. Every pharmaceutical prescribed has significant risk. Does this stop the physician from prescribing them if that medication was indicated? Supplementation by a practitioner who understood these issues and can guide individuals accordingly will decrease this risk. How is this different to highly toxic pharmaceutical compounds that are 62,000 times more likely to cause an adverse side-effect (please refer to the chapter on supplements). Any pharmaceutical has to be used cautiously and guided by a practitioner that understands the pros and cons of using these drugs. This is no different to a supplement!

Reductionist thinking - The small versus big picture

I am a classically trained medical practitioner from Sydney University, and as a medical practitioner, I was taught a reductionist and interventionist model of disease causation and control. It is not to say that this reductionist model does not have its place in treating illness, as it does, and you may one day depend on this to save your life if you ever suffer a severe traumatic injury, a severe infection or a metabolic problem that needs absolute urgent intervention.

However a much more enlightened approach would be to use a preventative or integrative approach for chronic disease states that by stealth sneaks up on an individual and where preventative measures early in the piece, can prevent future medical disasters that can change the life of a human being, severely and irreversibly.

Early intervention is key. Using both a nutraceutical and a pharmaceutical intervention approach in synergy makes a great deal of sense and doctors need to have these nutritional interventions in their 'tool-kit' when they deal with patients. These are not mutually exclusive interventions! Indeed, they are highly concordant, synergistic and mutually beneficial approaches in clinical care if the same thought and care went into nutritional approaches as it does for pharmaceutical treatments.

There is a sheer lack of nutritional understanding at the grassroots level of medical practice, and this needs to change dramatically and change soon. It is not the fault of doctors at the front-line of medicine but of the system that has been fixated on magic-bullet, reductionist and pharmaceutical molecular fixes as if one single mechanism is involved in the creation of chronic disease states. The prevailing thought is that if you can simply fix that one molecular issue with one magic bullet, then all is well and that chronic illness is cured or controlled! This thought must be so enticing for pharmaceutical companies. Just think about the sums of money involved in creating a molecular fix for say obesity or diabetes two huge problems in society currently. How can this single magic-bullet solution become a reality when the problem with chronic illness is multifactorial?

There are a staggering number of inputs from genetics to the microbiome to micronutrient deficiencies, other environmental factors and dietary and lifestyle choices that have a powerful impact on the evolution of a particular chronic illness. The problem with pharmaceutical fixes is that by modifying one molecular component you modify many other interconnected molecular pathways and this is the cause of many of the side-effects produced by pharmaceutical interventions. Just view 'The Metro Analogy' described in this book which is an analogy of the complexity of micronutrient and molecular interconnectedness.

On the other hand, you have brilliant minds in medicine that are providing ground-breaking research into micronutrient deficiencies, nutrition in general and cutting-edge research on the microbiome to have a greater understanding of their role in health and disease. A much more enlightened approach to illness is emerging within my University, Sydney University, investing in the Charles Perkins Centre. On their website they state;

"Traditionally, the majority of initiatives addressing obesity, diabetes, cardiovascular disease and related conditions have approached them as medical conditions, concentrating on their complex biology at the levels of genes, cells and organs. While these are important areas for research, the causes and consequences of these diseases are much more complicated than biology alone. These are complex problems that require a new and complex solution which is why we have brought together scholars from a range of disciplines to explore the interconnectedness of our environment, our food and our health." (Charles Perkins Centre, Sydney University)

You can see how minds are changing about health and disease. An integrative approach is the only way forward regarding chronic illness like diabetes or heart disease, many cancers, osteoporosis, allergies, autoimmunity, dementia, hypertension, asthma and inflammatory bowel disease. These make up a large burden on the health system. An amazing 6 out of 10 deaths in New York, USA are caused by chronic diseases and responsible for 23% of all hospital admissions and where 40% of New Yorkers suffer a chronic illness. (Health N.Y. 2016)

The problem is the time it takes to change the minds of those who practice medicine at the coalface where doctor-patient interactions occur, and treatment decisions are made. Being conservative in how we manage disease in the face of compelling new evidence is foolish! Medicine is never static. It is a dynamic and evolving discipline and rigid minds in the face of inevitable change and new findings, have no place in the practice of modern medicine.

Adapt or perish, would be an apt warning for those in the medical world that cling rigidly to outdated paradigms and who do not embrace dynamic change in a scientific world where the pace of change and emergence of new scientific disciplines in medicine is simply astounding! I am proud of not only the many colleagues I work with but the multitudes of my colleagues that attend diet-related seminars and conferences who know the importance of diet and exercise in health but do not have the necessary understanding to move forward in this regard in a practical sense. These medical professionals educate themselves and move forward.

The mindsets of new generations of young doctors will change because of universities like Sydney University. This university has invested a huge sum of money in establishing an institute like the Charles Perkins Centre. Sydney University will no doubt ensure medical graduates are privy to the incredibly important nutrition-related knowledge emerging in medical science from not only that centre but the burgeoning number of similar research centres sprouting up across the planet in the most prestigious of universities and independent research centres of excellence.

The findings from these research facilities will shatter the way we currently deal with illness.

Running out of our soil and running out of phosphorus!

The human population seems to be increasing in numbers unabated, and perhaps this is the folly of humankind. Each new human being will need to eat and excrete and thus place a burden on this fragile planet. With limited and mostly non-renewable resources, augmentation of the human population will only put us at risk of extinction as a species. Population growth assumes unlimited and infinite planetary resources.

'What If the World's Soil Runs Out?' was the title of an article written in Time Magazine in 2012. This article was written in collaboration with the World Economic Forum and soil science expert, Professor John Crawford from Sydney University who made the following statement:

> *'A rough calculation of current rates of soil degradation suggests we have about 60 years of topsoil left. Some 40% of soil used for agriculture around the world is classed as either degraded or seriously degraded – the latter means that 70% of the topsoil, the layer allowing plants to grow, is gone. Because of various farming methods that strip the soil of carbon and make it less robust as well as weaker in nutrients, soil is being lost at between 10 and 40 times the rate at which it can be naturally replenished. Even the well-maintained farming land in Europe, which may look idyllic, is being lost at unsustainable rates.' (Time, 2012)*

> *"The Nation that that destroys its soil destroys itself" Franklin D Roosevelt 1930's*

That soil is critical to our survival as a species is an incontrovertible fact and yet so little is known about this existential threat. When asked 'Why haven't we heard more about this?' Professor John Crawford's response was *'Probably because soil isn't sexy'.* Whether sexy or not it affects all of us. Poor soils mean poor nutrition and ultimately poor health for every single person on this planet. Chronic diseases from malnutrition as a result of chronic micronutrient deficiencies will soar, as will the cost of healthcare to treat the multitudes with complex chronic illnesses caused by, or exacerbated by these deficiencies that sadly, could have been prevented through better stewardship of population growth and the management of non-renewable resources like soil.

> *'the world that secures its soil will sustain itself' (Koch, McBratney et al. 2013)*

Running out of phosphorus

Soil degradation and loss are of major concern but to add to these woes is the fact that we are running out of phosphorus which is critical for plant and animal health. In fact, Phosphorus is essential for life and is a component of DNA, RNA, ATP and phospholipids which are incorporated into cell membranes.

Without phosphorus, life cannot exist!

The Institute of Science in Society stated the following in an online article titled 'Phosphorus Starvation Threatens the World'

> *"Phosphorus is a limiting nutrient for humanity. Phosphorus is key to the storage of genetic information in DNA and RNA; it plays a crucial role in cell membranes and in practically all energy transactions through ATP (adenosine triphosphate) and other organic phosphate molecules. Phosphates are ubiquitous in life chemistry as they are involved in just about every function" (Institute-Science-In-Society, 2014)*

In 2008, the price of phosphorus ore skyrocketed by 800% and this will put an absolute strain on developing nations as food quality and scarcity will have to follow due to the lack of this critical element for growth of plants and animals. Could this trigger wars? Many a war has been fought for land and resources.

Two of the most avid consumers of phosphorus, China and the United States of America will have exhausted their phosphorus reserves in 50-60 years and it is stated that *"by the end of the next century nearly 90 % of all reserves of phosphates, which are important for the production of food, will be controlled by one country – Morocco."* (Institute-Science-In-Society, 2014)

I cannot believe that the massive amount of money spent on space exploration is simply to satisfy our curiosity. Hopefully, the Moon and Mars will have plenty of phosphorus to keep humanity alive from the existential threat of topsoil and phosphorus depletion. Who needs a massive asteroid to take us all out? We are doing a great job in the name of self-extinction ourselves! For now, the lucky few generations ahead have enough phosphate for our biological needs.

Choline deficiency and Schizophrenia

Phosphatidylcholines make up a major component of cell membranes, and as the name suggests, they need both phosphate and choline to form these compounds. However, because of the typical Western diet, we are not getting enough of choline, an essential nutrient which is classed as a vitamin but technically is not strictly a vitamin but should just be called an 'essential nutrient'.

For anyone planning a child, and for anyone with a fatty liver or diagnosed with prediabetes, Type-2 Diabetes Mellitus (T2DM) or the Metabolic Syndrome, the following information is extremely important but is also important for anyone wanting to maintain optimal health. Of interest is that fatty liver is a very common finding in general practice and the consensus of thought among general practitioners who find this problem, often incidentally while investigating something else, is 'what do I do with this now?' In keeping with the theme of micronutrient deficiencies and the devastating effects these can cause, here is another very new finding of how a deficiency in choline may result in schizophrenia if it was deficient during the critical period of intrauterine brain development.

Professor Robert Freedman is a Psychiatrist and researcher into the molecular basis of mental illness at the University of Colorado, Denver. He believes that choline, a compound grouped under B-complex vitamins and a precursor to a very important neurotransmitter, acetylcholine, may prevent many childhood behavioural problems and schizophrenia if this compound was supplemented in the same way folic acid is in the prenatal period and during pregnancy when the brain is being formed and vital neural connections are created. Choline was officially recognised by the Institute of Medicine (IOM) as an essential nutrient in 1998 (Zeisel and Da Costa 2009).

What is shaping up to be extremely important, and yet often ignored in medical research, is the crucial aspect of ***timing***! Providing a nutrient at the right time in the development of an organ system will determine the long-term consequences in that individual. In assessing the importance and effectiveness of any nutrient, timing as a critical variable should be tested at various stages in the development of a foetus or at different ages in individuals. Not considering timing as a variable, has probably resulted in a huge number of negative findings in nutritional research which then taints the minds of skeptics and holds back valuable insights that could make a massive difference in society regarding health outcomes.

Choline, Methyl Groups & Epigenetics

Of interest is choline's role in homocysteine metabolism and we know that elevated homocysteine levels are very toxic to tissues even in the low-normal range. The other very important role of choline is the formation of methyl groups through the homocysteine pathway (Fischer, da Costa et al. 2010). Methyl (CH_3) groups are an important part of the epigenetic switching mechanism that turns genes 'on' or 'off'. Epigenetics plays a critical role in cell differentiation in foetal development instructing stem cells to form the various tissues and organs at different times during foetal development in utero. You can easily see that if these epigenetic mechanisms are impaired at a time the brain is being developed, then neural pathways would be affected which in all probability would be irreversible.

These quantitative and qualitative changes in neural connections could then determine the mental outcome of an individual. The integrity of cell membranes and cell signalling also depends on choline and its metabolites (Fischer, da Costa et al. 2010). So here is another mechanism that could cause havoc in cell differentiation and development through poor cell signalling mechanisms.

Rarely will one mechanism be the sole causative factor of any illness. Most disease states are multifactorial, and this means numerous inputs causing a defective endpoint. Humans can produce small amounts of choline through the biosynthesis of phosphatidylcholine, but this is not enough for optimal health. The enzyme that is involved here in choline synthesis is oestrogen dependent. For this reason, 80% of men and postmenopausal women (oestrogen deficient) will suffer from liver and muscle damage, but still, 43% of premenopausal women will all have these effects when choline deficient (Fischer, da Costa et al. 2010). A paper that Professor Robert Freedman co-authored indicated that choline in amniotic fluid activates the **alpha-7 nicotinic receptors** in the foetus and that this facilitates cerebral inhibition. This effect of cerebral inhibition implies a dampening down of certain neurological pathways which may help prevent hardwired mental illness states becoming established and all through micronutrient (choline) sufficiency. The authors stated that choline supplementation in pregnancy:

> *"...represents a paradigm-shifting approach to the prevention of psychiatric illness. It was a finding like this that led to the now routine regimen for pregnant women to take folic acid supplements" (Ross, Hunter et al. 2013)."*

Preventing mental health problems

Just think of what it must be like to be schizophrenic or to have a child that suffers this condition. Consider all those dreadful psychotic episodes resulting in the use of medications to prevent them. Choline, through the support of acetylcholine production, may prevent many childhood behavioural problems and schizophrenia if this compound was included in prenatal supplementation in the same way folic acid is in the prenatal period and during pregnancy when the brain is being formed, and vital neural connections are made.

Choline was officially recognised by the Institute of Medicine (IOM) as an essential nutrient in 1998 (Zeisel and Da Costa 2009). What is shaping up to be extremely important, and yet often ignored in medical research, is the crucial aspect of *timing*! Providing a nutrient at the right time in the development of an organ system will determine the long-term consequences in that individual.

Antipsychotic medications can have a dramatic adverse impact on the quality of life and increase the risk of metabolic disease such as Non-Alcoholic Fatty Liver Disease (NAFLD) and diabetes as those suffering mental health issues also suffer from poor nutritional habits, and micronutrient/macronutrient deficiencies and choline will be one of them.

Medications blunt the mind diminishing creativity and energy. Imagine the tremendous limitations placed on the individual with a mental health disorder just to survive in society and the individual's chance to live a full and productive life. Can one simple teaspoon of lecithin before and during pregnancy significantly decrease the risk of Schizophrenia and other forms of mental illness? Ensuring choline sufficiency in pregnant women and ensuring adequate diets in this group may well prevent so many physical and mental impairments in the long run.

Why isn't this being studied intensively rather than worrying about mental health support in the community when simple nutritional measures may decrease the overall incidence? Shouldn't governments look at this in-depth?

Preventative health care may involve financial input initially but just look at the savings long-term not only in financial savings due to the diminished incidence of chronic mental illness, but also saving society from so much emotional pain due to the effects of mental illness felt by everyone in the community directly or indirectly. Choline supplementation would cost just cents a day, but it is not just choline insufficiency that needs addressing we need to ensure the sufficiency of a range of micronutrients and macronutrient ratios. Ensuring nutrient sufficiency in populations will count the most regarding long-term physical and mental state outcomes.

Choline and Prenatal formulations

Two of the most commonly used prenatal supplements in the Australian market have no choline in the formulation. At least iodine is now a well-entrenched addition to these supplements. If schizophrenia or childhood behavioural problems can be prevented or diminished by simply consuming high-choline foods or supplementation at the recommended intake levels, then it is a shame that this vitamin-like compound is not added to prenatal formulations.

In fact, it is irresponsible that choline is not added to prenatal supplements as this is an essential compound and provided it is consumed in amounts recommended daily, is very safe. This supplement like any nutritional intervention has to be tested till the cows come home until sense prevails but pharmaceuticals that are 62,000 times more likely to create a side-effect can be rushed through to populations with the research on toxicity being done in real-time while people are using them.

That this real-time testing of pharmaceuticals is an absolute fact cannot be challenged as in my 30 years of practising at the coalface of clinical medicine, I have seen pharmaceutical after pharmaceutical withdrawn due to horrendous side-effects and countless deaths from complications like an acute liver failure or kidney damage or damage to a variety of different organ systems.

Once again, I am not anti-pharmaceutical as the pharmaceutical industry is simply trying to find solutions to existing medical problems although shonky business is also rife in the industry. What I am against is a ridiculous double-standard where 100's of thousands of critical adverse events can occur due to pharmaceuticals for various reasons, but if just one liver-related injury is due to a supplement, then this makes front-page news in medical newspapers as if the world is coming to an end.

It is known that men need a higher choline requirement than postmenopausal women and that postmenopausal women need a higher choline intake than premenopausal women (Zeisel 2004). As fate would have it, the National Health and Nutrition Examination Survey (NHANES) in 2005, found that only 2% of postmenopausal women consumed the recommended daily intake of choline.

Choline requirements

When rat pups were given supplemental choline during development in utero or during the second week of life, they had lifelong memory enhancement (Zeisel 2004).

> *"Foods highest in total choline concentrations per 100g were beef liver (418 mg), chicken liver (290 mg), and eggs (251 mg) (Zeisel 2004)."*

Wheat germ is also high in choline as well as lecithin. A small amount of liver is not an issue regarding animal protein consumed, but eggs have their inherent problems as I have discussed in this book. Egg yolk may be rich in choline, but there is a plethora of research out there that challenges the wisdom of consuming eggs due to many nutritional problems such as a very high omega-6 to omega-3 ratio. Is it likely that pregnant women will eat liver? People who are trying to watch their cholesterol levels may be avoiding animal products, and those that consume much alcohol may be at risk of choline deficiency. Strict vegetarians and those involved in endurance exercise on a regular basis may be at high risk of choline deficiency. Anyone that eats a highly processed diet may be at risk.

The use of non-solvent extracted lecithin from non-GMO plant sources that are unbleached forms of lecithin will provide the choline needed for optimal health. Worrying about taking an essential nutrient as a supplement makes no sense if taken at the RDA for this compound. It is no less safe than the plethora of foods out there tainted with preservatives, herbicides, pesticides, colourings or food chemicals consumed daily by children and pregnant women.

According to established dietary guidelines, adults 19 years and older need 550 mg/day for males and 425 mg/day for females with a slight increase to 450 mg/day during pregnancy and 550 mg/day during breastfeeding. Around 5 grams of lecithin (phosphatidylcholine) will provide around 550 mg of choline. Large intakes of choline are not advised as a compound called TMAO can increase the risk of cardiovascular disease due to specific bowel organisms that can convert choline to TMAO and this is discussed further in the chapter on protein. Choline is an essential nutrient, and so the intake of choline on a daily basis is not negotiable as all essential nutrients need to be acquired through diet.

A lack of choline can lead to fatty liver and muscle damage. What we are trying to avoid is a choline deficiency or insufficiency in the prenatal and pregnancy period and early life. We are not using choline as a pharmaceutical agent but simply ensuring that there is an adequate supply at a critical time. **We all need this recommended daily intake of choline**. Have you ever considered this in your dietary planning? How much choline do you get in each meal? One teaspoon of lecithin is all you need per day, and this could easily be sprinkled on salads or added to a blended drink.

Fatty Liver - What is your risk?

Fatty liver is a very common finding in general practice and yet choline deficiency causing this is rarely ever considered. An estimated 6 million people in Australia are affected by chronic liver disease (Strasser and Pattullo 2017) and so in a country of 24 million people, this makes 25% of the population suffering from this serious disease. 90% of chronic liver disease is due to non-alcoholic fatty liver disease (NAFLD), and according to a report by the Gastroenterological Society of Australia (GESA), if you are 40 years of age or older, you have a 40% chance of suffering from NAFLD.

Choline deficiency, non-alcoholic fatty liver disease (NAFLD), insulin resistance and the metabolic syndrome (a pre-diabetic state), is tightly linked (Corbin and Zeisel 2012). Insulin resistance (prediabetes) can speed up the fatty liver formation, and this can lead to cirrhosis of the liver. If you have a large waist circumference then in all probability, you have a higher than normal level of intra-abdominal fat, which is associated with a higher risk of insulin resistance.

Waist circumference measurements that increased metabolic risk are over 94 cm in men and over 80 cm in women (WHO 2008). A BMI of only 27 increases your risk of NAFLD (Lai and Liao 2013).

Choline insufficiency or deficiency will increase your risk of developing NAFLD which can potentially lead to cirrhosis of the liver and even liver cancer (Corbin and Zeisel 2012). With 60% of the Australian population and similar figures in Western world's being overweight or obese, a lack of choline in susceptible populations should be a public health concern, but nutritional approaches to preventative health care that should be a number one priority stay on the backburner. Huge numbers of people, as a result, are put at risk.

For those that love their sugar and carbohydrates like rice, pasta, wheat-based products, pancakes, maple syrup, honey and a range of other sweet products may be putting them at risk of liver injury. They may want to read the study that showed the extent of fatty liver and liver fibrosis (scarring), was 'indistinguishable' when compared to equal amounts of alcohol consumption. This study stated, *"An adequate supply of dietary choline or its precursor methionine (either free or in casein) protects the liver; neither excessive deposition of lipids nor fibrosis could be detected in any of the rats receiving lipotropic supplements."* (Best, Hartroft et al. 1949).

Isn't this amazing that it may not be alcohol itself having a direct toxic effect on the liver but the fact that poor nutrient intake and a lack of choline may be the culprit behind the effects of alcohol. Someone that likes their alcohol may be able to substantially decrease risk by ensuring an optimal micronutrient, fibre and phytochemical intake including an optimal intake of choline.

Gout, High Uric Acid Levels and NAFLD

High uric acid levels that can cause gout are also very prevalent in society. There is a strong correlation between high uric acid levels and insulin resistance and the pre-diabetic condition called the Metabolic Syndrome (Kuo, Yu et al. 2010). In fact, 23% of those with gout also had NAFLD, and the risk of more aggressive NAFLD was higher in patients with gout and evidence of insulin resistance and the Metabolic Syndrome (Kuo, Yu et al. 2010). Worse still, the MRFIT (pronounced 'Mister Fit') trial known by virtually every doctor showed a 26% increased risk of acute myocardial infarction (heart attack) with high uric acid levels (Kuo, Yu et al. 2010).

Too often an elevated uric acid level in an individual who undergoes a blood test is downplayed by the medical practitioner who does not correlate the uric acid level with the ALT level which is a part of liver function tests. Uric Acid and liver function testing (LFTs) are often a part of what is known as the Multiple Biochemical Analysis (MBA20) which also includes renal function. The ALT is highly correlated with fatty liver (Kuo, Yu et al. 2010), and this should never be ignored as progression to cirrhosis of the liver and cancer of the liver can occur. You may suffer from these consequences, long after the doctor that ignored the results has retired or succumbed to the same fate.

Of great interest for anyone with insulin resistance, the Metabolic Syndrome, Polycystic Ovarian Syndrome (PCOS), high uric acid levels and gout and anyone with diabetes, both Type-1 and Type-2, is that fact that just a 6 week supplementation program with choline can help reverse fatty liver (Buchman, Dubin et al. 1992, Arslan 2014). Free choline can help increase the amount of VLDL (very low-density lipoprotein) that increases transport away from the liver (Arslan 2014).

Choline & Bowel Dysbiosis = Poorer Outcomes

It is important to note that if you have a bowel dysbiosis where abnormal gut bacteria are prevalent, that choline can convert to toxic compounds that can make matters worse (Arslan 2014). However, this is not a reason to avoid supplementation with lecithin. What this is saying is that the Western diet is tremendously damaging to the gut microbiota and this has profound implications about overall health and not just abnormal choline metabolism.

Any research looking into the effects of choline on NAFLD will be doomed to failure if it does not take into consideration bowel dysbiosis. They cannot assess treatment modalities in isolation of the effects of the holobiome on research end-points. Ensuring you add choline supplementation to as optimal a diet as you can achieve, and this includes probiotic supplementation, then you can offset this concern and help decrease the risk of dreadful complications of NAFLD.

From a nutritional perspective N-Acetyl Cysteine (NAC) (see Appendix 7) and Vitamin E has shown significant benefits on liver function (Angulo and Lindor 2001). Vitamin E at 800 IU/Day, showed improved liver histology results in those with non-alcoholic steatohepatitis (NASH) a complication of NAFLD (Strasser and Pattullo 2017).

So, you can see by consuming a Western diet and being even slightly overweight with excess fat in the abdominal area, that this excess abdominal weight can put you at great risk for liver damage. Add to this a regular consumption of alcohol, sugar and carb excess along with micronutrient deficiencies such as choline and you have a recipe for disaster.

Tremendously important nutritional interventions that are vastly safer than any drug out there are being ignored to the detriment of millions of people. The potential to save lives or prevent adverse health or mental outcomes through optimal health and supplementation, is enormous, saving communities untold sums of money. Such interventions are being held back for reasons I'm sure you can guess. What a shame!

Did Carrie Fisher die from magnesium deficiency?"

Carrie Fisher, who played Princess Leia in Star Wars, will long be remembered for this movie part in one of the most successful movie franchises in history. Her name was well known at the time of her death at the end of 2016, 40 years after the first film appeared in 1977. She will no doubt be remembered long into the future. The title above appeared in a 2017 Medscape article by Dr George Lundberg. He rightly points out that vast numbers of people die suddenly in the United States of America with a massive figure of 300,000 to 400,000 cases of sudden death each year. (Zipes and Wellens 1998). Fisher's death may have been due to many comorbid issues, but micronutrient shortcomings may place anyone on a knife's edge for an acute event like an arrhythmia when things go wrong.

In this article, it was hypothesised that magnesium deficiency could have played a role, as magnesium deficiency affects more than 300 biochemical reactions in the body. It is involved in genome stability, DNA maintenance and repair, supporting numerous steps during the synthesis of DNA and RNA and also supporting protein synthesis. Even the vitally important synthesis of glutathione a critical innate antioxidant compound in the body that we discussed regarding the autoimmune thyroid problem, Hashimoto's Disease, is dependent on magnesium (see NAC, Appendix 7).

Magnesium also affects insulin sensitivity. Low levels can impair Vitamin-D activity, and magnesium has a role in systemic inflammation. Magnesium has a vital role in ion transport across membranes and shifts of magnesium, potassium and calcium across nerve, cardiac and muscle cell membranes cause impulses to propagate and muscle contraction to occur. So you can see that deficiencies in magnesium could easily trigger off an abnormal cardiac rhythm.

Magnesium is involved in both aerobic and anaerobic energy generation involving the formation of adenosine triphosphate (ATP). Thus low magnesium will affect the amount of ATP (energy) generated in all cells including cardiac (heart) cells. Lowered cellular energy levels and suboptimal magnesium levels create the perfect storm for a fatal heart rhythm (arrhythmia) that can result in sudden death. Remember, a chronic magnesium deficiency is most likely sitting alongside established cardiovascular disease, perhaps coronary artery blockages, endothelial dysfunction and in all probability, exists in conjunction with a range of other micronutrient deficiencies at the same time.

An important article in the Australian Doctor, 2017 pointed out the importance of considering magnesium supplementation in anyone with atrial fibrillation (AF) or strange heart beats (ectopic beats). This is excellent advice for anyone with an abnormal heart rhythm.

Anyone taking magnesium depleting medications such as diuretics, or using recreational drugs and anyone with cardiovascular disease may be far more susceptible to underlying magnesium deficiency triggering off an abnormal heart rhythm.

To hold back on supplementation makes no sense when supplementing magnesium at around 400 mg per day would be very safe with the Linus Pauling Institute supporting the RDA of 400 – 420 mg/day for men and 310 -320 mg/day for women.

How can someone suffer from magnesium deficiency?

This deficiency affects vast numbers of people, and the extent often underestimated. Medicine seems to look for gross deficiencies, and yet serum concentrations may not reflect true intracellular magnesium status – i.e. the amount of mineral inside a cell. A doctor may view a blood magnesium result, sees that it is within the reference range and then pat you on the back saying, 'good news the result is normal'. Such assurance may be far from the truth. The Sonic Healthcare owned, Douglass Hanly Moir laboratory states in their online manual available to medical practitioners;

> *"Less than 1% of body Mg^{2+} stores are extracellular, so serum levels are an imperfect reflection of total body status. There is limited and slow exchange with large pools in muscle and bone, so full replenishment of body Mg2+ deficiency can take up to several weeks."*

With fruit and vegetables cultivated for yield and not nutritional value, there has been an established 'dilution effect'. The amount of minerals and protein in plants is sacrificed for yield and not nutrient density. In agricultural circles - yield is King! It is as if the philosophy is that we just need to produce food to put in the mouths of expanding world populations. It does not matter what the nutrient content of that food is as long as something is put in their mouths.

There is an inverse relationship between crop yields and mineral content of the food (Davis 2009). This inverse yield-mineral content was tested directly through the growth and comparison of high-yield cultivars of broccoli and grains, and the results were consistent with lower levels of minerals and protein in these high-yield foods compared to low-yield cultivars of the same foods grown (Davis 2009). In Australia, whenever you read an article on a nutrient deficiency, a rosy picture is always painted, and you are told to go and eat that mythical optimal diet for all your nutrients.

How on earth can you get these minerals in your food if the soils are deficient and if you are using high-yield cultivars at the expense of nutrient sufficiency? Countries do this not only to feed more and more mouths on the planet but to export food for income and economic benefit?

One paper stated that in Australia 14% of men and 12% of women consumed less than 70% of the recommended daily intake of magnesium. Now, in a country of around 23 million people in Australia, this equates to around 1.6 million men and 1.4 million women having suboptimal magnesium intakes. It is a huge 3 million people in a small country like Australia, with a relatively small population, which is suffering from magnesium deficiency.

So, when you look at the millions just in Australia with dietary intakes of less than 70% of the recommended daily intake (RDI), then this statistic is quite frightening. One study found that for those who consumed less than 75% of the recommended daily intake of magnesium, there was a staggering 76% increased risk of pancreatic cancer (Dibaba, Xun et al. 2015). There seems to be a pancreatic cancer rate increase worldwide, and magnesium could certainly be a significant part of this risk through all the mechanisms we discussed already. This same study indicated that

> *".. dietary magnesium intake alone may not be sufficient." (Dibaba, Xun et al. 2015)*

So you can see that even if you took a great interest in meal composition that you can still be deficient in a vital mineral like magnesium. So food (dietary) intake may fall far short of the mark regarding magnesium sufficiency. We are not living in a perfect world, and we have to consume imperfect food from imperfect soils and imperfect plants bred for yield, not nutritional value. So tell me, where can I find that mythical optimal diet again?

So is a Multi-Vitamin and Mineral supplement hopeless?

How in the world could nutrition ever have an impact on health in the slightest? I often wonder if this statement is the way many researchers and individuals in the medical world seem to think. Such an anachronistic way of thinking similar to the flat-Earth notion or the idea that we are the centre of the universe. Hopefully understanding the triage mechanism theorised for the shuffling of nutrients from non-essential tissues to vital organs provides this framework of understanding of how micronutrient deficiencies can inflict long-term tissue and organ damage. The many interactions between micronutrients when one or more is insufficient or deficient is complicated. Taking a multivitamin may just be that 'insurance policy' you need to ensure you have optimal levels of all the essential micronutrients necessary for efficient cellular and organ function.

The impacts of a nutritional deficiency happen long-term and long before you become aware of it or where it can be measured. You are now aware, these micronutrient insufficiencies and deficiencies are designated long-latency diseases. Short-term (acute) effects do occur such as an iron deficiency from a gastrointestinal bleed but most chronic nutrient deficiency states leading to ill health and chronic disease happen over a long period.

So are multivitamins of benefit or is your hard-earned money simply going down the toilet?

Well, we need a hard and fast scientific, reliable and reproducible test to see if there is any worth. Importantly we have just the thing to help us, and these are your telomeres. I have written a whole chapter in this book on telomeres, so please refer to this chapter for more information on this extremely important and highly researched surrogate marker for your overall physical and mental health.

Telomeres are like shoelace caps at the ends of chromosomes that ensure these chromosomes stay intact with every cell division that is undergoing replication and where DNA in chromosomes are redistributed to new cells. These telomeres shorten with every division of a cell. Telomeres also shorten due to many inputs from poor diet and exercise to poverty and low socio-economic stresses and even living in a threatening environment such as a dangerous neighbourhood (Blackburn 2017).

Telomeres distinctly reflect your state of physical and mental health and also reflect how long you will enjoy your healthspan or the years you will suffer in your disease-span. The disease-span is how long you will have to put up with a chronic illness in your lifetime.

The longer your telomeres, the better off your health and increased longevity. From studies on a range of nutrients, we know that Vitamin-D, Vitamin-B9 (Folate), Vitamins C & E and Multivitamins (mixed evidence) are associated with longer telomeres (Blackburn 2017). These findings were published in the book 'The Telomere Effect' by no less than Dr Elizabeth Blackburn a Nobel Prize winner on telomerase and telomere length.

A study published in the American Journal of Clinical Nutrition (AJCN), showed a 5.1% increase in telomere length in those women who took multivitamins daily and longer telomeres in those taking Vitamin-C and E even in those not taking multivitamins (Xu, Parks et al. 2009). So here you have a measurable and reproducible parameter that is highly correlated with health or disease depending on telomere length and shortening.

Multivitamin Intake - an associated 8% decreased cancer risk

A large study published in the Journal of the American Medical Association (JAMA), and based on Harvard University's Physicians' Health Study (PHS) II which provided data from almost 15,000 physicians. The authors of this study stated:

> *"In this large-scale randomized trial of 14 641 middle-aged and older men, a daily multivitamin supplement significantly but modestly reduced the risk of total cancer during a mean of 11 years of treatment and follow-up. Although the main reason to take multivitamins is to prevent nutritional deficiency, these data provide support for the potential use of multivitamin supplements in the prevention of cancer in middle-aged and older men."*

They found a 'modest' reduction in cancer risk of around 8%, but I think the authors were modest in underestimating this reduction in the real world. In the United States of America, it is estimated that over 1.6 million new cases of cancer are diagnosed each year. An 8% reduction in risk means that 128,000 cancers are prevented! This result does not sound that modest to me but indicates quite a significant reduction in risk. This study did not show a reduction in prostate cancer from the use of multivitamins, but it did not show an increased risk of the disease either.

"Enough is Enough: Stop Wasting Money on Vitamin and Mineral Supplements"

Was the title of an article written to discredit the use of multivitamins looking at studies on chronic disease (Guallar, Stranges et al. 2013). They chose studies on chronic disease i.e. well established, long-standing disease states whose metabolic processes have caused significant damage to cellular, vascular and organ systems, and then decided to look at studies that 'threw' multivitamins and minerals at these well-established diseases in the inane belief that they will magically reverse all this entrenched cellular and tissues damage by a simplistic pharmacological approach to nutrition and long-latency disease processes caused by micronutrient deficiencies.

When these multivitamins and minerals do not restore function back to normal, it is heralded as a disastrous outcome and enough to discredit the use of multivitamins and minerals by individuals. For multivitamins and minerals to work, they need to be used in the infancy of a disease process and not in the late-stage. Micronutrients are used to prevent chronic disease from the beginning or to hinder their progress by rectifying micronutrient deficiencies that drive pathological metabolic processes in the body. This study angered many of the heavyweights in the nutrition research community that included Balz Frei, chairman of the Linus Pauling Institute, Oregon State University, Professor Walter Willet from Harvard University, Jeffrey Blumberg from Tufts University and Professor Bruce Ames of Children's Hospital Oakland Research Institute.

Professor Ames is the one who came up the Triage theory of nutrition hypothesis. These highly respected researchers were staggered by the ignorance of such a study and penned a rebuttal stating that the article;

> *"...ignored decades of nutrition research and diet monitoring of the U.S. population to reach this misleading conclusion." (Frei, Ames et al. 2014)*

The fact that we are purely an amalgam of chemical processes requiring an optimal intake of a multitude of essential nutrients for cellular function is absolutely irrefutable scientifically and yet, the thought of cellular processes becoming defective because they lack a nutrient component necessary to drive metabolic pathways seems strange and alien to many researchers and many in the medical profession. These professionals make it their life's ambition to fight the thought that we require nutrients from food or supplementation for our bodies to work effectively and to avoid disease states. Statistics glaringly show that large numbers in the community do not consume an optimal diet and that genetics, illness, medication use, agricultural practices, socioeconomic and environmental factors all conspire to decrease nutrient sufficiency and these insufficiencies or overt deficiency states initiate and drive many a chronic illness.

One MD who responded to the journal that published the Guallar paper stated:

> *"I recommend that Guallar and colleagues be thought fools rather than put their opinions in print and remove all doubt. The authors cite a collection of poor studies that they claim to be factual. I recommend that patients who find a physician who states that persons receive all of the vitamins and minerals that they need from the food that they eat should find another physician. Enough is enough!"*

There would have to be a vested interest in trying to refute the benefits of multivitamins in the face of all the research out there and the fact that disease just does not occur because there is a shortage of a pharmaceutical in the food supply.

Vitamins, minerals, nutraceuticals or pharmaceuticals all can (and should) be provided ethically to people in need. Low-cost supplementation can obtain major impacts on positive health outcomes. The use of all of these interventions needs to be guided expertly and as such, supplementation needs to be regulated for this to happen professionally to protect people. There is a great need for guided nutraceutical interventions that have a rightful place in the treatment of disease processes.

Micronutrient deficiencies and cancer

A paper titled Micronutrient Deficiencies A Major Cause of DNA Damage by Professor Bruce Ames stated that:

> *"Deficiencies of the vitamins B12, B6, C, E, folate, or niacin, or of iron or zinc mimic radiation in damaging DNA by causing single- and double-strand breaks, oxidative lesions, or both. The percentage of the population of the United States that has a low intake (<50% of the RDA) for each of these eight micronutrients ranges from 2% to 20+ percent." (Ames 1999)*

So is damage to DNA a possible cause of cancer? Without a doubt! Cancer is the accumulation of many errors in DNA through cell replication or other environmental or micronutrient deficiencies that prevent adequate repair of DNA over time, and this eventually tips a cell into becoming a malignant rogue cell.

The feast signal and the AMPK/mTOR pathway I discuss in-depth in this book constantly bombards the body meal-by-meal through high caloric intakes, and this stimulates rapid cell multiplication resulting in DNA errors along the way. This feast signal is well within your power to control just by looking at what you have on your plate.

We must not forget that the Western diet is calorie-rich, yet micronutrient-poor. One only has to look around at friends and family suffering from so many cancers at an early stage in their lives or a chronic illness or look at the waistlines of the people in any suburb to know that dietary intake is not optimal. Trying to have an optimal diet but also realising that foods may be lacking in micronutrients and that a multivitamin is a very cheap insurance policy to avoid potentially damaging insufficiencies makes it an easy decision to supplement a few times a week and I recommend every 2nd day. See Appendix-20.

If there are scientifically researched improvements in clinical outcomes from preventing DNA damage to decreasing the risk of cataracts in the eye simply through popping a pill, then these are improvements in spite of horrendous Western dietary practices because these studies were done looking at how often someone took a multivitamin and then assessed their health outcomes. The researchers would not have ensured every individual also consumed the mythical 'optimal' diet. So these effects are in spite of terrible Western diets.

Imagine the outcomes of a tightly controlled diet that managed to implement all the dietary guidelines in this book including intraday fasting to dampen down AMPK/mTOR signalling for cell repair and maintenance and then, on top of this ensuring an optimal supply of all the micronutrients through a multivitamin and mineral supplementation programme, what would the outcomes then be? I think these would be staggeringly good. I for one do not believe we can get an optimal intake from diet no matter the makeup of our diet. ***Even if you are doing all the things recommended in this book, there is still a chance you could be deficient in a vitamin or mineral because so many things conspire to undermine nutrient sufficiency as I have discussed.***

In a world where the risk of a micronutrient deficiency is high for various reasons discussed, taking a multivitamin and mineral supplement is a small, cheap and easy price to pay for good health.
See Appendix 19.

Can a multivitamin be harmful?

Anything can be harmful if you have too much. It is important not to overdo it by going beyond recommended daily doses, but this may be an issue if you are taking some other supplements at the same time (poly-supplementation). If we compare the risk of a multivitamin in comparison to a pharmaceutical, you would have to take many times the RDA of the various components in the multivitamin for it to become toxic. If we look at a pharmaceutical, toxicity can occur with even mild increases beyond the therapeutic dose.

The body can excrete most of the multivitamins or minerals you take in excess beyond your needs. The fat-soluble vitamins can be toxic in high doses or where the synergy and ratios of the fat-soluble vitamins – A/D/E/K, are abnormal. However, even fat-soluble vitamins require high doses for toxicity to occur and a well-constructed multivitamin formulation will never contain these toxic doses. Many supplements may have similar components found in the multivitamins, and thus there is a risk of going beyond the safe limit if you combine numerous supplements in your regimen of supplementation. Practitioner-guided supplementation can significantly reduce this risk by targeted approaches and simple advice.

One of the problems with nutritional supplementation is that people choose the least costly product. Many products are found to be lacking, and indeed it is often said that 80% may not meet regulation standards (Australian Doctor: 17 February 2017)

The therapeutic goods administration (TGA) in Australia has announced in 2017 that it will perform laboratory checks on complementary medicine and this is a great step forward. By stamping out shonky practices, nutritional medicine can move forward and save countless lives. I feel that the shonky end of this business has tainted the minds of many a person who then uses a 'shotgun' approach to nutritional interventions blaming the whole discipline for the poor practices of a few.

GORD (US: GERD) and Proton Pump Inhibitors (PPIs)

Powerful medications exist that suppress stomach acid very effectively. Acid-suppressing drugs are important medications for those who suffer from severe heartburn due to oesophageal (US: esophageal), reflux caused by a hiatus hernia or in people who are overweight or obese or consume foods that increase the likelihood of reflux such as caffeinated drinks, chocolate, smoking or medications such as calcium channel blockers for hypertension.

I have no hesitation in prescribing this medication to someone who has Barrett's Epithelium, a precancerous condition of the oesophagus that can undergo a highly malignant transformation. However, I am not blind to the dark side of PPIs that can interfere with protein and micronutrient absorption significantly and where PPIs can decrease the acid sterilisation of bacteria and other microorganism-riddled food that enters the stomach. PPIs increase the risk of disrupting the bowel microbiota with pathogenic strains including a potentially lethal infection called Clostridium difficile that can cause pseudomembranous colitis and may result in severe ill health or death.

The first stage of protein digestion is the conversion of pepsinogen to pepsin, and this occurs due to the high acid state of the stomach that is vital in this conversion process. Inhibition of pepsinogen to pepsin conversion can lead to protein-energy malnutrition (PEM) putting the individual at risk of sarcopenia and osteoporosis in the long-term. Protein makes up 50% of bone volume and one-third of its mass (Heaney and Layman 2008). Keeping in mind all your structural proteins from cells to organs is due to the amino acids from protein, thus inhibiting the absorption of protein through the use of PPIs will affect every cell in your body, your enzyme systems and your neurotransmitters, muscles, tendons and ligaments. You are being programmed for weakness and risk many chronic illnesses by the long-term use of PPIs. It is absolute folly, and essentially it is irresponsible, unprofessional and unethical to put people at risk by not discussing these potentially devastating side effects. Remember, the uses of PPIs need to be balanced by the clinical need for these medications.

Iron and Vitamin-B12 absorption can be significantly impaired in a low acid stomach environment (Aymard, Aymard et al. 1988) and zinc absorption (Sturniolo, Montino et al. 1991) may be affected by acid suppression. Interestingly, these studies were carried out on the much weaker H2 antagonists that do not suppress acid secretion as strongly as the PPIs.

Iron has to be in its heme form or in its reduced ferrous state (Fe^{2+}) to be absorbed effectively, and this is achieved through hydrochloric acid or even Vitamin-C (Ascorbic Acid). All minerals need to be dissociated from proteins or food components or from the supplement form taken such as a mineral carbonate or citrate or sulphate combination, by hydrochloric acid to facilitate absorption (Gerber).

Chronic kidney disease and the role of PPIs

To add to the problem of PPIs that are so commonly prescribed and available across the counter without a script is an increasing awareness that PPIs are damaging kidneys. PPIs are linked to both acute kidney injury (AKI) and chronic kidney disease (CKD). The exact mechanism is not known but a paper published in the Journal of the American Medical Association (JAMA), stated that there is a 20-50% increased risk of CKD with PPI use (Lazarus, Chen et al. 2016). Such a staggering figure and so anyone using PPIs long-term, and at high doses - you have been warned! Are we priming our babies for long-term CKD by using PPIs so early in life?

Thus use in the elderly where 30% (or perhaps more), have acid secretion that is already lower than young healthy individuals, are having their acid suppressed even further by the use of PPIs for GORD symptoms or dyspepsia. Susceptible elderly individuals who already have a well established risk for protein-energy malabsorption, are being put at greater risk for lowered protein absorption and utilisation due to suppressed acid secretion vital for protein digestion as discussed and even worsening vitamin and mineral absorption by the acid suppression beyond the already present 30% decreased acid secretion level creating an iatrogenic (doctor-induced) malabsorption state.

In a study of 60-80 year-olds on long-term PPIs, 75% were deficient in Vitamin-B12 (Ito and Jensen 2010). A low Vitamin-B12 puts an individual at risk for a megaloblastic anaemia, high homocysteine levels and central nervous system damage.

40% of the American population suffers from GORD (GERD) (Ito and Jensen 2010). So this is a major public-health problem with the dilemma of trying to find ways to help these individuals without doing any irreparable harm long-term. At least long-term H2 antagonists (Tagamet; Tazac) is not associated with kidney damage. Safer still would be alginates that create a 'raft' of soothing anti-inflammatory gel. Even safer still would be to remove the underlying potential cause for a lot of the reflux problems and that is being overweight or obese and avoiding foods that cause reflux.

Hopefully, you see how micronutrients and macronutrients like protein can be profoundly affected by medications. The ageing process is associated with decreased physiological functions, and diminished gastric acid secretion is one such physiological function that you have now discovered, that declines as you age and this has a natural impact on protein, and micronutrient absorption made worse by PPIs.

This is why the mantra of 'eat a balanced diet' directed to everyone by qualified nutrition 'experts' is absolutely illogical and inane, when factors that include, but are not limited to, age, medications, chronic illness, lifestyle factors (smoking, alcohol, drugs, medications) the amount and intensity of exercise, genetic makeup, and the gut microbiome is never taken into consideration.

Paediatric use of Proton Pump Inhibitors (PPIs)

Of great concern is the use of PPIs in babies thought to be suffering from reflux. These little humans have rapidly multiplying cells for growth and tissue development, and we are giving them powerful acid suppressants that will significantly impact protein digestion and mineral absorption. Once again, PPIs that are given to a baby needs to be used in a specific clinical context and not just a knee-jerk prescription. These PPIs should be used short-term if needed and used after careful consideration!

It is interesting that acid secretion in a newborn is low (Mason 1962) and this may impair protein digestion. In the elderly, 30% or more may have low acid production as discussed above due to both a loss of parietal cells in the stomach that secrete acid as a result of ageing and attrition and also a reduced capacity of existing parietal cells to produce acid (Champagne 1989). It very interesting that PPIs are then used in these two populations of humans – the old and newborn where both these groups have low acid levels and are treated by the most powerful of pharmaceutical agents that suppress acid extremely effectively. It makes no sense and puts these groups of individuals at extreme risk of protein-energy malnutrition and a markedly diminished mineral bioavailability due to the lack of acid in the stomach.

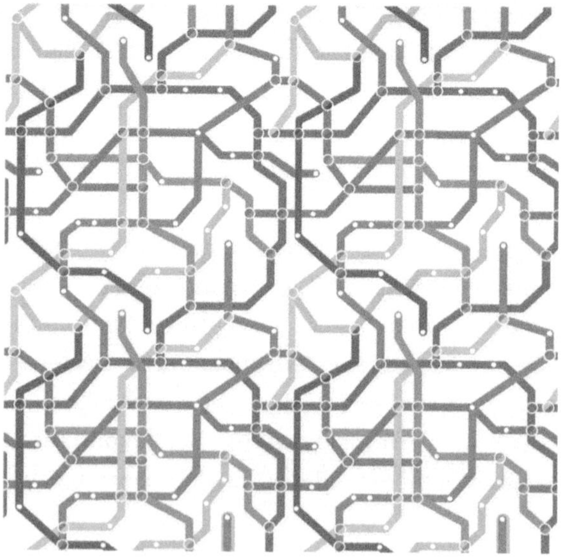

The metro grid analogy

I liken micronutrient deficiencies to a metro grid. If one track gets blocked, it will have an impact on many other tracks that criss-cross that affected path. If multiple tracks are impaired the whole grid (think the whole body), will become extremely sluggish and may even grind to a halt. Certain tracks that become affected will determine which other related (intersecting) tracks become troubled in this maze of interconnectedness, not unlike an urban metro system.

The same complexity is associated with a micronutrient deficiency impacting on cellular functions in a broad array of cellular and organ systems where one system affects another in the network or grid known as the 'body'. One micronutrient deficiency may compound the effectiveness of another micronutrient that could either be deficient or insufficient due to synergistic effects. Thus one micronutrient may be at an optimal (sufficient) level and yet be affected by the deficiency of a synergistic micronutrient as is seen with Iron and Vitamin-A or Zinc and Vitamin-A.

If we have a nutrient deficiency that affects an endocrine gland which produces a vital hormone and this could be let's say the thyroid gland, producing the essential thyroid hormones T4/T3, this micronutrient deficiency and resulting endocrine gland dysfunction will ultimately have an impact on the whole body.

So what I suggest is not to try and pick or choose which micronutrients to use in isolation unless you have been found to have a significant deficiency in a micronutrient due to blood testing as mentioned earlier. It is important to try to optimise your diet with nutrient-dense foods meal-by-meal and to supplement with a broad array of vitamins and minerals a few times a week. For micronutrient sufficiency the composition of each meal is paramount. I will discuss supplementation shortly, and this is not a negative as you will see.

Illogical ideas about supplementation have no place when someone's health is at stake and supplementation is vital in many medical circumstances with dire consequences if these deficiencies are not corrected. Indeed it would be absolute malpractice not to correct these! Just think about what you have just learnt about one essential micronutrient like choline and the drastic effect this could have on the liver if deficient. Just be aware that doctors have a very scant understanding of nutritional concepts.

Dirt poor! Can nutrient deficient soils provide us nutrient dense foods?

If the micronutrient is not in the soil, then it will not be incorporated in the fruit, vegetables and plants we eat grown in that soil. These micronutrients will not be found in the animals that eat the plant matter derived from those deficient soils. If we genetically modify or choose cultivars for yield and not nutrient values, then we will all suffer from declining micronutrients in our plant food and in the animals that eat these plants. A true slippery-slope.

A comprehensive paper published in the American College of Nutrition in 2004 by Donald Davis from the Bio-Communications Institute, Wichita, Kansas and the Biochemical Institute, The University of Texas, Austin, Texas; looked at 43 garden crops from 1950 – 1999. The researchers assessed the changes in food composition of these foods in the USDA database. This study found 'reliable declines' in the following nutrients: Calcium, Vitamin-C, Riboflavin (Vitamin-B2), Iron and Phosphorus that occurred over half a century (Davis, Epp et al. 2004). Other micronutrients not assessed in 1950, but assumed to have declined, included Magnesium, Zinc, Vitamin-E and Vitamin-B6.

With more and more mouths to feed and as the Earth's soils become depleted of their nutrients, then as a species, we need to find ways to increase yield from poor soils. Add to this climate change and warming temperatures, and we have a recipe for disaster.

That the environment can change the composition of our plants is undeniable. Increasing temperatures or indeed increasing carbon dioxide in the atmosphere can cause a change in protein and starch content, and this impacts the quality of the starch produced in grains like wheat. It is interesting that the protein gliadin increases when environmental temperatures are high at 35 degrees Celsius and above, affecting the gliadin producing regions of the grain genome but not the glutenin peptides thus increasing the gliadin: glutenin ratio (Blumenthal, Barlow, & Wrigley, 1993).

It is the gliadin component that individuals with Celiac Disease (CD) react to. Wheat is one of the major cereal grains of the world. There appears to be a spectrum of reactivity to gliadins from the increasingly recognised, non-celiac gluten sensitivity, to the full-blown autoimmune reaction in celiac disease that can destroy the small bowel lining and lead to severe malabsorption and even small bowel cancer if not treated effectively by total gluten avoidance in the diet.

Many third world countries are changing from the non-gluten containing grain rice, to wheat in the so-called 'Westernisation of the Asian diet' (Pingali, 2007). This convergence of third world countries towards a Western diet and the increasing use of wheat in a globally warming scenario can only mean more and more Celiac Disease, or nonceliac gluten sensitivity will begin to rear their ugly head's creating sicker and sicker individuals and more and more malnourished people on the planet. This concern about gluten will affect those in Western countries greatly where a huge proportion of packaged and fast food is wheat based.

To add to the woes of wheat, when carbon dioxide levels rise, the proportion of protein will diminish, and the amount of starch will increase. Environmentally-induced change in food composition will increase the risk of protein-energy malnutrition (PEM) in those countries that are highly dependent upon cereal grains for energy and protein.

Ideally, you want to move away from cereal grains or limit their use and perhaps move away from cereals that contain gluten or wheat which has a high level of fructans. Fructans are a polymer of a large number of fructose molecules strung together. Individuals with irritable bowel syndrome (IBS) are often sensitive to fructans which can cause significant bowel discomfort, abdominal distention and diarrhoea in people sensitive to fructose. Another good reason to avoid wheat.

Many nutritionists blame gluten for all the woes caused by diet and gluten indeed may be a significant problem for many. However, this is not the only mechanism that causes cellular injury as you have found out in the probable causation of Hashimoto's Disease for example. It may simply be a selenium and iodine deficiency that triggers off an autoimmune reaction to attack the thyroid gland and not due to problems of increased intestinal permeability as some suggest as the sole cause of autoimmune disease.

The proposed mechanism of damaged bowel lining and increased intestinal permeability allows food components or intestinal organisms to enter the lymphatics and bloodstream triggering off cross-reactivity between antigens (molecules that trigger off an immune response) and normal body components such as the thyroid or joints and other tissues. This increase in intestinal permeability and molecular mimicry may well be a part of the story, but we need to look at the significance of micronutrient deficiencies in the food we consume as a major contributor to ill health, autoimmunity and early death. The mechanism may be bowel damage leading to poor micronutrient absorption that could be a trigger for autoimmunity.

Blood tests. Are they helpful?

You could and perhaps should go to your doctor and ask for some tests to assess if you have anaemia. Check your iodine status, B12, iron and thyroid function and perhaps hormone levels. It is unlikely a comprehensive set of tests will be approved by a doctor as they are hesitant to order an extensive battery of tests and indeed, governments are hesitant to pay for many important tests. Appendix-3 provides you with a list of blood tests that outline a broad coverage of blood markers. These markers will point to overt signs of micronutrient deficiencies in your blood. Remember, this type of testing does not discover early changes of micronutrient insufficiency; they are simply markers of late-stage deficiency states. Once again, this reinforces what I have said about modern medicine about chronic disease states, that it uses reactive and interventionist actions rather than preventative ones. What we hope for in an enlightened world is that technology has advanced far enough is to find very early stages of micronutrient insufficiencies and stop this in its tracks before cellular harm occurs.

Should we try to target specific micronutrients?

The answer is 'Yes' and 'No'. I have indicated that some tests can be done to see if you are grossly deficient in a micronutrient (see Appendix 3). These gross deficiencies impact your biochemistry and haematological parameters in particular ways. If you had say, a severe specific Vitamin-B12, zinc or iron deficiency, then you would try to replenish these deficient micronutrients as soon as possible and then embark on an optimal diet that is nutrient-dense to ensure this never happens again.

Some books provide a table of medical conditions, and the micronutrients thought to help prevent or treat these clinical problems, but the number of macronutrients and micronutrients impacting on those conditions are immense, and the highly complex interactions of micronutrients make such a condition-micronutrient list a very blunt instrument at best. We saw how micronutrients work is such a synergistic way and how one micronutrient deficiency may have an impact on the function of others. So how do you work around this complexity? I have struggled with this answer for over two decades in designing diets for individuals using the best current dietary knowledge. It is only in the past few years that our knowledge has jumped exponentially in nutritional molecular understanding providing us wonderful new longevity pathways to guide us and the whole area emerging on microbiome research is showing that we need to keep our gut and hence immune systems happy or pay the price in health long-term.

The answer lies in a multi-targeted approach. We need to ensure probiotic diversity, consume a high fibre (prebiotic) diet along with the consumption of a wealth of phytochemicals coming from a range of multicoloured foods. We need to rotate our foods regularly on a daily basis and choose seasonal foods. Avoid red meat in particular as this is a known carcinogen and avoid other animal meats to a large extent, increasing your intake of plant protein but limiting protein to an optimal level and never consuming protein excessively. Include organic sea vegetables (kelp) that can provide a range of trace elements including iodine, 1 – 2 Brazil nuts a day provides us with the selenium we need daily and to ensure a wealth of lignans, gums and mucilage through seeds and other plant materials. All these factors are entrenched in the Activ8Health Plan-A and Plan-B diets. Look at those closely (Appendix 13, 14, 15, 16). Paid advice is available on the www.a8h.com.au website.

These diets like every other diet out there is at the mercy of agricultural practices that favour yield rather than nutrient density. Food nutrient composition is at the mercy of poor soils and at the mercy of all the practices in food handling from transportation, storage and cooking that leads to micronutrient depletion. Our own individual needs will differ from others. Genetic mutations in us may result in the consumption of far more nutrients than someone else. This is made abundantly clear in someone who has the Haptoglobin (HP-2) gene which is so common in society. Those with the HP-2 chew through Vitamin-C in that individual's body. This interesting HP-2 mutation is described in the chapter on supplementation at the end of this book. Throw a chronic illness into the mix and then add nutrient depleting medications, and you have a recipe for disaster regarding nutrient sufficiency.

For this reason, taking a multivitamin and mineral supplement (a practitioner-only product) along with a high-quality, practitioner-only omega-3 supplement should be the least you should do to try to avoid a slow kill due to a lack of valuable micronutrients in your body.

Key Points

- Most of the well-respected diets cannot provide the full range of nutrients needed
- Poor soils, poor agricultural practices, cultivars chosen for yield and not nutrient density, time in transportation and storage, cold-chain breaches, cooking, chronic disease, medications, genetic mutations and higher consumption of nutritional resources due to exercise, ageing, hard labour, pregnancy or breastfeeding – all conspire against us to produce micronutrient deficiencies.
- Micronutrient deficiencies are subtle and may be asymptomatic
- Micronutrient deficiencies cause long-term problems and create long-latency disease states such as cancer
- One micronutrient deficiency can compound the effect of another micronutrient
- Micronutrient deficiencies are constantly being looked for in medical practice such as iron, B12, Folate deficiencies
- You cannot reverse decades of neglect, cellular and organ damage just by popping a vitamin pill. Ensure that damage does not occur in the first place over your lifetime by supplementation early in life
- A pharmaceutical is 62,000 times more likely to cause an adverse event than a supplement
- Pharmaceuticals can save lives in those with existing disease states, but diet and exercise can prevent disease and nutraceuticals have their place in treatment as well alongside pharmaceutical interventions.
- Practitioner-guided nutrient interventions should be appropriately prescribed as per pharmaceuticals, after considering an individual's clinical situation, sensitivities, allergies, drug-nutrient interactions etc.

CHAPTER 3

The Amazing AMPK/mTOR Pathways

Protein, Insulin, IGF-1 and diseases of the Western civilisation

Ensuring you keep Insulin/IGF-1 levels low through dietary approaches described in this book will make all the difference between you ageing rapidly, or potentially developing common cancers often seen in Western populations or suffering a chronic illness early in life diminishing your healthspan and greatly increasing your diseasespan.

Chronic disease, so rife in Western worlds will prevent you from enjoying life in your mid to senior years and increase your risk for premature death. Oh, the joy you say! It is sad indeed to have countless millions of people around the world suffer from diseases that could have been prevented. Once you have developed an illness through dietary mismanagement, you now become fodder for the interventionist machine that is the medical model, which is not only costly but also exposes you to a range of other risks.

The interventionist model becomes necessary because dietary approaches described in this book were not implemented early enough in life to prevent the damage that occurs to your body's multitude number of cells, tissues and organ systems in the body.

Meal composition is your key to keeping Insulin/IGF-1 levels low. Let's take a closer look at the molecular signalling provided by AMPK, mTOR and Insulin/IGF-1 because understanding these metabolic pathways is vital if you want to live a long life and enjoy a long healthspan and avoid medical interventions for as long as you can! This molecular understanding is a powerful guide to your meal planning. Without this knowledge, meals are simply ad hoc piles of food components on plates!

The Laron Syndrome

Laron Syndrome describes individuals who have decreased growth hormone (GH) receptor sensitivity due to a gene mutation and Insulin-like growth factor-1 (IGF-1) deficiency. Growth hormone (GH) is a powerful anabolic hormone that stimulates cell reproduction and growth in the body and is very active in the growing phase of children and adolescents. In fact, it is not GH that is the growth stimulus, but IGF-1. GH stimulates receptors in the liver, and then the liver increases production of IGF-1. It is the IGF-1 molecule that exerts the powerful anabolic effects seen in the body.

So in Laron Syndrome, growth hormone and thus IGF-1 action is blunted, and so you would expect individuals who are born with this genetically determined syndrome are short people and this is the case.

The upside to being short is the huge benefit caused by decreasing this anabolic, cell proliferating effect of GH/IGF-1 and these benefits include a striking absence of Type-2 Diabetes Mellitus (T2DM) and an almost complete absence of cancer in those with Laron Syndrome (Melnik, John, & Schmitz, 2011). Perhaps the Laron Syndrome can teach us about the effects of the food we eat on our bodies and how to avoid disease.

What does the Laron Syndrome have to do with meal composition?

Meal composition can either stimulate the Insulin/IGF-1 axis through the amount of carbohydrate in the meal and the amount of protein in that meal likewise, can also powerfully stimulate insulin secretion. It is for this reason that consuming large amounts of protein in the diet is folly even though there are many high-protein diets recommended out there. There seems to be a lack of understanding of, or perhaps a total disregard for the effects of protein on the Insulin/IGF-1/AMPK/mTOR axis. Dairy is a particularly interesting food that I discuss in more detail in this chapter as dairy is a powerful driver of insulin secretion and hence human IGF-1 levels.

It is evidence gathered from genetic mutations like the Laron Syndrome and other research on small worms called C.elegans (Caenorhabditis elegans), by Professor Cynthia Kenyon that have given us a wonderful insight into how Western diets are killing people through the Insulin/IGF-1 axis. C.elegans is a very small worm as shown below.

Very clever and insightful research into this small worm where a defect in the DAF-2 gene was discovered and studied, showed that this gene encodes an Insulin/IGF-1 receptor (Kenyon, Chang, Gensch, Rudner, & Tabtiang, 1993).

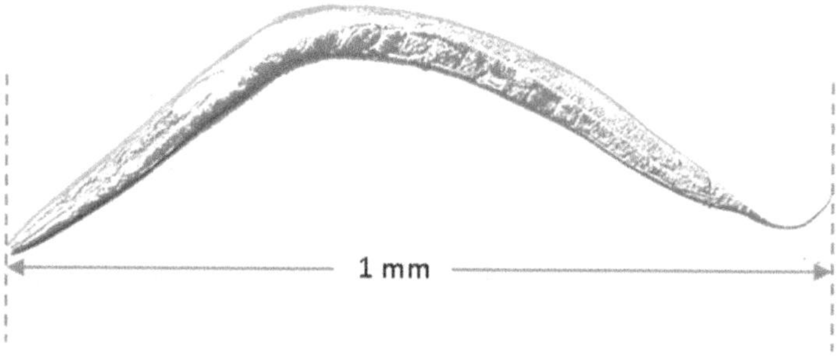

C.elegans graphic - The original uploader was Kbradnam at English Wikipedia (Original text: Zeynep F. Altun, Editor of www.wormatlas.org) - Transferred from en.wikipedia to Commons.(Original text: Donated by Zeynep F. Altun), CC BY-SA 2.5,https://commons.wikimedia.org/w/index.php?curid=2680458

When the DAF-2 (Insulin/IGF-1) signalling receptor is not functional, it allows FoxO, a protein transcription factor to enter the nucleus of a cell to attach to the longevity genes in the cell's DNA. FoXO triggers off a cascade of cell signalling events to ensure the cell is working in an optimal state and where repair mechanisms are called to action. In essence, the cells switch from frenetic cell multiplication driven by Insulin/IGF-1, to a far more subdued state of cell maintenance and repair. Low energy states as in fasting, allow FoxO to do its life-extending work as fasting keeps Insulin/IGF-1 levels low, and so mimic the effects seen in the Laron Syndrome and C.elegans.

So what does all of this have to do with meal composition?

Wouldn't you want to have cells in your body repair any damaged DNA which could lead to cancer? Wouldn't you want to lose weight, have damaged and non-functioning cell proteins fixed and have the cells function optimally? Well, all you need to do then is ensure you create a substitute for the DAF-2 gene defect in C.elegans or the lowered Insulin/IGF-1 signalling in Laron Syndrome by:

1. **Keeping Insulin/IGF-1 levels low** – do this by avoiding a massive intake of energy in the form of starchy carbohydrates, protein and dairy, all of which can produce significant surges in Insulin/IGF-1 after eating. High Insulin/IGF-1 levels are the exact opposite of what we want and the exact opposite of what is happening in C.elegans or the Laron Syndrome. High Insulin/IGF-1 levels are a stimulus of feast and for rapid cell multiplication. Do you want this massive stimulus for cell growth when you could be harbouring a cell DNA defect that could lead to cancer?

2. **Keeping cellular energy levels low** - by avoiding a large intake of food including fat you will keep calorie levels down. We want calorie restriction but optimal nutrition providing us with enough calories for our energy needs but at the same time providing us with all the micronutrients and Phytochemicals necessary for optimal health. Intermittent or intraday fasting does this if you have a solid plan for food intake. Fasting increases AMPK one of the major energy sensors in the cells that indicate an 'energy crisis'. AMPK is an energy signal. High AMPK warns cells that energy levels are too low to commence churning out more and more cells as much energy is required for protein synthesis, creating cell organelles, DNA and other molecules. So this energy crisis signal is one that gets FoxO into action activating all those wonderful longevity genes. We move from rapid cell multiplication pressures to a cell maintenance and repair mode.

Graphic:

FoxO is normally 'chained' to the cytoplasm of a cell. If conditions are right such as a low Insulin/IgF-1 level or if cellular energy is too low to produce things like proteins or cell structures or if there is a danger signal like oxidative stress (inflammation), then FoxO breaks free from its chains, moves into the nucleus and then attaches to gene elements in the DNA. This action then triggers off numerous repair factors as shown. This is your key to keeping cells youthful and functioning optimally and to repair damaged DNA or damaged proteins decreasing your risk for cancer.

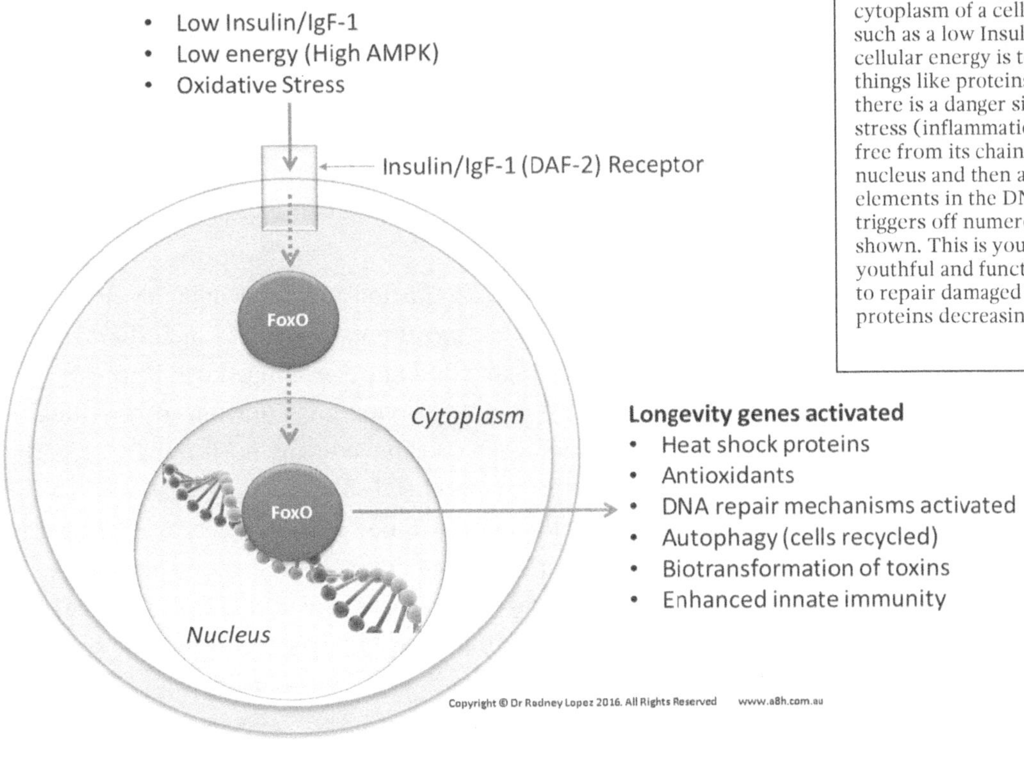

Feast and Famine Signalling

You can readily understand this concept by thinking of it as a feast or famine signalling process. One thing to keep in mind is the biological imperative of procreation and passing on your genes to the next generation. Our biology is hardwired for this imperative and evolution has shaped our response to food abundance with this generational gene transfer in mind. When times are good, and we have an absolute wealth of food around us, Nature's response is to prime us to produce babies and ensure genetic immortality. It does so by ensuring we increase our muscle mass, bone strength, and that our energy supplies are adequate for the task of producing, nurturing and protecting our progeny.

By channelling a good part of that food energy intake to body fat; it makes sure that mum and dad have enough strength and energy reserves, to do all that foraging and hunting needed to support those Super-Energy consuming processes of a developing foetus in the mother's womb and then to ensure you can support that baby after birth. You cannot produce a healthy baby without an optimal supply of dietary energy and nutrient sufficiency.

Feast signalling is essentially a time of high Insulin/IGF-1 levels in the body that drives cell multiplication in the mother, father, developing foetus and developing baby after birth. A large caloric intake will ensure you keep FoxO out of the nucleus. Keeping FoxO out of the nucleus and away from the DNA housed there will ensure you dampen the mode of cellular maintenance greatly and shift the cellular machinery towards cell multiplication at all costs. When we have a mad rush towards cellular multiplication, cell repair takes a back seat in this frenzy of activity. This mad rush to cellular multiplication is the typical pressure caused by high-energy foods in a typical Western diet and the fact that people are constantly eating and snacking and never allowing the body to move into the cell maintenance and repair mode!

The famine signal is also hardwired into us. When there is food scarcity, it is as if the body knows that this is not a good time to procreate. During times of decreased food availability, clever evolutionary design makes sure that high energy consuming processes like cellular multiplication and protein synthesis will dampen down and cell maintenance processes are ramped-up. Nature is keeping us fit and healthy during this bad time (famine), for when the good times roll again so that the baby making process can begin and can then be supported by nutrient and energy sufficiency in times of feast for foetal growth and infant care.

The famine signal is thus one of low Insulin/IGF-1 signalling allowing FoxO to enter the cell nucleus, attach to the DNA and trigger off all the wonderful molecular work it does.

Foods that boost Insulin/IGF-1 Signalling

As discussed, all starchy carbohydrates are converted to glucose in the body, and this includes rice, pasta, cereal grains, oats, bread, pastries, and potato, starchy tubers (yams, sweet potato, kumara and others). The larger amount (larger portion size) of these starchy foods, the higher and more prolonged will be the elevated blood Insulin/IGF-1 level. When do you ever see a Westerner having small portions of anything? Just look at the massive amount of fried potato chips or potato mash consumed in any meal along with garlic bread or other bread along with the chips followed by a dessert or sweet soda.

Having a lot of sweets, sugar or honey will also dramatically increase blood glucose levels, triggering off a high Insulin/IGF-1 response. Why? Because insulin is the main hormone that helps transport the glucose into cells for either conversion to energy in the form of ATP or storage as glycogen and more likely stored as fat if too much starch (glucose) is consumed. We seem to be a carbohydrate consuming society, and this seems to be encouraged by the powers that be with all those grains to be sold and money to be made.

Breakfast can be extremely toxic!

People often start their day with something that comes out of a box. Cereals are the most commonly consumed breakfast and all because advertisements tell everyone that this is the right thing to do. Breakfast in a box is the thing encouraged in any mainstream dietary advice as if starch and whole grains are an absolute necessity. There seems to be an irrational fear that if you do not consume a carbohydrate of some kind that you will die from a lack of energy. This assumption is blatantly false.

There is no such thing as an essential carbohydrate. You can produce glucose from glycerol found in stored fat, and from the many amino acids that can be converted to glucose through gluconeogenesis in the liver, and these sources can easily supply your body and brain with the energy they need. In an obesogenic world where 60% of populations are overweight or obese, there is a tremendous store of energy as body fat in most individuals, so no one is going to die because they do not eat starchy carbs in abundance!

The problem with breakfast cereals, is that they are packed with carbohydrate in the grains. These packaged cereals are then adulterated with highly processed carbs (sugars) that spike both glucose and Insulin/IGF-1. Blood glucose may stay elevated for many hours after consumption. This includes oats which are carb rich.

To add more insult, dairy (milk) is poured over these cereals and dairy you will soon find out, magnifies the insulin-producing effect of this deadly combination which starts your day off very badly.

Think about first principles when you consider meal planning

I often see a battle of the macronutrients and whether a low-fat, high-protein diet is better than a low-carb, high-fat diet with a range of other macronutrient ratios one can argue about. Such distinctions are illogical to me as one needs to consider the impact these macronutrients will have regarding caloric (energy) intake and how these dietary components will affect signalling molecules like hormones after consumption.

That any Dietitian or Nutritionist can think of macronutrients (protein, carbohydrates, fats and fibre), as purely sources of calories and not how they affect many signalling molecules and hormones is anachronistic now. Not all Dietitians and Nutritionists have this errant way of thinking. You just need to ensure the experts you use to guide you are a part of the modern world and current in their scientific thinking.

All calories matter and all macronutrients matter.

Cellular reproduction and proliferation essentially need two important signals as discussed on the next page. Balancing these signals can create a profound effect on the longevity pathways, i.e. the AMPK/mTOR pathways that drive cell multiplication or are dampened down to drive cell repair and maintenance.

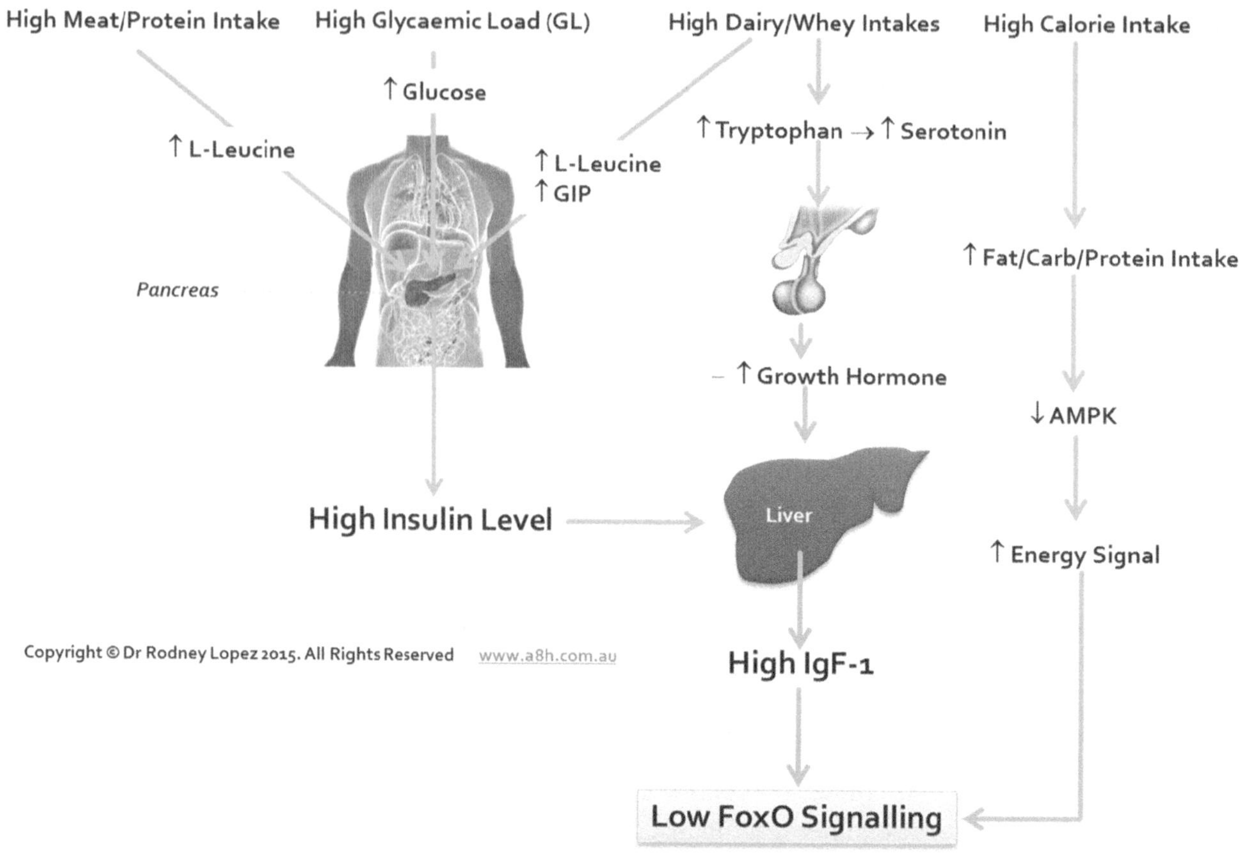

The two vital signals are:

1. **An energy signal** --- This signal is important to tell the body that there is enough energy available for cell synthetic (anabolic) processes to begin. We have already discussed such anabolic processes which include making proteins, creating DNA, producing receptors, forming signalling molecules, forming cell membranes and a host of other synthetic (anabolic) processes to form a fully functional, metabolically active cell. AMPK is a metabolic 'master-switch', and in essence, a vital energy sensor, informing the cells whether there is enough energy for anabolic processes to occur, or whether there is an energy crisis and thus anabolic (synthesis or building) processes should be dampened.
Low AMPK = High energy availability; High AMPK = Energy Crisis

2. **A protein adequacy signal (esp. L-Leucine)** --- Protein gets its name from the Greek word 'proteos' which essentially means "primary" or "taking first place" (Groff & Gropper, 2000). Thus consider protein as the starting point in every meal design - you need to consider your protein component first. You build every other macronutrient component (fats, carbs and fibre) in the meal around this protein content. Without proteins and the essential amino acids that these proteins supply, life is not possible. Every organ and cell membrane is dependent on protein and protein is critical to help form cell receptors, enzymes, many signalling molecules and Neurotransmitters in your brain. One of the most important signals for protein adequacy is the essential amino acid L-Leucine which is a mTOR activator, a critical molecular signal for protein synthesis.

The Master Energy Signal: Let's discuss AMPK a little more

AMPK is a master energy sensor (an energy signal) as mentioned above. For those not familiar with the biological sciences the body has a currency for energy, and this is called adenosine triphosphate (ATP). ATP drives muscle action, speech, cellular processes, repair and cell maintenance and a myriad number of cell 'housekeeping' processes. This ATP molecule is created when energy production occurs from fats or carbohydrates or even amino acids. ATP is thus formed, and as you can see in the image below, there are three phosphate (P) bonds.

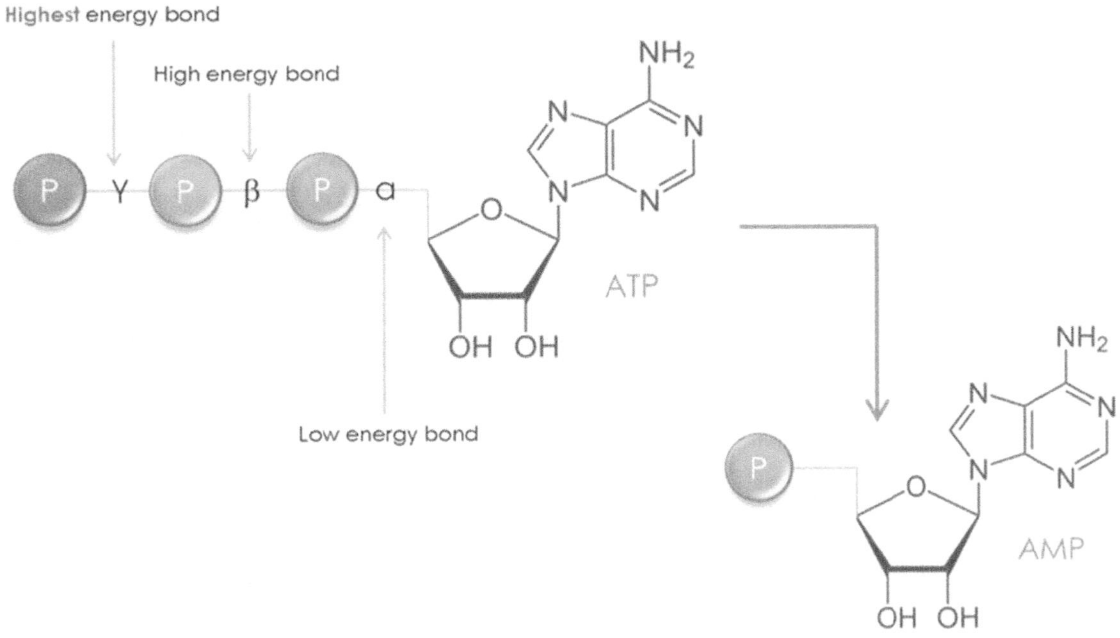

The phosphate at the very end is the so-called high-energy bond and the second phosphate from the end is also high in energy but lower than the first bond. Once both of these are cleaved off to release energy, what we are left with is the very low energy molecule called **adenosine monophosphate (AMP)**. An increasing AMP level is a signal of low cellular energy, and this now triggers off AMPK into action to re-establish the energy balance of the cell.

So how does this all work with AMPK?

The reason why AMPK is an extremely important energy signal is that this molecule is linked directly to the energy currency of cells – the ATP/AMP system. I have developed the machine-gun analogy to get across how ATP, AMP and AMPK work to provide energy and an energy feedback signal to the body. As mentioned, ATP is the energy power molecule, and the two end phosphate molecules are cleaved off by enzymes to release energy when your body needs this to produce cell components or to drive cell processes or produce any muscular movement of the body. If you go to the gym let's say and do an exhausting workout that requires a lot of ATP to fuel muscle contractions, eventually during the exercise, muscle ATP will start to decrease, and your AMP levels will rise. You have moved from a high energy state before exercise, to a low energy state during and towards the end of your workout. As you are now aware, the AMP molecules created are like spent bullets, all the power has been depleted and you are finding it difficult to give that weight one last rep or even run one last minute on the treadmill.

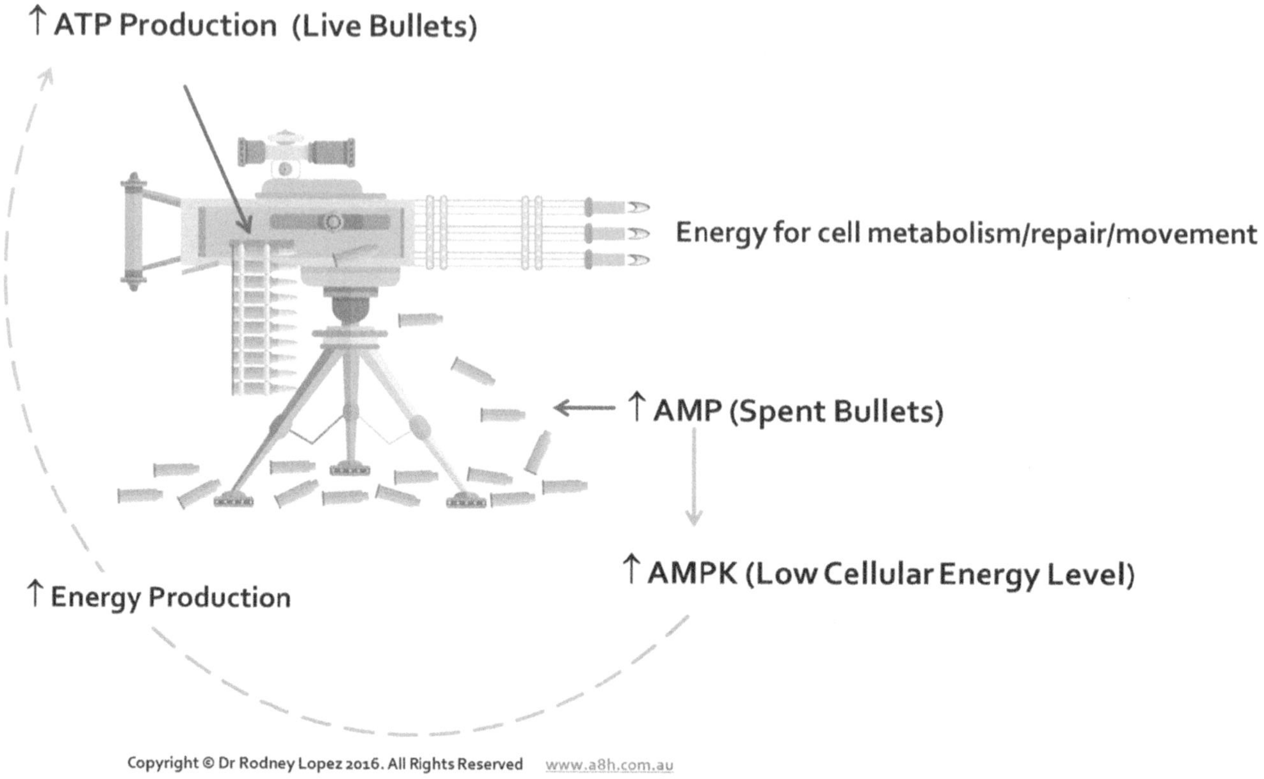

So ATP molecules are like the live bullets ready to be shot with all that power and force (energy) out of the barrel of that machine gun, and this energy is used for both anabolic (building) and catabolic (breaking down) purposes in the cell.

The spent bullets falling and gathering at the base of the gun are the AMP molecules left after the energy from each bullet has been discharged. As the spent bullets accumulate, this signals that we need to reload the machine gun with live, active bullets and this is exactly what AMPK does. It senses the low energy (high AMP or spent bullets) and calls into action processes such as the burning (oxidation) of fats in muscle cells or increasing glucose uptake in cells to create energy and restore the energy balance of the cells to the pre-exercise state.

High AMPK may be ramping up energy producing processes to build up stores of ATP, but at the same time high AMPK levels signalling low cellular energy, will decrease any anabolic processes such as protein synthesis or fat formation as these take energy and if AMPK levels are high, this signals that there just isn't enough energy available to perform the cell or muscle building (anabolic) tasks (Dreyer, Fujita et al. 2006).

Fasting and exercise increase AMPK which then dampens down mTOR action and allows FoxO to now move into the nucleus of the cell, attach to the cell DNA and take effect for cell repair and maintenance. The intraday fasting regimen I recommend in this book is a great way to take advantage of this mechanism of action. The intraday fasting both lowers energy (increases AMPK) and decreases Insulin/IGF-1 levels allowing your body to rest and relax from all that incessant eating that Westerner's engage in for the most of a day.

A protein adequacy signal: Let's talk about mTOR

We have discussed the AMPK energy signal; now let's take a closer look at the protein adequacy signal. Remember, for cell multiplication to proceed in earnest, we need 1) an energy signal and 2) a protein adequacy signal. We are now discussing the important second signal that seems to be ignored by those who propose high-protein diets. These signals do not work in isolation. They enhance certain pathways and inhibit others.

A critical part of this protein adequacy signal is mTOR; a protein kinase complex called the **mammalian target of rapamycin** also known as the **mechanistic target of rapamycin.** It is interesting that we owe the discovery of mTOR to Easter Island. In 1964, a team of researchers from McGill University went to Easter Island which was called Rapa Nui by the natives. They wanted to study the flora and fauna before civilisation encroached even more onto this intriguing island. Many visitors wanted to view those mysterious monolithic stone statues but in ever-increasing numbers. These visitors would change and contaminate that pristine environment.

Many animal and plant samples were collected by the McGill research team including blood and saliva from the 949 residents there at the time of the research project (Stipp, 2012). It is interesting that one of the biggest scientific prizes came from a small test tube of Easter Island soil. This soil sample had a microorganism called *Streptomyces Hygroscopicus* that produced a macrolide antibiotic compound called **rapamycin.** Like all good researchers, they had a molecule called rapamycin and now wanted to know what the target of this new molecule was and hence the discovery of the mammalian target of rapamycin (mTOR). This molecule revolutionised our understanding of the molecular basis of longevity as mTOR has a central role in a myriad number of cellular functions. For those wanting to read an excellent article on mTOR, please read 'A New Path to Longevity' by David Stipp, Scientific American (Stipp, 2012)

It was in 2009 that researchers discovered that rapamycin extended the lifespan of mice by inhibiting mTOR activity. This was a revolutionary finding as it was the first time a pharmaceutical intervention was shown to extend life by decreasing cellular growth and multiplication. Once this was shown, the race was on to explore the mysteries of mTOR, Easter Island's gift to the world. mTOR described as a 'Jekyll & Hyde molecule' responds to energy signals and nutrient levels to either ramp up protein, lipid and cell production in times of plenty (feast) or to conserve resources in times of scarcity (famine).

What happens when mTOR is overly stimulated?

Overstimulation of mTOR is a feast signal stimulus! Plenty of food is getting past those lips into the body and this causes the cell producing 'industrial mTOR complex' to ramp up production of all the 'factory components' that are necessary to make cells. The good times are rolling in with an abundance of food all around and as we have discussed about biological imperatives, this is obviously a good time to have babies.

So high mTOR signalling is priming your body to produce babies whether you are at an age to do so or not. Excessive cell multiplication will occur as a result, and you will get fatter and fatter storing all that energy to look after your brood. It is unimportant whether you can have babies that need to be cared for or not as evolution has created this system to store energy in your body for not only procreation but as a means of ensuring an adequate energy supply to get you through leaner times. Remember, there is nothing special about being a human being.

We are not above evolutionary design or evolutionary pressures. We are programmed just like any other animal, and we will respond to environmental stimuli in ways we are pre-programmed to do so, and this is exactly what is happening when people eat as if there is no tomorrow, and then pile on the weight. I will keep on reiterating this that we need to keep in mind that 60 percent of people in many Western populations are overweight or obese including Australia. Many people may not look overtly overweight or obese but tend to store fat deep in the abdomen which is called visceral fat. These people are thin on the outside and fat on the inside (TOFI's).

The problem with overstimulation of a cell production line through AMPK/mTOR signalling is the creation of abnormal cells. The appropriate analogy here is a factory that produces a huge number of cars for the masses at the lowest price possible. What suffers from this type of business model is that quality control becomes secondary to quantity. It is the number of units produced that counts not how well those units function.

If we look at very expensive cars, and I'm sure you can think of many that fit this bill, the numbers produced are small in comparison to those mass produced and thus quality control now is paramount and every aspect of that car is checked and checked again because people are paying a lot of money for them, and expect a high-quality unit for that purchase price.

Poking a 'stick' at a potentially vicious abnormal cell in the body

Constantly prodding a cell with a 'stick' that is on the verge of becoming a cancerous cell is absolutely daft. We all have as adults an abundant variety of damaged cells that could easily become malignant. Why stir them up?

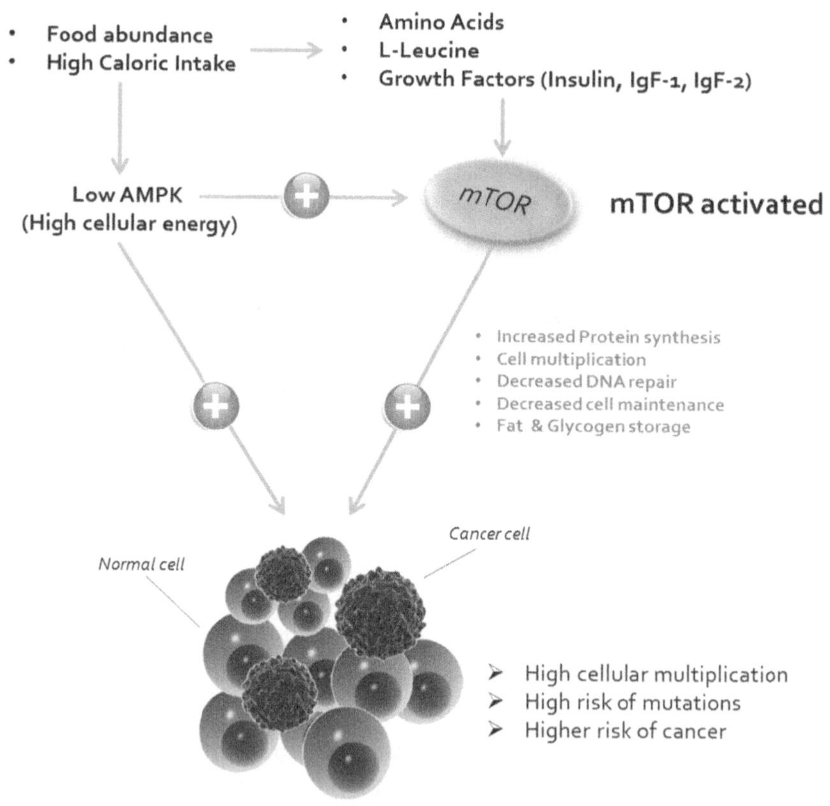

So overstimulation of mTOR is essentially creating cell units in a mass production 'AMPK/mTOR factory' where quantity counts at the expense of quality and the reverse is true when there is decreased stimulation of mTOR because of low energy and low protein intake. If there is a shortage of energy yet an optimal intake of nutrients, mTOR now becomes a factory that produces smaller numbers of high-quality cell units and ensures those units are checked again and again for errors in the DNA or in proteins such as enzymes or structural components and repairs them. Fine-tuning occurs in a low energy and optimal nutrient environment.

However, we are talking calorie restriction but optimal nutrition where we have all the nutrients we need for cells to be created and repair themselves but we are restricting the energy part of the equation that dampens down the frenetic production of defective cell units.

What happens to abnormal cells that are already present in the human body with mTOR overstimulation?

So when you think of all those calories being consumed creating an abundance of growth factors like Insulin/IGF-1 or protein adequacy signals like amino acids and L-Leucine driving mTOR into a cell producing frenzy, that this can't be a good thing for abnormal cells that already exist in human bodies that are too old to reproduce and where this procreative evolutionary imperative being driven by excessive food intake is totally inappropriate.

One interesting study comes to mind regarding prostate cancer. Keeping in mind 80% of the most common cancers - breast, prostate and bowel cancer can be prevented by diet. A paper published in the British Medical Journal stated;

"Diet is one of the most important lifestyle factors and has been estimated to account for up to 80% of cancers of the large bowel, breast, and prostate (Cummings & Bingham, 1998)."

A study in 1986 where 180 consecutive autopsies were carried out on men 40 years and older who died from various causes other than prostate cancer, revealed some frightening statistics on prostate health in men (Billis 1986). The authors found that 25% of these men already had latent prostate cancer and this incidence increased with the age of the men, and 85% of these men had atypical cells that could lead to cancer as there is a direct relationship from atypia to cancer.

So from the age of 40 at least and possibly much younger, men were harbouring abnormal cells in their prostate gland long before prostate cancer becomes apparent.

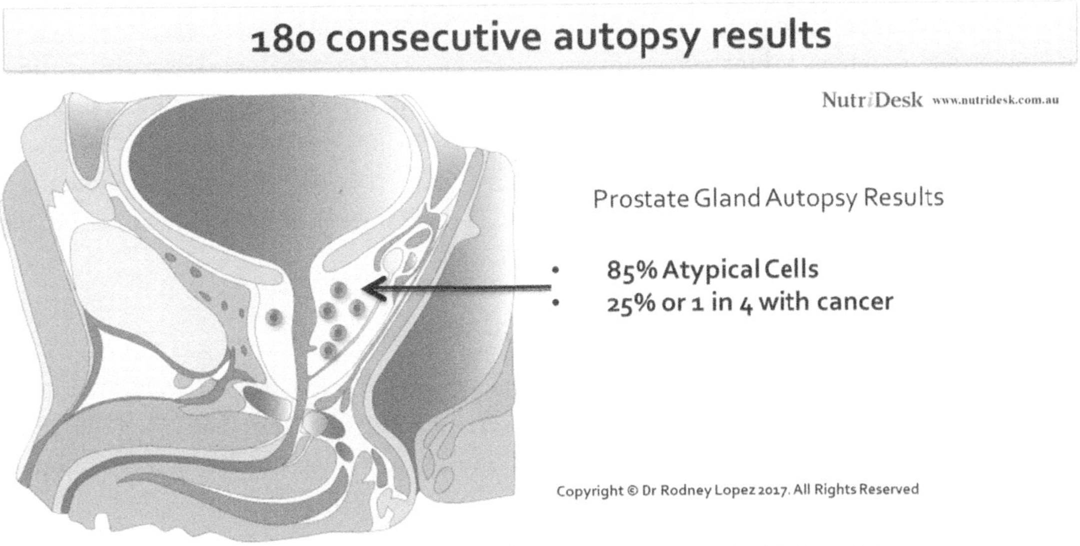

Billis, A. (1986). "Latent carcinoma and atypical lesions of prostate An autopsy study." Urology **28**(4): 324-329.

So with this study by Billis et al. showing hidden and unknown prostate cancer and abnormal cells that can lead to prostate cancer to the extent of 85% of men in the study, do not you find this a staggering discovery?

If you are a man, this must surely scare you as prostate cancer is so common among men out there and this can manifest in your 40's and 50's at a time in your life where you may have a family and a thriving career and a healthy sex life with all of this potentially threatened by the onset of prostate cancer that has the potential to spread, maim and kill.

So regarding mTOR and high energy stores (low AMPK) in the body through merciless feeding rituals a few times a day and 365 days a year, you constantly drive the pathways towards cell multiplication, and you are constantly prodding these abnormal cells with a metabolic 'stick'. I am hoping you see that this relentless growth stimulus will also fall on these abnormal prostate cells and latent prostate cancers. Keep in mind the study above was in ostensibly healthy men who died from a variety of causes other than prostate cancer but just had their prostates examined in that research project.

85% of men in this study were a part of these amazing negative prostate statistics, and remember, your odds are small indeed that you have a normal prostate with no cancer hiding in that glandular tissue. Do you want to annoy these cells and pour fuel on the fire by constantly eating and snacking especially on high energy, high protein foods? Do you still want to pile food on the plate? Seconds or thirds anyone? Dessert?

So, you can see that meal composition which includes the quantity of food consumed in any given meal is vital to ensure you dampen down mTOR signalling. Meal composition will be discussed in more detail later but knowledge is key to understanding why you need to do things from a dietary perspective to protect yourself from disastrous health consequences at a time you should be enjoying life and the fruits of your hard work.

Women and breast cancer risk

In an Australian study on 207 consecutive autopsies of women in Melbourne with an age range from 15 years to 97 years of age, who had their breasts assessed histopathologically (tissue analysed under a microscope), it was surprising that 84.6% of these women had epithelial proliferations of various kinds with 13% having carcinoma in situ and 1.5% with occult invasive breast carcinoma (Bhathal, Brown et al. 1985). So like the prostate study, we have hidden pre-cancerous lesions waiting for a signal to go rogue.

Always remember the Cummings & Bingham statement that 80% of cancers of the breast, prostate and bowel, which are the most common of cancers in the Western world, are driven by dietary and lifestyle forces. Smoking and high alcohol consumption are obvious lifestyle drivers of many cancers but not the only ones. We need to look at the diet of the individual as a whole and take seriously the dietary components that drive the AMPK/mTOR/Insulin/IGF-1 axis. If you have a strong family history of breast, bowel or prostate cancer and indeed any cancer, you now know what you need to do.

Bowel Cancer in Younger and Younger Age Groups

Colorectal cancer (CRC) is increasing dramatically in younger age groups. In particular, Generation-X (born 1960's to early 80;s) and Millennials (born early 80's to early 2000's) (Hackethal 2017). It has been predicted by researchers at the University of Texas, Anderson Cancer Center, that by 2030, cases of bowel cancer in the 20 – 34 year age group will increase by a whopping 90%! (McMillen 2016).

The author himself has seen some people recently in their 40's, diagnosed with colorectal cancer. Unfortunately, this potentially deadly cancer unless treated early, will have already undergone metastatic spread in this younger age group and this could be for various reasons. This younger group may dismiss symptoms, are too busy to see a doctor or the doctor does not think of this diagnosis because of their younger age. Any sudden change in bowel habit or any bleeding or mucus in the stool should be assessed medically as soon as possible.

There is compelling evidence that insulin and IGF-1 are involved in driving bowel cancers. An article in the journal 'Frontiers in Oncology', stated:

> *"The insulin/insulin-like growth factor (IGF) system is a major determinant in the pathogenesis and progression of colorectal cancer (CRC)." (Vigneri, Tirrò et al. 2015)*

Colorectal cancer is very common in Western societies, and the age at which this is occurring is getting younger. This phenomenon is driven in no small part due by the obesity epidemic.

Grains and dairy are consumed in large quantities, and I will discuss dairy shortly. The concern is the elevation in Insulin/IGF-1 with these types of foods driving cancer incidence and propagation.

Bowel cancer is now the second most common cancer in Australia in 2016 behind prostate cancer with prostate, bowel and breast cancer the top three in that order. Bowel cancer risk increases in the 40 – 44 year age group and then it gradually increases in incidence as one gets older. However, as I have stated, just look at the future figures for the 20 – 34 year age group, and this is frightening. Many parents will be burying their children unless society does something about this reckless dietary intake that is ignored by governments and just fuelled by qualified nutrition advisors that are preened by vested interests to muddy the waters with tainted research and articles that suggest otherwise.

It is known from studies that abdominal adiposity in particular and obesity in general, are factors associated with adenomatous polyps which are precursors to bowel cancer (Lee, Park et al. 2008). Many Asian countries are now adopting Western diets, and obesity is on the rise in these countries with a consequent increase in bowel cancer rates.

IGF-1 is not only a strong cancer driver it is also strongly anti-apoptotic. Apoptosis is cell death, and so anything that stops the normal cell-death cycle will only cause damaged cells to live longer, and these damaged cells may be precancerous or cancerous. Thus producing high Insulin/IGF-1 levels by eating dairy, protein or high carbohydrate loads will prevent damaged cells from dying. It is known that IGF-1 is involved in many aspects of cancer formation, progression and metastatic spread (Lee, Park et al. 2008).

No one factor will be the answer, but one huge factor is the overall diet with multiple sub-factors under this dietary umbrella. Micronutrient poor foods are resulting in micronutrient insufficiencies/deficiencies which can cause DNA damage and a long-term risk of cancer. Eating processed meats even occasionally such as bacon, hot dogs, salami etc. and poor fibre intakes can all drive cancerous change in the bowel.

Driving cell multiplication only increases the risk of random DNA mutations and malignant change. Constantly driving the mTOR pathway and suppressing FoxO is never clever. To think that diet has a small role in all of this is naïve in the extreme and it is the elephant in the room that needs to be addressed by governments. They need to take a greater role in preventative health care. Changing your diet through meal planning would have to be one of the smartest moves you can make to decrease your risk of many cancers.

The trouble with dairy: The GI-Insulin Dissociation

It has long been known that milk has a low glycemic-index (Low-GI) but produces a high insulin response. It is known as the glycemic-index (GI) - Insulin Dissociation or **GI-Insulin Dissociation.** This disparity is not driven by carbohydrate but by growth factors in dairy. Both whole milk and skimmed milk with has much less fat, produce a similarly **potent increase** in insulin in **healthy normal subjects** and found to be the result of a protein component of the milk (Hoyt, Hickey et al. 2005). It is important to note that apart from cheese all other dairy products that include whole or skimmed milk, yoghurt, fermented dairy products ice cream and cottage cheese all produced this potent insulin response (Hoyt, Hickey et al. 2005).

GI-Insulin dissociation may seem unusual but understandable if one considers that milk is designed for a newborn baby and designed to stimulate growth in that infant. However, is this a clever idea for adults or those with insulin resistance, to consume dairy products as the pancreas is already struggling to supply enough insulin in Type-2 Diabetes Mellitus? Dairy has been shown to help prevent Type-2 Diabetes Mellitus in some studies, but dairy may also hasten beta cell burnout in those with labile diabetes where the pancreas is on its last legs or in insulin-resistant states that demand more and more insulin from a struggling pancreas. Remember, with overweight and obesity rates and large waistlines in society; insulin resistance and diabetes is quite a common problem.

Do adults need a growth factor long after their growing days are over? As Professor Loren Cordain states, humans are the only animals that continue to consume milk-based products long after they have been weaned. Sure, this is not human breast milk that humans are consuming long after weaning, but it is the milk produced by a mother of another animal with the same physiological purpose, and that is to stimulate growth in their babies. We have already discussed the Insulin/IGF-1 pathway and mTOR signalling, and here we have food that produces a high insulin response after consumption.

These abnormal cells just need that one last DNA mutation to make it fully-fledged cancer and how do you produce this one last DNA mutation? You drive these cells to multiply through Insulin/IFG-1 bombardment! Every cell multiplication cycle increases the risk of DNA errors (mutations). Your telomeres also shorten with every reproductive cell cycle. Adults also have latent cancers in the prostate, breast or bowel and elsewhere as I have pointed out that are yet to manifest in the body. Somehow, your body is suppressing these cancers from spreading, and so this is a fine balancing act produced by the immune system.

This immunity balancing act can easily be disrupted by massive caloric intakes that drive the AMPK/mTOR pathways or the overconsumption of growth factors like Insulin/IGF-1 from dairy consumption that have a powerful impact on those pathways and hence cell multiplication. If you simply went to the PubMed portal and typed in 'dairy and cancer risk' you will see a plethora of studies that show risk. Looking at just one of these studies, the authors stated,

> *"..whole milk intake in men contributed to elevated prostate cancer mortality risk significantly. Furthermore, a linear dose-response relationship existed between increase of whole milk intake and increase of prostate cancer mortality risk (Lu et al., 2016)."*

A linear response is meaning the more you have, the greater the risk! It is interesting that dairy has been found to have some protection against colorectal cancer and that this may be due to the calcium content of dairy binding bile acids in the bowel, but this is too great a risk for other forms of cancer like breast and prostate. You can get an abundant supply of highly bioavailable calcium from dark green leafy vegetables, so you do not need dairy for this. Seeds like sesame and better still black sesame seeds are calcium-rich. Black sesame seeds and black tahini are packed with cancer reducing anthocyanins, and calcium. Is dairy essential? The answer is NO!

Virtually all breast cancer cell lines have IGF-1 receptors (Outwater, Nicholson, & Barnard, 1997) and if there is one thing we know, it is that the length of time the breast is exposed to oestrogen activity will determine breast cancer risk.

Starvation pressures and the emergence of dairy in the diet

Dairy, in an evolutionary sense, has never been a part of the food chain but became so as a result of the food scarcity pressures around 5,000 years ago. Some bright spark in Europe saw baby animals thriving on milk from their mothers and so risked life and limb to milk a beast far removed from the docile cows now used for dairy production or milked other less ferocious creatures to survive like those baby animals.

For those individuals who could tolerate lactose they endured, but for those who were lactose intolerant because they lacked the enzyme lactase to break down this milk sugar, they starved regardless due to gastrointestinal problems and malabsorption. For those with lactose intolerance forced to either consume dairy or starve, the result was similar in that chronic diarrhoea and malabsorption, as a result, ended up killing them slowly ultimately.

Famine has been the norm in our time on this planet, not feast. Death from episodic starvation has killed countless millions of people over millennia. Dairy was one way out during times of starvation. It saved lives or took lives, but now dairy keeps on taking lives due to the very nature of dairy as a growth stimulant. Cancer is one of the common killers in the world, and we need to keep in mind that an individual's diet is a powerful driver of many cancers and this is not an arguable point, it is a fact borne out of a huge database of research.

Dairy and Bovine IGF-1

Insulin increases the number of growth hormone receptors in the liver, and as a result, it stimulates an increase in IGF-1, its evil cousin to do all the growth functions associated with insulin action. Insulin also increases the bioavailability of IGF-1 (Sandhu, Dunger et al. 2002).

Thus dairy stimulates the beta cells in your pancreas to increase your human insulin which in turn increases your IGF-1 level, but there is a twist, bovine dairy which is the most commonly consumed dairy, is also rich in bovine IGF-1, so you get a double-whammy. Your axis of Insulin/IGF-1 production is stimulated through bovine growth factors but you now also get the additional bovine IGF-1 absorbed in your digestive tract adding fuel to the fire. It is extremely interesting that complete amino acid sequencing of bovine IGF-1 and human IGF-1 has been carried out. Importantly, the finding is that bovine IGF-1 is identical to human IGF-1 – not even one amino acid in this bovine IGF-1 protein is different from the human version (Francis, Upton, Ballard, McNeil, & Wallace, 1988).

Remember, IGF-1 is a powerful anabolic (building) molecule, and it dampens down protein breakdown and ramps up protein synthesis and **potently prevents apoptosis** (cell death) (Sandhu, Dunger et al. 2002). Apoptosis is important to get rid of damaged and perhaps dangerous cells in the body. What some of the naysayer's state is that bovine IGF-1 gets destroyed in the stomach or small intestine by acid or small bowel enzymes. However, studies have shown that Epidermal Growth Factor (EGF) which has a similar molecular weight to IGF-1, when accompanied by casein protein in milk, can protect the EGF from digestion by inhibiting enzyme action thus protecting EGF. Infant studies have shown that intact EGF is absorbed. Bovine IGF-1 could similarly be protected and absorbed in the body (Outwater, Nicholson, & Barnard, 1997).

It is important to realise that hormones are very powerful signalling molecules and that only infinitesimally small amounts are needed to exert powerful post-receptor effects (Cone 2012). So even if small amounts of intact bovine IGF-1 were absorbed after consuming dairy, the effects would still be potent.

What we must not lose sight of is the fact that most of the effect of dairy will be via the body's own Insulin/IGF-1 axis with stimulation of the body's intrinsic IGF-1 being produced in the liver to exert the powerful anabolic and anti-apoptosis effects in the body. Milk was designed to do exactly this, i.e. to stimulate growth in a developing baby. Having this powerful cell growth stimulus in a fully-grown adult who could in all probability harbour abnormal cells, is simply madness when dairy is not essential to survive and where many foods can provide the same nutrients less dangerously.

Dairy and Type-2 Diabetes Mellitus (T2DM)

Type-2 diabetes mellitus is the most common type of diabetes in the Western world affecting 85 – 90% of all those with diabetes and millions suffer this form of diabetes around the planet. It is estimated that by 2020, there will be 3 million Australians with diabetes (Shaw & Tanamas, 2012). According to the American Diabetes Association (www.diabetes.org), in 2012, 29.1 million people had type-2 diabetes, but the sad fact was that an estimated 8.1 million people were undiagnosed.

The statistics for prediabetes is even more frightening in that 86 million Americans aged 20 years and over had prediabetes, and thus the total of pre-diabetics, diabetics and undiagnosed diabetics equals 123 million people out of a population of 324 million in total. Thus around 1 in 3 Americans is either diabetic or pre-diabetic. In Australia, around 16.4% have prediabetes over 25 years of age (Twigg, Kamp, Davis, Neylon, & Flack, 2007).

The same common denominator is insulin resistance in prediabetes and Type-2 diabetics. Insulin receptor resistance results in the pancreas pouring out more and more insulin to overcome this obstacle as if sending out more and more troops to find a way through the impasse. It is important to note that pre-diabetics have a high risk of progression to frank diabetes and a high cardiovascular risk. Around 30% of those presenting to an accident and emergency department with an acute heart attack had pre-existing prediabetes or diabetes (Jessani, Gangopadhyay, Patel, Lip, & Millane, 2007)

The worry is that the pancreas is already under siege in pre-diabetics and people with diabetes. The pancreas is already struggling to produce insulin, and by consuming dairy, we are demanding more and more insulin from the beta cells that are finding it difficult to cope with the stimulus to produce this hormone. Do people with insulin resistance states like prediabetes, diabetes, PCOS and the Metabolic Syndrome need this powerful action of dairy growth factors stimulating the pancreatic beta cells? Is it irresponsible not to tell patients that this is what is happening when they are consuming dairy products? As has been pointed out in a research paper:

> *"Except for cheese with an insulin score of 45, all dairy products (whole milk, skimmed milk, yoghurt, ice cream, cottage cheese and fermented milk products) have been shown to have potent insulinotropic properties that may have far-reaching health effects, given the hypothesis that insulinaemia is a modulator of insulin resistance." (Hoyt, Hickey, & Cordain, 2005)*

It is important to note in the quote above the term 'potent' was used by these researchers. The term 'insulinotropic' means influencing the production or activity of insulin. So dairy **potently** affects the pancreas and insulin production.

White Lies

An excellent, in-depth paper on dairy titled 'White Lies' can be downloaded as a PDF on the internet and is highly recommended reading (Butler, 2014). Food is a double-edged sword and yet so much about its dangers are hidden and all for commercial and political reasons. Just look at what highly respected researchers like Cornell University' s Professor T Colin Campbell a professor emeritus and author of The China Study, a joint project with Oxford University, states in this White Lies report,

> *"It is not that these various dairy effects are independently proven to be true beyond doubt, any more than tobacco use is independently proven to cause lung cancer and heart disease. Rather, it is the weight and breadth of the evidence, along with its biological plausibility, that should determine the reliability of the*

evidence. Using these criteria, there is no doubt that this evidence on dairy is sufficient, at a minimum, to question the rather specious claims of health for cow's milk that have been made by the industry and its supporters and apologists."

Dairy and oestrogen

The other concern for both men and women is the oestrogen content of dairy and the link to many hormone-sensitive cancers such as breast, prostate, ovarian and uterine cancer. One paper described the concern of the authors about the oestrogen content of milk and the risk of many common life-threatening cancers in society. They stated:

"The continued increase in incidence of some hormone-related cancers worldwide is of great concern. Although oestrogen-like substances in the environment were blamed for this increase, the possible role of endogenous oestrogens from food has not been widely discussed. We are particularly concerned about cows' milk, which contains a considerable quantity of oestrogens. When we name cows' milk as one of the important routes of human exposure to oestrogens, the general response of Western people is that "man has been drinking cows' milk for around 2000 years without apparent harm." However, the milk that we are now consuming is quite different from that consumed 100 years ago. Unlike their pasture-fed counterparts of 100 years ago, modern dairy cows are usually pregnant and continue to lactate during the latter half of pregnancy, when the concentration of oestrogens in blood, and hence in milk, increases." (Ganmaa & Sato, 2005)

The industrial machine has changed the nature of milk composition. I have already discussed previously, that there is a linear response between milk consumption and prostate cancer mortality. We know that both androgens like testosterone and oestrogen are required for cancerous changes to occur in the prostate (Risbridger, Bianco, Ellem, & McPherson, 2003). Oestrogen drives prostate hypertrophy (enlargement), and this is a known quantity (Wilson, 1980). Enlarged prostates are a very common problem in men. Why risk this? In women, one known constant about breast cancer is how long those breasts are exposed to oestrogen.

Anyone for milk and biscuits? I am hoping you see how powerful meal planning is. It is not only about what to put on the plate but what to exclude!

Why starting your day with cereal and milk is not a great idea!

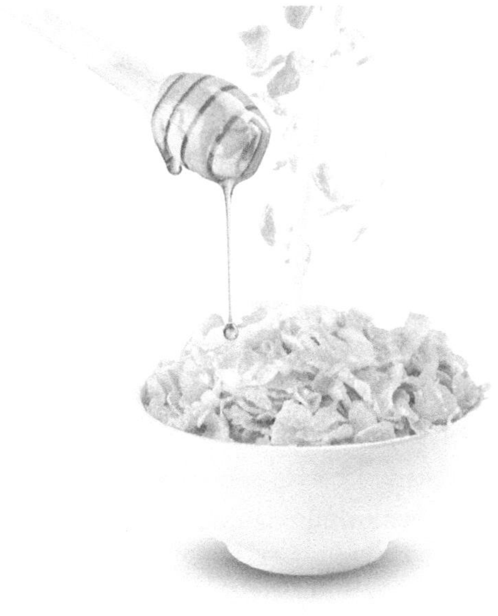

The insulin responses of many foods have been calculated in an Australian study where various foods with the same energy value were tested for their insulin response, i.e. how much insulin was produced and how much glucose each food generated (Holt, Miller, & Petocz, 1997). For those who love their white or wholemeal bread, the sad news is that these foods along with the potato were the highest insulin-producing (insulinogenic) foods on the list.

The researchers stated;

"Collectively, the findings imply that typical Western diets are likely to be significantly more insulinogenic than more traditional diets based on less refined foods."

Cereal breakfasts like All-Bran® and oats produced lower insulin scores than breakfasts consisting of Cornflakes® or Honeysmacks® or Special-K®.

However, you need to take into consideration the glycemic index and how much of that carbohydrate you are consuming, i.e. the glycemic load (GL) and consuming large amounts of a carbohydrate-containing food will result in high glucose and Insulin/IGF-1 responses and will keep them elevated in the postprandial state for 6 hours or more. For those with insulin resistance, these elevations may be 24/7 in the blood!

Consuming a high carbohydrate load at breakfast along with cow's milk and honey or agave is a toxic combination and toxic load and is not how you want to start your day. The cereal itself is an incomplete food that lacks essential amino acids and nutrients with highly bound, poorly bioavailable minerals. High glucose generation from the cereal and added sweeteners stimulate Insulin/IGF-1 profoundly.

We are already stimulating Insulin/IGF-1 by the carbohydrate in the cereal but to add even more insult; we pour milk into this cereal and milk as you are now aware, has a powerful Insulin/IGF-1 stimulating effect.

High fructose sweeteners such as table sugar, honey and worse still, agave syrup added to breakfast cereals, worsen the toxicity. We discussed that glucose glycates (damages) proteins and yet fructose is 8 – 10 times worse than glucose in glycating (damaging) all the proteins in your body (Levi & Werman, 1998, McPherson, Shilton, & Walton, 1988).

Table sugar is a 50:50 glucose-fructose combination. Honey has a higher level of fructose than table sugar. Agave syrup has an even higher level of fructose than honey. A large analysis of 19 agave syrups from 3 major production areas and four productions facilities were analysed for their content of major carbohydrates, polyols and oligosaccharide profiles. In this analysis of agave syrups, the finding was that the average fructose concentrations in these syrups was an astounding 84.29% (Willems and Low 2012)

So, even though fructose does not stimulate insulin release from the pancreas, it damages your body through glycation, by increasing triglycerides in your blood, through blood vessel-damaging triglyceride-rich VLDL and increases uric acid levels. Uric acid is an independent marker for heart disease and a pro-oxidant, i.e. it stimulates oxidative stress and can damage your kidneys. See Appendix-21.

There are important issues with cereals

1. Every meal counts! Glycemic load (GL) essentially accounts for the glucose response produced by each gramme (US: gram) of food. This Australian study supported the concept of a higher GL being associated with insulin resistance (O'Sullivan, Bremner, O'Neill, & Lyons-Wall, 2010)

2. The Tehran Lipid and Glucose study showed a significant association between dietary insulin load and developing insulin resistance (Mirmiran, Esfandiari, Bahadoran, Tohidi, & Azizi, 2016).

Choosing an Activ8Health Plan-A type meal (solid or blended) as a breakfast choice is the best thing you can do for your immediate health, healthspan and longevity.

Rethink what breakfast should be! Move away from food in a box including all mueslis and oats and everything packed into a cardboard box and promoted as a healthy breakfast. Healthy breakfast in a box is essentially an oxymoronic statement. An Activ8Health Plan-A diet or Plan-B diet will be 'just right'! Pun intended.

Key Points

- Thank God for Easter Island, a speck in the ocean that provided an amazing insight into the molecular basis of longevity through rapamycin and the mammalian target of rapamycin (mTOR). We discovered the powerful anabolic (cell building) effect that growth hormones like Insulin/IGF-1 have on mTOR
- A constant feast signal through the energy sensor AMPK and protein sufficiency signals via amino
acids especially L-Leucine, trigger frenetic cell multiplication via mTOR
- Producing more and more cells through a feast signal only increases the risk for DNA mutations and cancer risk.
- The more a cell divides, the shorter the telomeres at the ends of chromosomes and the shorter will be our healthspan and lifespan.
- A high intake of carbohydrates, dairy and even protein will lead to high Insulin/IGF-1 levels that help drive the AMPK/mTOR pathways. pathway.
- High carbohydrate loads from cereal foods increase Insulin/IGF-1 and glucose levels in the blood
- Milk and most dairy products are potent stimulators of Insulin/IGF-1 a well-established, incontrovertible scientific fact.
- Cereals and dairy are not essential, and all the nutrients and fibre in these foods can easily be obtained through eating vegetables, fruits, nuts, seeds and low-starch tubers and non-red meat protein sources including fish and shellfish
- Supplementation should be seen in the context of worsening food supply systems and nutrient loss between paddock to plate, poor and worsening soils worldwide, high-yield cultivars with diminished
nutrient values, personal genetic mutations, personal lifestyle factors, personal ill health and micronutrient depleting medications, all conspire against optimal micronutrient sufficiency.

CHAPTER 4

Sirtuins & NAD^+

Sirtuins are Nicotinamide adenine dinucleotide (NAD^+) dependent enzymes that remove acetyl groups (deacetylate) on histones, DNA or proteins and as such, they are extremely important players in the epigenetic process that switch genes 'on' or 'off'. NAD^+ is shaping up to have a vital role in biological ageing, and this molecule is vital cellular energy transfer processes which diminish as we age. People growing older often suffer an 'energy crisis' and NAD^+ will have a role in this.

> The Silent Information Regulator 2 (SIR2) protein was the first sirtuin to be discovered in yeast. In mammals, SIRT1 is similar to yeast SIR2 (Casey 2012). To date, there are 7 members of this family identified in mammals and labelled SIRT1-7, where some are located in the nucleus (SIRT1, SIRT6, SIRT7), the cytoplasm (SIRT1 in some cell types & SIRT2), or in the mitochondria (SIRT3, SIRT4, SIRT5) (Merksamer, Liu et al. 2013, Bonkowski and Sinclair 2016)). Collectively they are called Sirtuins.

SIRT1, for example, removes acetyl groups (deacetylates) several transcription factors that are responsible for activating antioxidant genes. SIRT1 also activates several of the FoxO members, and this is something we discussed in the chapter under AMPK/mTOR pathways. FoxO you may remember is activated when you provide a fasting signal such as the intraday fasting signal recommended in this book. FoxO then activates several stress-response genes for cell repair and maintenance.

The Sirtuins are linked into this process, and **Nicotinamide adenine dinucleotide (NAD)** is the **Vitamin-B3** related **master of the Sirtuins.**

NAD (graphic) exists in the oxidised (NAD^+) or reduced (NADH) form. Without Vitamin-B3 and NAD life does not exist. These molecules are involved in redox (electron transfer) reactions, and I will discuss this shortly.

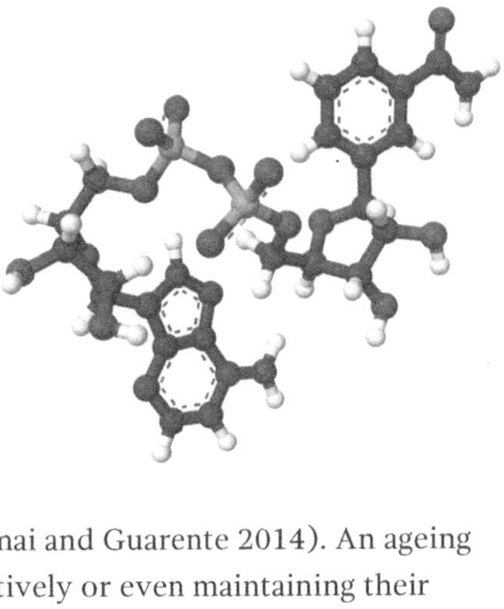

The energy crisis as you age

There is a decline in NAD+ with ageing, and this may be due to the age-related defective biosynthesis of this important compound (Imai and Guarente 2014). An ageing individual often feels lethargic preventing them from exercising effectively or even maintaining their motivation, mobility and balance. This lethargy may often be misdiagnosed as depression and treated as such in older individuals. Ineffective production in ATP, the molecular currency of energy in cells drops as you age, and by supplementing with NAD+ precursors, nicotinamide mononucleotide (NMN) or nicotinamide riboside (NR) you can help restore NAD+ levels so that critical energy generating processes keep on working optimally in your cells. With dropping levels of NAD^{+} as you age, mitochondrial functionality will be affected, and mitochondrial numbers will diminish in cells making matters worse (Gomes, Price et al. 2013).

We are discovering a wonderful interplay of many proteins and signalling molecules that interlink to provide an orchestrated response to environmental cues about cell repair processes, cell maintenance and longevity. Your dietary intake is a major environmental cue that turns on or off such pathways, and thus dietary regulation primarily determines your destiny regarding health and longevity.

What you eat, and the number of calories you consume with each meal is well within your control. Dietary management on a daily basis is the most powerful tool you have at your disposal to avoid premature illness and extend your healthspan and in all probability, extend your lifespan.

An Australian study on skin cancer showing the power of Nicotinamide

A phase 3, double-blind, randomised, placebo-controlled trial (Oral Nicotinamide to Reduce Actinic Cancer [ONTRAC]) study was conducted in Australia at the Royal Prince Alfred, and Westmead hospitals on individuals with sun damaged skin and a history of skin cancer (Chen, Martin et al. 2015). These individuals already had at least two (2) histopathologically confirmed non-melanoma skin cancers diagnosed in the past five years so were high-risk individuals for further skin cancers. The research participants received either 500 mg or 1500 mg of the Vitamin-B3 amide (nicotinamide), which is a precursor of NAD. The findings were that individuals taking daily 500 mg nicotinamide doses, had a 29% reduction of actinic keratoses - sun damaged spots that can give rise to basal cell carcinomas (BCCs) or squamous cell carcinomas (SCC's) – both of which are non-melanoma skin malignant cancers. There was a 35% reduction in actinic keratoses in those taking 1500 mg of nicotinamide (Chen, Martin et al. 2015).

> Risks – An individual with a high risk of insulin resistance should not exceed 2 g of Nicotinamide per day as insulin sensitivity may be affected and not to increase Nicotinamide over 3 grams per day as liver toxicity may occur.

Keeping in mind that non-melanoma skin cancers affect around 50% of the Australian population and that BCCs can locally infiltrate tissues and SCCs can metastasise (spread). Both could lead to horrific disfiguration as a result of possible heroic surgery needed to preserve life or death if these cancers were ignored. These skin cancers are thought to result in at least a $500 million burden to the Australian nation regarding treatment costs and lost productivity.

In the United States of America, this cost is thought to be 4.8 billion dollars (Chen, Martin et al. 2015). The ONTRAC study did not look at preventative aspects but only studied individuals at high risk of skin cancer with significant sun-damaged skin in an advanced state of ultraviolet-induced DNA damage, and yet the Nicotinamide had such a powerful effect in preventing the precursor solar (actinic) keratoses.

So in a country with around 24 million people, the reduction in premalignant actinic keratoses could affect 4 million people and save lives and save a substantial cost to the nation. So just ensuring you have an adequate intake of Vitamin-B3 from food and supplementing with Nicotinamide and in particular, Nicotinamide Riboside could help stave off skin damage and cancer in this sunburnt country or indeed in any country as skin cancer is so common worldwide.

Nicotinamide, when taken in recommended doses, is very safe. To worry about the risk of supplementing in the setting of advanced UV skin damage is downright irrational and dangerous exposing those individuals to possible unnecessary medical interventions and disfigurement. Let's not forget the enormous emotional toll on an individual who fears the worst with skin cancer and who has to have regular surgical excisions. The risk is always balanced with benefit and is no different to any pharmacological treatment.

It may become a medicolegal issue if a doctor does not suggest a relatively safe treatment to a high-risk individual for skin cancer.

Sirtuin-Activating Compounds (STACs) and longevity

That a vitamin can have such a powerful effect on skin cancer must rock the world of those that think pharmacological (drug), or surgical approaches are the only way to treat disease. Preventative measures are obviously not even on the radar in the minds of such individuals. This effect on skin cancer by Nicotinamide can now be seen in the context of Sirtuin activation as this provides a mechanism of action that ties in with AMPK, mTOR, FoxO and Calorie Restriction (CR) to help repair and maintain cells in an optimal, youthful state.

In a joint research project carried out by Harvard University and the University of New South Wales (UNSW), Australia, Nicotinamide mononucleotide was given to mice to see if DNA damage as a result of ageing or radiation could be repaired. A lead researcher, Professor David S Sinclair from UNSW, stated:

"The cells of the old mice were indistinguishable from the young mice, after just one week of treatment."

NAD$^+$ & Oxidation-Reduction (Redox) Reactions

Oxidation-Reduction (Redox) reactions involve the transfer of electrons between two chemical species such as NAD$^+$ and NADH in the body. Most of the energy in mitochondria are derived from these oxidation-reduction reactions. NAD$^+$, the oxidised form, accepts electrons and becomes reduced in the process to form NADH. So your cellular energy depends upon this 'hot-potato' catch-and-throw interplay of electrons between these chemical forms. Cells can have thousands of mitochondria which extract energy from food to create Adenosine Triphosphate (ATP) to drive cellular reactions and muscle movement. The problem arises if a molecule like NAD$^+$ diminishes. To prevent this NAD$^+$ insufficiency, a naturally occurring precursor of NAD+, Nicotinamide riboside, comes in handy. Nicotinamide riboside is a NAD$^+$ boosting STAC. This compound is an important restorer of NAD$^+$ in ageing individuals.

As humans age, their levels of NAD$^+$ decrease as the body's ability to produce NAD$^+$ from the kynurenine pathway cannot keep pace with the need. The kynurenine pathway is where NAD$^+$ is created from the essential amino acid tryptophan.

A high dose of 100 mg to 1,000 mg nicotinamide per kg, per day was administered to rodents for more than six months with no apparent side effects (Bonkowski and Sinclair 2016). These are extremely high doses indeed, and so supplementation at RDA's or the level of 100mg given to an individual weighing around 70kg is a significantly smaller dose by many magnitudes in comparison to the animal study described above.

For those who are in their senior years who want to ensure their NAD$^+$ stores are adequate, then around 100mg of Nicotinamide Riboside may be all you need but if you have a high risk of skin cancer, then taking higher doses may be necessary. The research should guide this (Chen, Martin et al. 2015), and by your practitioner who will assess your risk for insulin resistance (a pre-diabetic state) and ensure that your liver is healthy, to begin with, and perhaps to follow-up high-dose treatment with checks on liver function (LFTs).

The interplay of Sirtuins, NAD⁺, FoxO and mTOR

There is a great deal of complexity regarding these pathways with many inputs that either activate or suppress them.

Following the recommended intraday fasting protocol in this book, and keeping to an Activ8Health Plan-A type diet that **does not increase** Insulin/IGF-1 signalling (IIS), you will activate these pathways that have been proven to not only prolong life but increase your healthspan.

SIRT1 can activate (deacetylate) FoxO or inactivate it depending on metabolic circumstances, but the consensus that is emerging is that SIRT1, by deacetylating and thus activating FoxO, allows FoxO to induce a set of genes that promote cell repair or maintenance (Greer and Brunet 2005). Factors involved are shown in the graphic. NAD^+ boosters (STACs) have the potential to boost all seven sirtuins (Bonkowski and Sinclair 2016).

Calorie restriction is a powerful booster of NAD^+.

By increasing Insulin/IGF-1 signalling through a massive intake of carbs, protein, dairy and essentially excessive calories, FoxO stays phosphorylated and locked in the cytoplasm of a cell. Decreasing this IIS signalling through dietary measures and intraday fasting will remove these phosphate molecules which are 'chaining' FoxO to the cytoplasm and allowing FoxO to enter the nucleus and promote transcription of all those wonderful life-extending factors (Greer and Brunet 2005). Once in the nucleus, SIRT1 a predominantly nuclear protein (Bonkowski and Sinclair 2016), can exert its deacetylating effect on FoxO and other proteins.

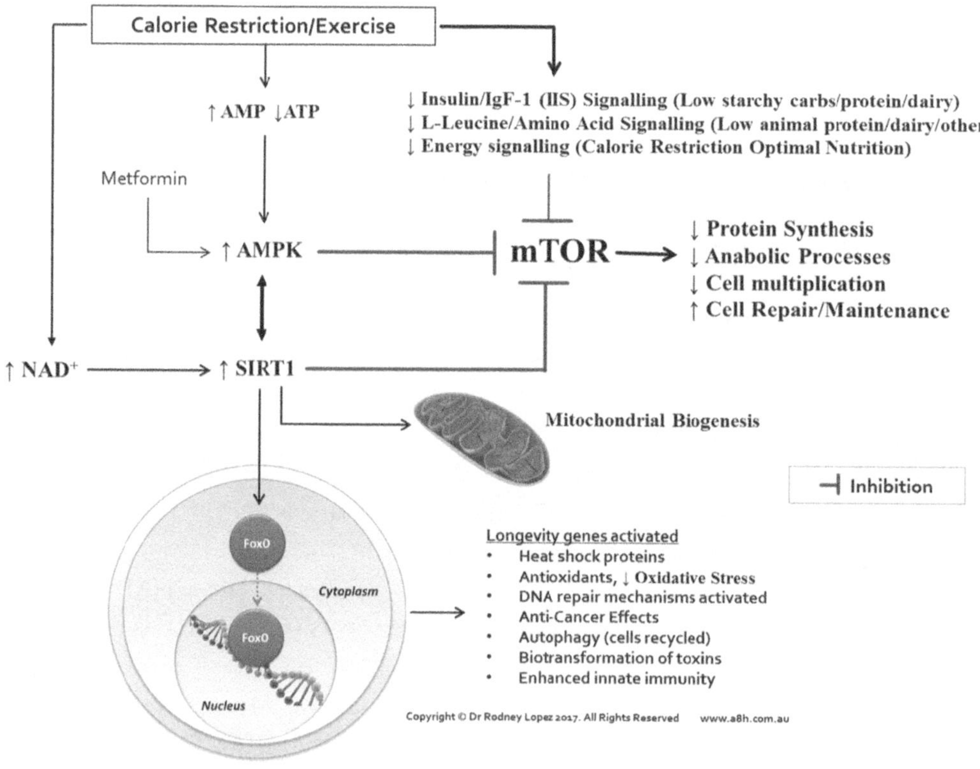

Calorie Restriction NOT starvation

Remember, we are talking about calorie restriction and not starvation. Starvation is destructive and can result in cellular and organ damage. **Calorie restriction but optimal nutrition** (CRON) is an entirely different concept. We are not bombarding our bodies with a mass of calories and growth factors that diminish NAD^+ and prevent the Sirtuins and FoxO from doing their wonderful work. What we are trying to achieve through diet and supplementation, is a nutrient and caloric intake that facilitates optimal cellular functioning promotes cell repair and maintenance and shifts cells to a youthful state.

It is easy enough to see how people are eating themselves to a diseased state and early death all due to that primal instinct to eat and store energy as fat for that possible famine around the corner. In this age of abundance, these physiological mechanisms are now killing millions of people prematurely every year.

That spending more of our time in a diseased and unhealthy state has been studied, and in the United Kingdom, it was calculated that the percentage of a man's lifespan spent in poor health has increased from 20% in 1995 to 40% in 2006 (Bonkowski and Sinclair 2016).

You as an individual are living a blessed life in a highly scientific and technological world. You are privy to the tremendous strides, knowledge and understanding of these longevity pathways and the STACs that can help drive known longevity pathways like NAD^+, Resveratrol, Calorie Restriction Optimal Nutrition (CRON) or even Metformin a diabetes drug known to activate AMPK. You now have the knowledge and power to change your destiny by simply ensuring every meal you consume has meaning and is not riddled with poor dietary choices. What may seem healthy in a food court or shopping mall could have devastating effects postprandially (after-eating). Knowledge counts and this book is all about providing you with tremendous insight into healthy diets.

Ageing, NAD^+, Preventing Disease

We know that Vitamin-B3 is essential to life and we know that Vit-B3 is a precursor to NAD^+ and we know the safety profile of this supplement from decades of research and where to take care regarding dose.

Waiting for every morsel of information to come through before implementing any treatment modality whether this is a pharmaceutical or nutraceutical agent is nonsensical as we will never have all the pieces of the puzzle in place. Our knowledge in 100 years, 1000, years or 10,000 will be vastly different to our molecular knowledge now. Do we have time up our sleeves to wait for all this knowledge to emerge or do we use the knowledge we have right now? Waiting for every bit of information to surface is an illogical notion and may well see the end of your life by acute or chronic disease and all because therapeutic approaches that have an evidence-base are not being implemented early enough.

In comparison to pharmaceuticals, natural compounds such as vitamins and minerals are 62,000 times less likely to create an adverse effect (ANH 2012), so why ignore them based on such an infinitesimally small risk. This risk comparison between nutraceuticals and pharmaceuticals is expanded upon in the section on supplements at the end of this book.

Niacin or Vitamin-B3 has been used for lowering cholesterol by the medical profession, and this effect known since the 1950's.

If the adult RDA for Vitamin-B3 is 16mg/day we need to take **125 times** this dose (125 x RDA) to equal the 2 grams suggested as a risk for insulin resistance and **187.5 times** the RDA (187.5 x RDA) for liver toxicity to manifest, as suggested by the Linus Pauling 'Micronutrient Information Center'.

So, taking 100 mg of a NAD^+ precursor falls incredibly short of the high doses known to put someone at risk, in fact, 20 – 30 times below the doses of concern. What an incredibly large therapeutic safety margin for this naturally derived compound, in contrast to extremely narrow therapeutic windows for the vast majority of drugs where even a small deviation from the therapeutic dose beyond the upper range can result in adverse reactions and possible lethal effects.

Ageing, tiredness and sarcopenia

A part of growing older is that feeling of tiredness that can prevent individuals from participating in a sport or other leisure activities and seniors can find it difficult to get through a workday. NAD^+ plays an important role in energy extraction from the metabolism of fatty acids, protein, alcohol and glucose. All this energy generation occurs in the mitochondria, the energy-producing powerhouses of cells. Lack of energy can manifest as depression, and the lack of energy is a disincentive to exercise thus promoting weight gain, in the central abdominal region (visceral fat) possibly triggering insulin resistance or Type-2 Diabetes Mellitus. Weight gain is a trigger for many chronic illnesses.

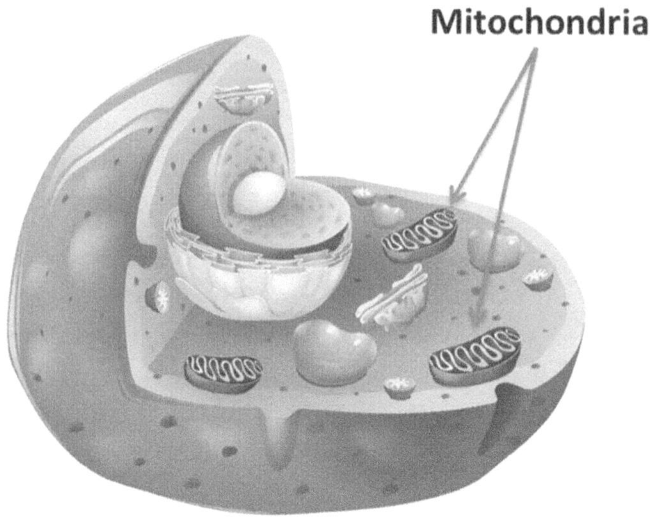

Supplementing with around 100 mg of nicotinamide or nicotinamide riboside which is 20 times lower than that 2-gram threshold discussed above, may just give individuals in their senior years the boost of energy they long for.

Sarcopenia, or a loss of muscle as we age, is also the result (and cause) for many a chronic illness as the metabolic rate greatly diminishes because muscle is a highly active tissue. With a loss of active, energy-consuming skeletal muscle (sarcopenia), comes higher postprandial (after-eating) spikes in glucose that stay high because this glucose-consuming tissue has been allowed to disappear simply.

An individual is put at great risk of falling and fracturing bones because muscle strength and balance is compromised as a result of ongoing muscle loss. Nicotinamide has been shown in mice studies to restore mitochondrial function to youthful levels, to improve insulin sensitivity if used in the right dose, to increase the high energy compound ATP, to protect against DNA damage and to protect against muscle wasting (sarcopenia) (Bonkowski and Sinclair 2016).

Sirtuins can be activated at any age through calorie restriction which has the effect of increasing NAD+ levels (Bonkowski and Sinclair 2016). Once again this reinforces the importance of intermittent fasting and what I suggest in this book, intraday fasting 2 – 3 times a week as tolerated while consuming the Activ8Health Plan-A diet at other times.

Other STACs

Resveratrol is a plant polyphenol the concentration of which increases in that plant with a stress of some kind such as ultraviolet radiation, crushing, or injury from temperatures like a cold climate. It is the reason why the cold-stressed Pinot Noir, a cold climate grape and wine, has a higher concentration of trans-resveratrol. Numerous studies have shown that resveratrol is a potent activator of SIRT1, but there is some controversy whether this is a direct or indirect action (Casey 2012). Through the action of sirtuins, resveratrol mimics the effects of caloric restriction. In essence, dietary restriction (DR) in a pill. Metformin the antidiabetic drug also does this through AMPK activation, and this may be one of the reasons that people with diabetes on Metformin do not have a high incidence of cancer or diabetic complications. Resveratrol and Metformin theoretically should have great synergies.

Pterostilbene is a compound found mainly in blueberries and is an analogue of resveratrol (Cheng, Di et al. 2016). Pterostilbene has been studied for its effect on longevity, and it produces a calorie restriction (CR) effect by action on the three main pathways involved namely, AMPK, Sirtuins and mTOR.

Pterostilbene has been shown to upregulate SIRT1 and FoxO and thus exert its calorie restriction mimetic effect.

No doubt other STACs will emerge as time goes on. You have enough information to choose ways to stimulate these longevity pathways from intraday fasting, calorie restriction optimal nutrition (CRON) through the achievable Activ8Health Plan-A diet strategy to the supplementation of Nicotinamide or Nicotinamide Riboside +/- Pterostilbene and the odd glass of Pinot Noir wine.

Metformin has also been used 'off-label' at a low dose for this purpose. Even a low dose could be worthwhile, and studies are underway on this diabetic medication to see what kind of effect it has on longevity and other chronic disease states.

One word of warning with Metformin, even though it has a great safety record, is that if you have a severe gastroenteritis or you do not drink enough fluids on hot summer days for example, and thus you are likely to dehydrate, then lactic acidosis may occur which is a potentially deadly outcome. Doctors and everyone else should never be scared of this side-effect but remember the warning. Metformin is worthwhile medication! When has a side-effect ever prevented a doctor from writing a script or a patient taking medication? We just need to make informed decisions.

If you think intraday fasting will decrease your metabolic rate, think again!

Starvation will decrease the metabolic rate dramatically as I have pointed out in the chapter on intraday fasting but not calorie restriction (CR). With CR you are not starving yourself. It is all about limiting unwanted calories and ensuring you have all the micronutrients you need for optimal health. Guidance is thus paramount to achieving this. Calorie restriction in fact increased mitochondrial numbers (mitochondrial biogenesis) and activity (Guarente 2008).

It has long been theorized, that calorie restriction exerts its effect by decreasing energy extraction in the mitochondrial respiratory chain, i.e. the electron transport chain. So the thinking is that by reducing energy extraction from food you decrease free radical production and damaging reactive oxygen species (ROS), both produced by energy extraction from food. This makes perfect intuitive sense doesn't it but is not true. In fact, we all have ageing mitochondria and roadblocks in the mitochondrial respiratory chain that prevent electrons from passing through effectively. These roadblocks in the mitochondrial electron transport chain allow masses of free electrons to escape and damage not only the mitochondria where they come from but other cellular structures around them injuring cells and ultimately, organ systems that house these cells.

When energy is extracted, free electrons are produced predominantly at Complex-1 and Complex-III in the electron transport chain (respiratory chain) and this is now widely accepted (Guarente 2008, Pamplona and Barja 2006). Ubiquinone (CoQ10) is also a major site of free radical generation (Scientific American 2006). If these free radicals are not quenched, they can damage the mitochondria themselves and cellular structures around them.

Calorie restriction (CR) indeed increases mitochondrial numbers (increases mitochondrial density in cells). Calorie restriction also helps repair those 'roadblocks' in the respiratory chain complexes. You may be guessing how this occurs and you may have guessed that all of this happens by dampening down the AMPK/mTOR pathways and triggering cell maintenance and repair processes through FoxO.

So CR does not slow energy extraction (respiration) it upregulates mitochondrial function and improves energy generation efficiency in mitochondria (Guarente 2008).

Leonard Guarente from the Department of Biology, Massachusetts Institute of Technology, Cambridge USA wrote an excellent article titled 'Mitochondria —A Nexus for Aging, Calorie Restriction, and Sirtuins?' The article outlines how this molecular effect and efficiency occurs in greater detail if you want to know more about the biochemical complexity of this change that occurs with CR. It is important to simply understand that calorie restriction is all about allowing the body to get rid of damaged proteins or to repair ineffective systems by shifting your metabolic framework towards your younger self. Why wouldn't you want to take advantage of this? Is food that much of a driving force that you are willing to put your health at

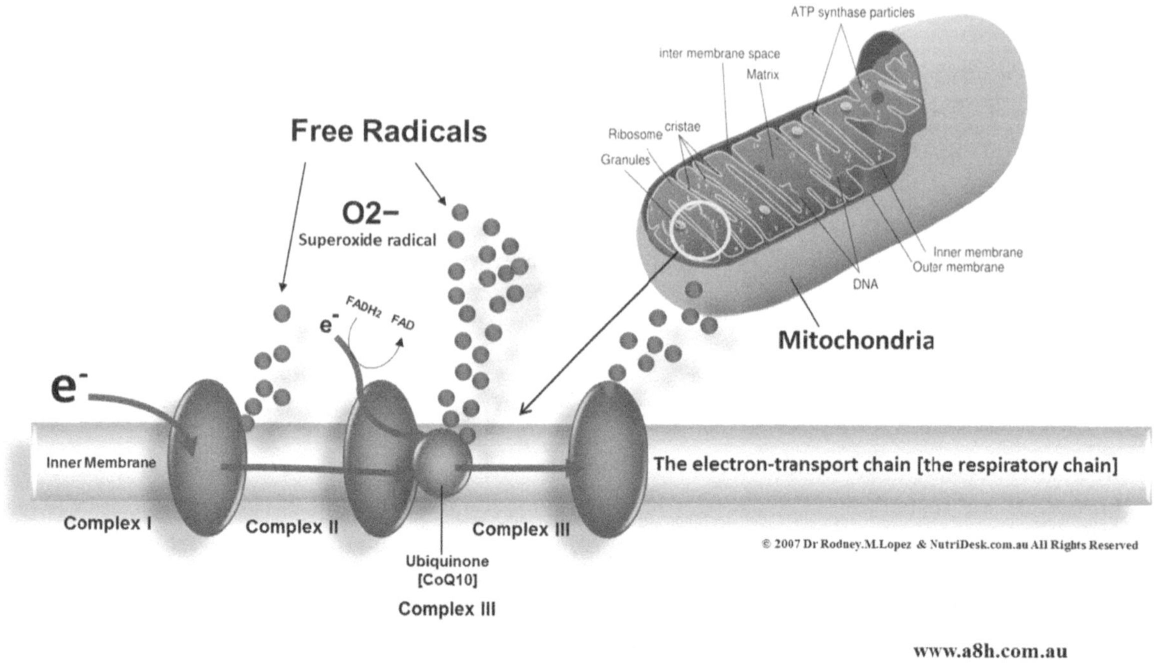

risk for a few minutes of taste satisfaction? Optimising meal composition is vital to upregulate these wonderful mechanisms towards a more youthful you!

Nitric Oxide (NO) Driving Mitochondrial Biogenesis and Citrulline as a driver of NO

The lining of your blood vessels throughout body is called the endothelium. It is the largest endocrine (gland) organ in the body and has been estimated have a surface area of around 400 square metres. Astounding! It has 1.2 trillion cells can respond to internal and external factors through the production of chemical mediators, unlike a hormonal gland like the thyroid (Änggård 1990)

Nitric Oxide, not to be confused with nitrous oxide the laughing gas, is a powerful vasodilator meaning it increases the diameter of blood vessels. Endothelial cells line the entire vascular system (Alberts, Bray et al. 2013) and this endothelium is vital for your blood vessels to function optimally.

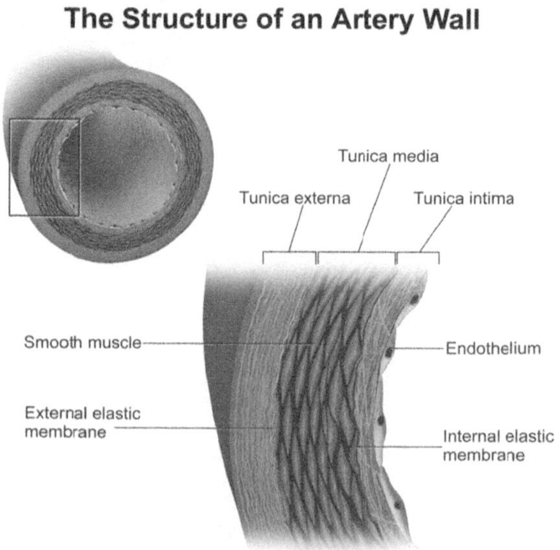

your and not

A lack of vasodilation capability will increase resistance in blood vessels and increase blood pressure and. Poor vasodilation is associated with atherosclerosis (cholesterol-laden plaques) which can lead to heart attacks and peripheral vascular disease.

Nitric Oxide (NO) levels decrease with age (Lyons, Roy et al. 1997), and there may be many mechanisms involved including the enzymes involved in producing nitric oxide to a lack of the substrate L-Arginine needed for nitric oxide production in the body. Of interest is the fact that endothelial nitric oxide (eNOS) can activate SIRT1 and increase mitochondrial biogenesis.

The increase in cellular respiration (energy production) and the increase in mitochondrial numbers per cell (mitochondrial biogenesis) is dependent upon endothelial nitric oxide synthase (eNOS) and nitric oxide, which has been shown to activate SIRT1 in cultured cells (Guarente 2008).

An important contributor to nitric oxide (NO) levels is the inorganic nitrate found in food with rich sources being beetroot and greens such as Baby Spinach and Rocket (Arugula). With over 90% of the population getting nowhere near the recommended intake of fruit and vegetables, this important source of inorganic nitrate will result in diminishing nitric oxide production in the body, and this will only increase vascular risk as occurs in every ageing individual.

Vegetables seem to be anathema to some individuals, and if this is the case, then consideration should be given to taking a supplement such as Citrulline a superior donor form of L-Arginine and hence nitric oxide. The amazing benefits of Citrulline as a donor of L-Arginine is discussed in Appendix-23, and this should be of great interest to anyone with cardiovascular disease, a history of hypertension or stroke and any man suffering from erectile dysfunction or Peyronie's Disease (PD) of the penis or any other scarring disease.

Citrulline as a superior source of L-Arginine and hence Nitric Oxide (NO) generation

Citrulline, an amino acid, gets its name from Citrullus, which is Latin for watermelon. Watermelon is rich in Citrulline especially so in the rind. It is for this reason that I recommend watermelon in juice most days (See Appendix 4) and also because watermelon is low in carbohydrate. L-Arginine seems to have been the 'go-to' molecule if you wanted to stimulate nitric oxide synthesis. Citrulline is not an essential amino acid but could be classified as 'conditionally essential' meaning, if there is an insufficient supply to meet the needs of the body, and the body cannot produce enough of it, then there may be harmful effects on the individual. However, L-Arginine is avidly taken up by the liver and converted to urea (Curis, Nicolis et al. 2005). Urea overload can be a problem in anyone with existing kidney disease as this would be an increased burden on the kidney to excrete nitrogenous compounds like urea putting the kidney at further risk.

> *".arginine is liable to cause excessive ureagenesis, since it acts as a catalyst of ureagenesis" (Curis, Nicolis et al. 2005).*

Ureagenesis is the creation of urea. High L-Arginine intakes leading to increased urea production is a real problem if the kidneys are functioning poorly. Prediabetes and diabetes are now leading causes of chronic kidney disease, and so this will need to be taken into consideration as prediabetes and diabetes are very common in society.

Citrulline avoids oral first pass liver metabolism unlike oral L-Arginine

Often the problem of silent chronic kidney disease is not taken into consideration when L-Arginine is recommended or taken by sports people. One clever way around this is to use Citrulline regarded as a 'masked-form' of L-Arginine. By 'masked' is meant that it is for all intents and purposes, L-Arginine but in the guise of Citrulline. Indeed Citrulline is converted to L-Arginine in the kidney thus by-passing the liver and increasing blood and tissue levels of L-Arginine – a much safer way of increasing L-Arginine and hence Nitric Oxide. Curis et al. noted in their detailed paper on Citrulline, that if it weren't for Citrulline, L-Arginine would be almost entirely taken up by the liver and converted to urea, leaving very little to form Nitric Oxide (NO) in the rest of the body. In the light of this understanding, it would seem illogical to use L-Arginine to increase Nitric Oxide in the blood vessels.

L-Citrulline as a Nitric Oxide booster for erectile dysfunction (ED)

The image on the next page and Appendix 23 provides an overview of Citrulline metabolism. What is poorly understood by many men who take Viagra® or Cialis® for erectile dysfunction is that Nitric Oxide (NO) is the vital first step for an erection to occur through the activation of Soluble Guanylate Cyclase (sGC).

When a man is aroused, nitric oxide is released from the parasympathetic nerve endings dilating the blood vessels in the Corpora Cavernosa (Dean and Lue 2005). Nitric Oxide released from the parasympathetic nerve endings, activates soluble GMP (sGMP) which then converts GTP to cGMP which in turn leads to PKG activation, a protein that lowers calcium in penile smooth muscle cells, leading to relaxation (vasodilation) and engorgement of the Corpora Cavernosa and hence an erection.

Viagra® or Cialis® by blocking the enzyme that degrades cGMP, i.e. inhibiting the phosphodiesterase-5 isoenzyme (PDE5) enzyme keeps cGMP levels high which in turn keeps on acting on PKG to maintain the erection. Ageing men may have lower arousal intensity than younger individuals, and the fact that they have erectile dysfunction indicates underlying vascular injury. More often than not, erectile dysfunction is due to endothelial dysfunction. The damaged endothelium through years of poor dietary choices, postprandial glucose and triglyceride elevations, inadequate nitrate intake vegetables or through smoking or sedentary lifestyles.

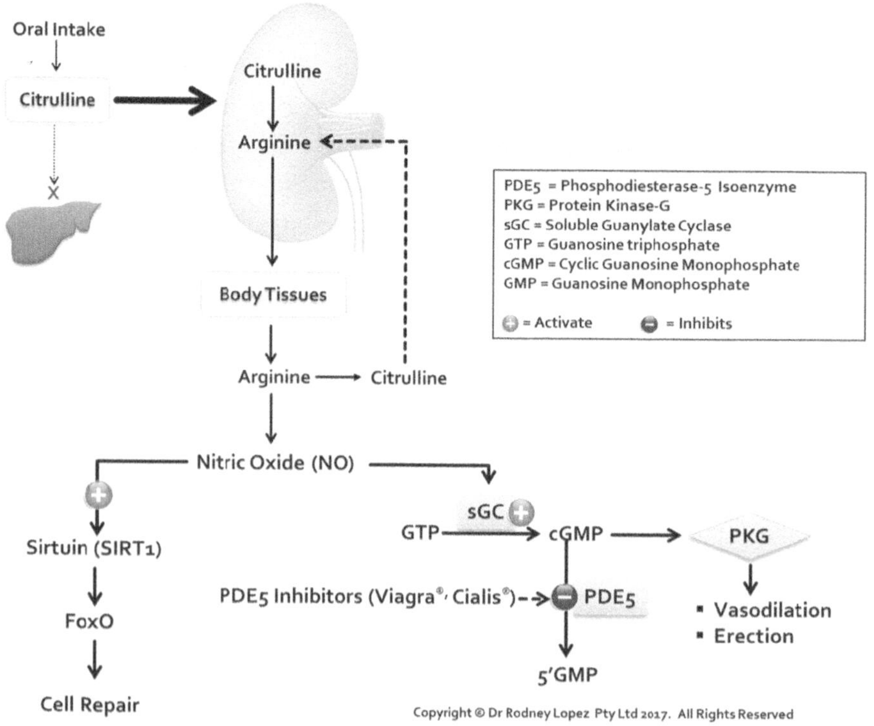

The first stage of an erection is arousal that sends impulses along the parasympathetic nerves which releases Nitric Oxide (NO) at the nerve endings in the Corpora Cavernosa leading to dilatation of the blood vessels there and engorgement. NO is critical for the activation of Soluble Guanylate

Oxidized-LDL damages the endothelium and this damaged endothelium upregulates (increases) arginase the enzyme that converts L-Arginine to ornithine preventing the L-Arginine forming nitric oxide (NO). Many men with erectile dysfunction also have vascular disease and risk factors such as hypertension, insulin resistance or diabetes. It is for this reason that 30 – 40% of men with erectile dysfunction do not respond to PDE5 inhibitors like Viagra® or Cialis®. These valuable medications can only function if there is enough cyclic GMP (cGMP) available to keep on stimulating PKG as you can see in the graphic. Without enough Nitric Oxide (NO) available, this will not happen thus diminishing the benefit from these medications (Pizzorno 2016).

Using Citrulline Makes Great Sense

Standard medical therapeutic interventions can be so much better than simply writing a script for a PDE5 inhibitor! If only medical practitioners understood this complex but critical need for Nitric Oxide (NO) to drive the process along, then perhaps the massive number of despondent men, some of which may be suicidal because they cannot function sexually, can be helped. Imagine the raft of interpersonal problems and emotional distress avoided by just providing a PDE5 inhibitor along with Citrulline.

Citrulline is incredibly safe and effective, and as a bonus, nitric oxide can help improve underlying cardiovascular disease and help repair processes through the Sirtuins and in particular SIRT1 and FoxO. Citrulline should be used in the context of an excellent diet that can also provide dietary nitrate donors such as the Activ8Health Plan-A and Plan-B diets. See Appendix-23 for some valuable information on Citrulline.

Integrative measures that provide such wonderful synergistic benefits should never be discarded as these are compounds that can be made in the body and so they are not alien to humans. These compounds like so many others can diminish with age or impaired functionally for a large number of reasons. We know that vital Nitric Oxide diminishes with age and needs a steady supply of L-Arginine for its production. Hopefully, enlightened medical practitioners will become aware of this wonderful synergy. The Activ8Health diets provide a rich source of plant nitrates, antioxidants and phytochemicals which assist nitric oxide (NO) generation. A more detailed graphic is provided in Appendix-23

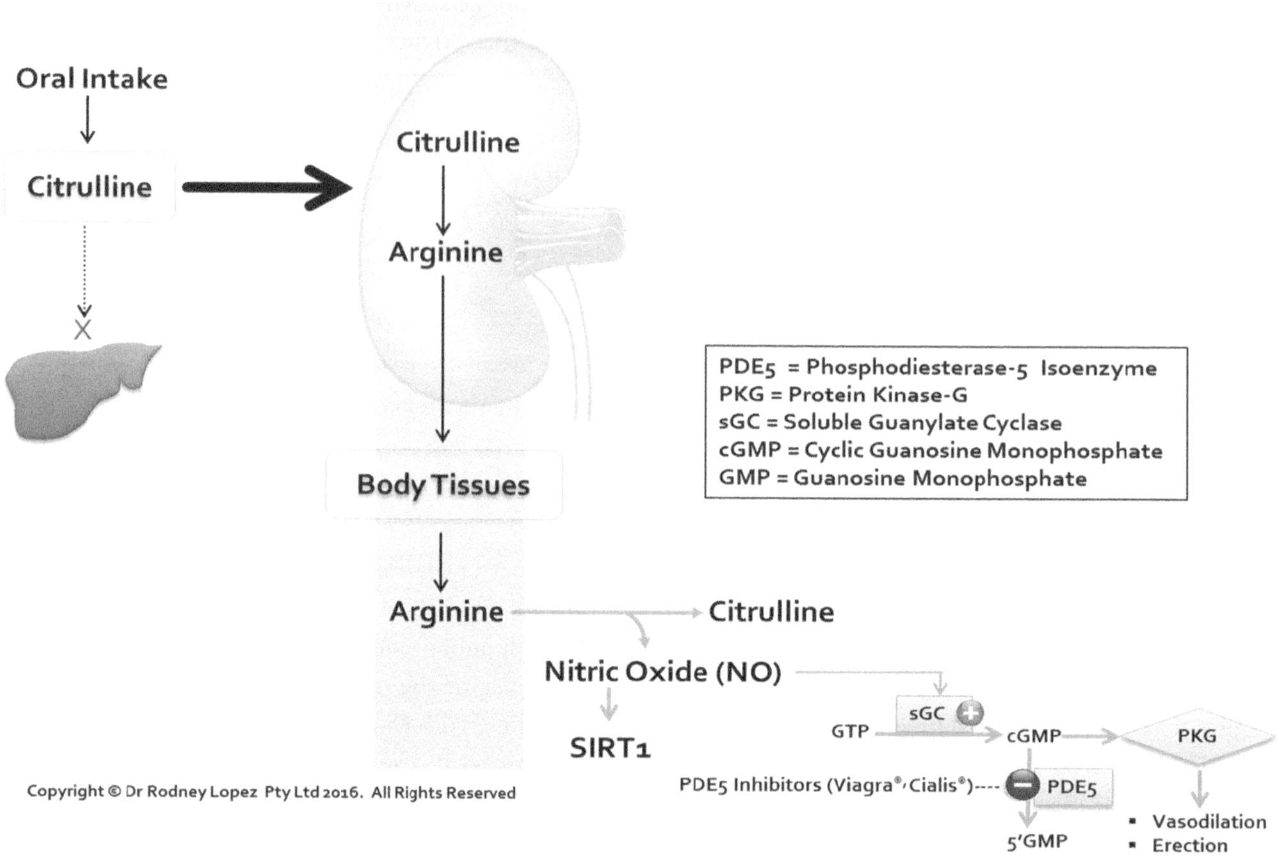

Graphic: Oral Citrulline is shunted to the kidneys where it is converted to L-Arginine and then distributed to the body through the circulation. This is unlike oral L-Arginine that is absorbed in the gut and carried to the liver in the portal circulation. The liver avidly takes up L-Arginine and converts it to urea. So the use of Citrulline as a 'masked' L-Arginine molecule is extremely clever medicine and thus provides the body with an abundance of L-Arginine to convert to Nitric Oxide (NO) so vital for your vascular endothelium and as an adjunct to the use of PDE5 inhibitors in erectile dysfunction. Not only are you creating a wonderful synergy with the PDE5's, you are helping to repair the underlying cardiovascular damage through the stimulation of SIRT1 and FoxO.

CHAPTER 5

Postprandial (after-eating) effects

Cardiovascular disease begins in childhood!

The ELEPHANT IN THE ROOM about cardiovascular health is the Western diet and in particular, the never-ending damage caused by every meal on a daily basis and over your lifetime.

As an individual, one of your greatest risks in life is a cardiovascular disease where you suffer a heart attack or stroke or peripheral vascular disease where arteries in your legs or neck (the carotid arteries) become blocked. What adds tremendously to this risk is your diet and lifestyle with diet a huge factor increasing your risk for these major killers in society.

Spikes in blood glucose and blood fats after eating will increase your risk for a multitude of common diseases which include diabetes, cancer, heart and vascular disease and the feared dementia as we all age. Your diet is well within your power to control. It is your choice to decide between the love of food or the love of life and in particular a healthy and long life that is disease-free for as long as possible. You can't have it both ways!

It is becoming more and more obvious that cardiovascular disease starts in childhood. We can prevent 90% of cardiovascular disease through preventative measures. You must be thinking this sounds like an outrageous statement, but it is an absolute fact, and a lot of this prevention will hinge on your risk factors in childhood and whether you were exposed to dreadful diets, sedentary lifestyles and if you were overweight or obese as a child. These factors will essentially determine your destiny in a cardiovascular sense as an adult – atherosclerosis should be thought of as originating in childhood with progression to symptomatic disease in adulthood (McGill, McMahan et al. 2008).

If we step back even further to a time before childhood, we can see a tremendous window of opportunity regarding the prevention of vascular risk. We diminish risk by ensuring optimal maternal and intrauterine nutrition, and by doing this, we can exert a profound positive impact on the genesis and progression of cardiovascular disease in childhood and adulthood. We discussed this concept under the Barker Hypothesis in the chapter on the Triage Theory of nutrition. Your mother's diet essentially will determine your cardiovascular destiny. Undernutrition during foetal development has dire consequences on childhood and adulthood cardiovascular risk. The absence of a major risk factor for example - high blood lipids, hypertension, prediabetes or diabetes by the age of 50 years of age has been shown to decrease your lifetime risk of cardiovascular disease by 90% up to age 95 years of age (O'Keefe and Bell 2007).

That we allow our children to eat the most heinous of foods in restaurants, or at home, and we allow them to gorge on artery-damaging food at children's functions, parties and school cafeterias are unconscionable acts when we consider each deadly meal is contributing to a lifelong vascular risk.

There seems to be a myth propagated in the medical profession that multiple risk factors explain only half of the coronary heart disease (CHD) seen in clinical practice. In fact abnormal lipids, smoking and diabetes were present *in "more than 85% to 90% of subjects experiencing CHD"* (McGill, McMahan et al. 2008). McGill et al. indicate that the *"only 50% myth should be abandoned."*

"War, what is it good for? Absolutely Nothing!"

These are the lyrics for the song 'War' which was written in 1969 for the Motown label and originally sung by the wonderful group, the **Temptations** and re-recorded by Edwin Starr who made this song one of the most popular protest songs in history. The song was indeed powerful and an obvious anti-Vietnam war song whose heartfelt sentiment resonated with any sane, peace-loving person. However, the lyrics suggest that war is good for nothing but sometimes war can have sad yet unexpected benefits for humanity. Two military engagements, the Korean and Vietnam wars provided medical researchers with a grim bounty of young and ostensibly healthy casualties of war to study, and these studies revealed stunning and highly concerning findings of atherosclerosis incidence in very young cohorts.

The astonishing findings were that 77% of young men with an average age of 22 years already had advanced atherosclerosis! (McGill, McMahan et al. 2008)

That the progression of fatty streaks in childhood sets, the foundation for cardiovascular disease in adulthood was firmly established in the 50's and 60's (McGill, McMahan et al. 2008).

So why has this carnage not been halted where countless millions of lives have been lost from heart attacks, strokes and other vascular complications, decade-after-decade long before they should have due to dietary mismanagement in pregnancy and early in life? The findings truly beggar belief. It all makes sense if you think about the agricultural machine and the immense power Big-Food has on governments and dietetic institutions that depend on the export dollars or sponsorships and junkets that keep this circus rolling along.

Remember, the Korean and Vietnam wars occurred remotely to the age of ubiquitous fast food outlets. Their staples were grains, meat and dairy. Sure, smoking was rampant, and this would have an impact on epigenetic imprinting, but the diet of individuals would be the driver of any epigenetic programming.

Vascular damage in childhood made worse with each meal in adulthood

If you accept that the foundation for heart and vascular disease has been set while you were developing in your mother's womb and that by the age of 22 you may have advanced heart disease as was shown in two wars discussed above at a time when obesity wasn't anywhere near the epidemic proportions as they are now, then you may want to read carefully what follows.

This foundation of childhood vascular damage and existing plaque which almost occluded many coronary blood vessels in those young soldiers is only be made worse meal-by-meal if you do not prevent the huge surges in blood glucose and blood fats that occur after every meal. Special attention to the composition of the meal is vital to prevent progression of vascular disease in adulthood.

Postprandial dysmetabolism is the term used for abnormal changes that occur in your blood after eating. After-eating metabolic changes are a well-entrenched and highly researched mechanism for vascular damage in the hours after consuming a meal and this is an important reason why pre-diabetics and diabetics do not fare too well with regards to vascular risk and organ damage. Remember, these surges in blood glucose and blood fats create a large inflammatory wave that floods not only your blood vessels but immerse and damage every tissue and organ in your body meal-by-meal, and this includes your brain. Avoid blood vessel damage, many cancers and dementia simply by taking the same amount of interest in what you eat or drink as you do in any other aspect of life important to you. Most meals are simply the ad hoc piling on of whatever is available and such meals are highly deficient in many aspects of nutrition. Let's look at how after-eating blood changes can shorten your life dramatically.

Postprandial Dysmetabolism

You have to eat to live, but the interesting point about eating is the profound effect the composition of that meal has on your blood biochemistry long after you have put your knife and fork down and washed the dishes.

After-eating surges in blood glucose, free fatty acids and triglycerides, can produce a huge number of metabolic shifts that affect the entire vascular system of the body and these blood biochemistry variations after a meal includes some incontrovertible metabolic changes termed: **'Postprandial Dysmetabolism'**. **(Dys)** metabolism means abnormal metabolism.

This concept of after-eating metabolic shifts is a known quantity that is evidence-based and rigorously assessed. If your meal is carb-heavy, you will have a marked elevation in blood glucose and blood insulin levels after eating, and the amount of carbohydrate will determine how high and for how long that blood glucose and insulin will stay elevated.

A fatty meal consisting of fatty meats, cream or sausages or indeed any other fat-laden food from a food court or fast food outlet, will cause a marked elevation in blood triglycerides (blood fats). These fats floating around in your blood after eating are enough to make the serum cloudy if you drew blood and then centrifuged it to separate the blood from the serum. Worse still is a huge portion of carbohydrate that is soaked in fat like the glistening noodles you see in heating pans at food outlets or pizzas full of carbohydrate and fat that raise both glucose and fats after eating.

Protein will cause a significant elevation in blood amino acids, and these amino acids can also cause insulin increases in the blood. All of these nutrient components will orchestrate a range of hormonal and cytokine signalling effects in the body long after you stop eating.

How many times in a day do you see children with huge portions of French fries in front of them or massive servings of sugar-laden desserts that they devour? Think of the changes that are occurring in their blood after they eat these dreadful meals and the vascular and organ damage these meals cause in that child. This sets the foundation for adult vascular disease. How many adults keep on eating as if they were still kids?

Every meal you have will damage you a little at a time incrementally and cumulatively throughout your life irrespective of how healthy you think that food it. Food is simply a mix of chemicals that your body uses to function. How much damage occurs after eating will depend on the composition of the meal you want to eat.

Cell 'Factories' Processing Food Chemicals

After eating, blood glucose and fats are either burnt off as energy or stored as fat if you have consumed a surplus of energy. These nutrient components from food are used to extract energy in your cells or build cellular components. The cells are like factories in this regard and like most factories manufacturing products, they produce some form of pollution and environmental damage through the production process.

So too do the cell 'factories' produce a form of 'pollution' called **free radicals** which are the by-products of the creation or consumption of energy from those blood nutrients and these charged particles zoom around at lightning speed damaging everything in their path.

Reactive Oxygen Species (ROS) are the other form of damaging cellular 'industrial emission's'. So this cellular 'pollution' causes environmental damage to nearby intracellular structures (the organelles of the cell), the tissues that house those cells and the organs that house those tissues through oxidative stress and inflammation.

Other damaging inflammatory biomolecules like cytokines or dietary fat-induced blood lipopolysaccharide (LPS) are produced, and these can harm the lining of blood vessels called the endothelium resulting in **endothelial dysfunction.** This wave of inflammation causes damage to the dangerous low-density lipoproteins (LDL) floating around in your bloodstream at the same time. A change in LDL at this very time is simply collateral damage to the LDL.

The free radicals, oxidative stress and inflammation start to attack floating LDL molecules also known as the 'bad cholesterol' to cause **oxidised-LDL (oxLDL).** This altered LDL or oxLDL is far more toxic and can burrow their way into the lining of blood vessels to trigger plaque formation under the lining of blood vessels. The elevation in blood glucose after eating also causes the glycation of LDL to form **glycated-LDL,** and both oxidised-LDL and glycated-LDL are powerful determinants of atherosclerosis. They trigger immune cell responses and inflammatory processes in and under the lining of blood vessels eventually causing blockages (stenosis). Remember the bigger the meal, the greater the potential to produce oxidised and glycated LDL in the many hours after eating.

The plaques once formed, can become larger in a similar way to sediment building upon a river or ocean bed. The depth of this sediment is increased over the years. It is a similar process about plaque formation and growth. Stimulation of plaque growth occurs meal-after-meal. Small pieces of this plaque can break off and fly off in the circulation, and these small plaque fragments are called emboli. They can lodge in and block smaller diameter vessels further down the track sometimes resulting in significant tissue damage to your brain or retina of the eye or peripheral circulation in the limbs sometimes cutting off the blood supply to a finger or toe.

Most people in the Western world are in the postprandial(after-eating) state 24/7 (O'Keefe and Bell 2007), and this is due to the massive meals and snacks consumed throughout the day and the fact that it may take 6 hours or more for the after-eating blood glucose and fats to settle down. As a result, oxidised and glycated LDL is also being formed 24/7 all because people just do not stop eating. How often do people not eat in a 6 hour period?

Treating established cardiovascular disease is 'Secondary Prevention'

I am sure that most doctors think that treating someone with established heart disease in an adult is primary prevention, but this is not the case. Treating someone with vascular disease in their 40's and beyond is secondary prevention (McGill, McMahan et al. 2008). Atherosclerosis is already well established by adulthood as we have seen with the casualties of the Korean and Vietnam wars who already had advanced atherosclerosis in their 20's. People are naïve indeed if they think they are getting away with eating massive meal portions, packed with calories and deficient in micronutrients.

Vascular damage is occurring irrespective of how they are feeling and remember, there are no symptoms caused by early plaque formation.

Primary prevention begins in pregnancy and childhood not in adult life. The risk was set by the grandparents whose sperm and ova were a reflection of the diet and lifestyle they kept and the epigenetic changes in these germs cells passed on to your parents. If you are planning to have children, ensure you minimise the risk through the best diet you can muster, exercise regularly and avoid destructive practices such as smoking, taking drugs or drinking alcohol excessively. An optimal micronutrient intake including Choline pre-pregnancy in both partners may just ensure a physically and mentally healthy baby.

Not to say that you can't make an impact in your adult life through dietary and exercise management as you could have a great impact on life expectancy but only if you follow the guidelines in this book with maximum discipline. You cannot change your mother's diet, and you cannot go back in time to your childhood to avoid all those sweet foods, sodas, carb and fat-laden meals as you grew up that laid the foundation of atherosclerosis. What you can do is ensure your children do not succumb to this madness in the home, in restaurants, at children's parties or in school cafeterias by ensuring they also abide by the principles outlined here most of the time. Change their destinies through parental guidance.

Remember, your children too will have their kids, and healthy diets in their childhood will influence their germ cells (ova, sperm) and thus change disease risk in subsequent generations. As I have stated in this book the mother's wellness, weight and dietary habits will affect the next three generations and the father the next two generations. Such a tremendous responsibility to the hordes of people that follow us. There is no greater gift than the gift of health!

1st and 2nd Phase Insulin Release Postprandially

It is interesting that you have two phases of insulin release with eating. There is an early phase where a small amount of insulin gets released over a 10 minute period followed by a more prolonged release of insulin by the pancreas that is dependent on the carbohydrate load consumed, i.e. the glycemic load or GL (O'Keefe and Bell 2007). That early 1st phase release helps to blunt the glucose surge soon after eating, but a very early manifestation of Type-1 and Type-2 diabetes is the absence of this early phase of insulin release.

When this 1st phase of insulin release vanishes, the level of blood glucose and free fatty acids increase significantly after eating (O'Keefe and Bell 2007). A long-term follow-up study has shown that decreased first phase glucose clearance could be detected an amazing ten years before becoming diabetic and this predicted the development of diabetes (Martin, Warram et al. 1992).

So are you at risk? If you have a strong family history of diabetes or you are putting on weight in the abdominal area then yes, you are at risk! This abdominal fat increases your risk of having insulin resistance and prediabetes. Even those who are thin may have a high volume of intra-abdominal (visceral) fat that resides deep in their abdomens surrounding internal organs, and this puts them at risk of this blunted or absent 1st phase insulin response which results in much higher glucose and blood fats after eating.

Simply checking your waist circumference or having a DEXA body composition scan to assess your visceral fat level will let you know that you may be in trouble.

It is important to state that you can be lean and at very high risk and so the only way to find out is to have blood tests for fasting lipids, glucose and insulin levels.

Postprandial (after-eating) waves perceived as a 'threat' to your body

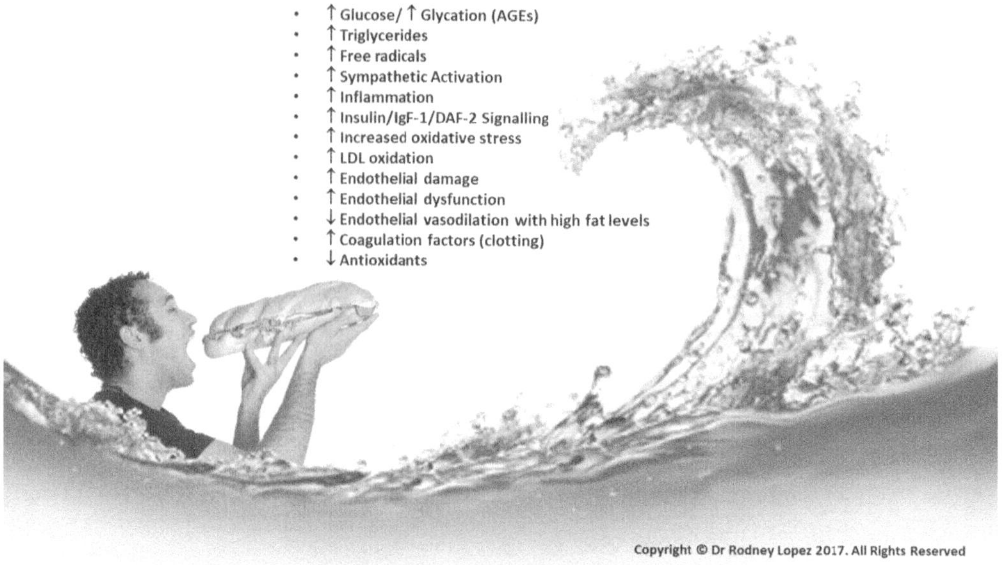

Professor Antonio Ceriello, a renowned diabetes researcher, has produced a wonderful visual image of these postprandial surges in glucose and fats in the blood. He sees these changes as a 'wave' that travels along the arterial conduits in the body with each meal causing wave after wave of biochemical changes leading to a marked inflammatory response in the entire body (Ceriello 2000).

According to other researchers, each meal is seen as a 'threat' to your body producing a frantic metabolic response to get your body back on track to a normal state in a process termed homeostasis. The mechanisms involved in the homeostasis process are simply a series of adjustments that try to get the body back to a normal resting state. In this postprandial state blood chemistry goes haywire after eating. A huge range or hormonal signals, receptor adjustments and cellular signalling responses, are called into play, They finely adjust to the *"stress of the postprandial state"* (Margioris 2009). These after-eating metabolic adjustments are highly orchestrated driving after-eating changes in the blood back to normal (homeostasis).

These blood nutrient surges (metabolic stressors), also greatly reduce the pool of systemic antioxidants leading to significant oxidative stress in the body after eating and this is the result of the trillions of free radicals produced with each meal and the need to 'quench' these damaging charged particles by antioxidant activity. The more antioxidants you have in your meal through plant-based phytochemicals, the more of a chance you will have of protecting this antioxidant pool after eating thus preventing dangerous dips in antioxidant activity that will then allow these free radicals to ravage the body in this after-eating state unrestricted.

Clotting factors are also affected, and this can lead to a heart attack or stroke as a result of eating just one heavy meal. How high your blood glucose rises after eating will depend on how much carbohydrate you have on your plate. Proteins **everywhere** in your body undergo damage by these high after-eating blood glucose surges, and this is called glycation. This glycation process ages you as glucose attaches to elastin and collagen in every tissue of your body increasing the wrinkling in your skin and also damaging these important structural proteins in tissues and organs, including your brain. Is it any wonder then that dementia is so common?

Relentless damage, meal-after-meal

Keep in mind; these surges are occurring meal-after-meal, and snack-after-snack, every day of your life for 365 days in a year and over your lifetime. The metabolic insult caused by an individual meal is small, but these small effects are incremental and cumulative over your life. You can see why meal composition is so vital.

The meals you eat will either produce small waves gently lapping on the 'shore' or produce a tsunami of metabolic damage caused by massive meals loaded with calories, carbs, fat and protein. Just look at what people pile on their plates in any home, restaurant or food court, and you can just imagine the metabolic tsunami about to occur and persist for 6 hours or more just from that one meal.

Is it any wonder that chronic diseases like obesity, diabetes, heart disease, Alzheimer's, cancers and a myriad number of other degenerative states have reached epidemic proportions? People are simply killing themselves with the quantity of food they eat of poor quality. People not only pile food high on any plate but go back for seconds or thirds and finish off their deadly meals with equally deadly desserts that add to the glycating effects through a massively increased blood glucose level caused by the carbs in the food and the highly processed carbs (sugar) in the dessert.

One meal can kill!

What if I were to say that a particularly heavy meal could be the end of your life? Sounds far-fetched to you? But research has shown time and again that many people have suffered from an acute cardiovascular event like a heart attack and ended up in a coronary care unit or indeed, died after a rich meal. In fact, there was a four-fold (4x) increase in the likelihood of an acute heart attack in the first hour after a meal (Lipovetzky, Hod et al. 2004; Tofler and Muller 2006). That this happens is undeniable as numerous research papers have shown that a rich meal has put an end to many a life as a consequence of multiple pathological metabolic mechanisms that manifest in the blood long after you stop eating. Please revisit the wave graphic to see a large number of changes that occur in the blood after a meal.

In essence, your life in the short or long-term depends on the composition of that meal. What constitutes that meal (qualitative factor), and the quantity (quantitative factor), will determine how long you will stay in your healthspan or how soon you enter the disease-span. The disease-span is how long you will be unhealthy and fighting off the devastating effects of chronic illness.

To this, we can add 'mindspan' because poor diets are associated with a higher risk of Alzheimer's and vascular dementia. If you are not a serious contender for an acute cardiovascular event, each meal you consume will put you closer to that life-changing or life-ending last meal. A meal may not end your life acutely, but it is a sobering thought that damage to your arteries and organs are occurring meal-by-meal and that this damage is cumulative over your lifetime. If you have never thought about food composition and the impact it has on your life, you may want to consider the following.

Interesting statistics based on our blood work

1. If you have a fasting blood glucose level of just 5 mmol/L - i.e. within the 'normal' range, it predicts that your 2 hour postprandial (after-eating) blood glucose can climb to a whopping 11.1 mmol/L which is essentially the diabetes cut-off point at 2 hours for a glucose tolerance test. These postprandial elevations have been shown in studies to lead to large vessel atherosclerosis (macrovascular complications) as well as small vessel disease (microvascular complications) (O'Keefe and Bell 2007). Ask your doctor to check your fasting blood glucose and fasting blood lipid levels. However, more and more research is showing that fasting blood glucose, and blood

triglyceride levels may be very deceiving as these are checked around 12 hours after eating. A better parameter would be to check how high your blood glucose and triglycerides are climbing after eating to ascertain risk.

2. In the United Kingdom Prospective Diabetes Study (UKPDS), it revealed that by the time someone was diagnosed with diabetes, 50% would have already suffered from diabetic complications (O'Keefe and Bell 2007). What this tells you is that the process is insidious, it develops over time and meal after damaging meal, and the damage can occur long before arbitrary cut-off points are reached and are occurring while you are symptom-free. The cut-off points in blood glucose used to diagnose diabetes in medicine is a late-stage marker and at a level that 'Blind Freddy' could pick up but long after early vascular damage occurs.

   It is difficult to reverse the late-stage vascular damage, where you now have to use stop-gap measures by putting stents in blocked arteries or doing by-pass grafting or try to pry open a stenosis through angioplasty. All plainly late stage interventionist medicine but makes sense for governments who do not consider preventing something in the future as worthwhile as this costs money and labelling prediabetes a disease means you now have to fund this new disease entity. It is wise to remember that you do not have to have prediabetes or diabetes to suffer all the complications that they do. They will simply get there a little earlier than you.

3. Two giant studies the Physician's Health Study (PHS) and the Multiple Risk Factor Intervention Trial (MRFIT trial pronounced 'Mr Fit') has also shed some light on the fats in the blood – the triglycerides.

   Sonic Health Care's cut-off point for a normal triglyceride level is less than 2.0 mmol/L in the fasting state. These two trials showed distinctly that for every 1.13 mmol/L increase in blood triglycerides, your risk of myocardial infarction (heart attack) jumped by a massive 40% (O'Keefe and Bell 2007). Triglycerides can increase greatly with a fatty meal where it is not uncommon to have a triglyceride level of around 7 mmol/L hours after a fat-containing meal (O'Keefe and Bell 2007). It is interesting that the higher the triglyceride level in the blood, the higher the level of lipoproteins like VLDL and chylomicrons that transport the fats in blood (Grønholdt, Nordestgaard et al. 1996). These lipoproteins block the formation of Nitric Oxide (NO) that dilates blood vessels (Ceriello, Taboga et al. 2002) and increases a molecule called endothelin

which constricts arteries

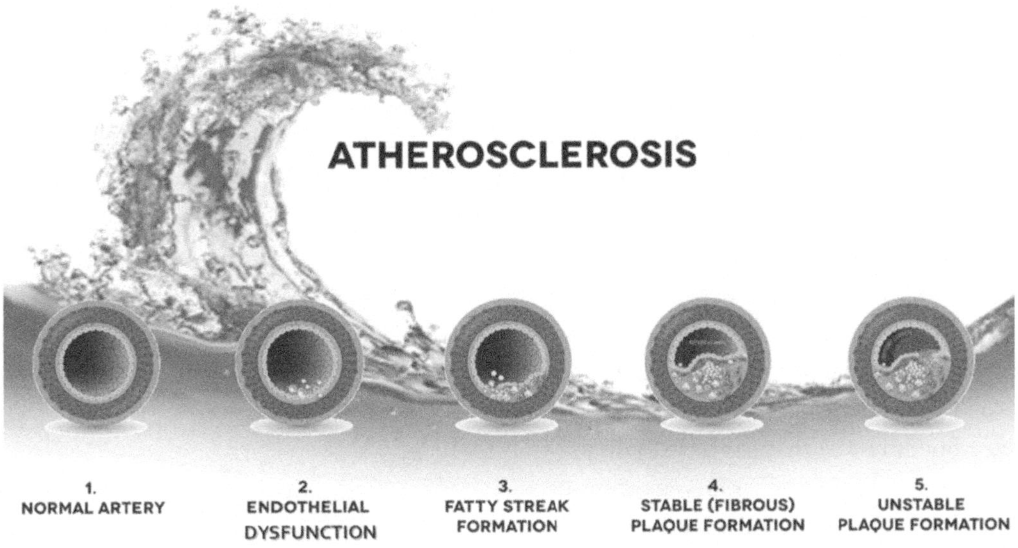

4

Cumulative effects of meals on atherosclerosis

As I have indicated, each meal adds to the effects of previous meals by causing progressive disease of arteries.

It all starts off with endothelial dysfunction where the lining of the blood vessels are damaged, and this can be due to all those postprandial effects I have discussed. Triglycerides are known to produce marked inflammation when they rise in the blood, and this inflammation weakens the endothelial lining of the arteries. A lack of dietary nitrates and a lack of Nitric Oxide (NO) formation in the arterial walls will prevent these blood vessels from dilating (enlarging), and thus they become stiffer and more damaged by shear forces caused by the blood pressure waves generated by heart contractions.

Poor meal choices only lead to more and more damage caused by the after-eating dysmetabolism causing plaque to build up and new plaque to form. Meals that are rich in plant-based foods like rocket (arugula), spinach and beetroot can provide high levels of nitrates that can boost nitric oxide production. So too can L-Citrulline (Appendix-23) provide a significant nitric oxide boost and N-acetylcysteine (NAC) Appendix-7, can help by providing the sulphur based amino acid cysteine to ensure an adequate supply of the powerful intrinsic antioxidant glutathione which then becomes available at meaningful levels to mop up those damaging free radicals produced from eating.

Calcium Artery Calcification

Inflammatory changes to the plaques will cause calcification to the layers under the endothelium of the blood vessels causing even more arterial stiffness and damage. Calcified plaque may be more stable than the soft lipid-rich plaque that can rupture due to shear stress and inflammation in the blood. The benefit of knowing you have a high calcium score is that it can alert you to a high plaque burden in the coronary arteries which means a high risk for an acute coronary event depending on the extent of the coronary artery calcification and other risk factors. For those of you who have a strong family history of heart disease, diabetes, prediabetes, premature cardiac death, abnormal lipids or glucose even in the normal upper range, you may want to consider Calcium Artery Calcification (CAC) scoring which is done in a CT scanner. Discuss this with your doctor. New cardiovascular risk calculators like the Multi-Ethnic Study of Atherosclerosis (MESA calculator at (https://www.mesa-nhlbi.org/MESACHDRisk/MesaRiskScore/RiskScore.aspx), can use this calcium score along with other risk factors to provide a 10-year risk of an adverse heart vascular event.

For anyone who has an existing cardiovascular risk, to just depend upon medication is not advisable as these medications cannot abolish the devastating postprandial effects of food and will just be a Band-Aid approach to treatment.

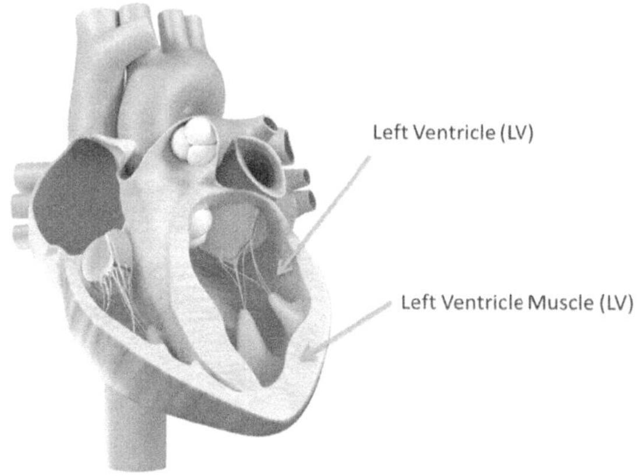

Combining medications if you have existing vascular disease with the strict dietary guidelines as suggested in this book will be of great help. You need your medical practitioner to keep an eye on medications as you undergo dietary changes and find a dietitian (see Appendix-17) that can assist you in analysing your diet and perhaps arranging other tests to guide dietary management. Find a medical practitioner who understands that these types of diseases are not the result of a lack of pharmaceuticals in the air or water; they are the result of poor dietary practices over a lifetime. Avoid practitioners who simply want to add more and more pharmaceuticals to your treatment without any consideration of the root cause of the disease process itself. In this day and age when diet and exercise-as-medicine are becoming *de rigueur*, this pure pharmaceutical approach to treating complex chronic diseases like atherosclerosis and heart disease is now seen as quaint and anachronistic by progressives in the medical game.

Sympathetic hyperactivity

This concept of sympathetic activation by a meal is alien to medical practitioners, but this is an established postprandial fact and a part of the dysmetabolism process after eating. The sympathetic and parasympathetic nervous systems are known as the 'autonomic nervous system', and the sympathetic system is involved in the 'fight-flight-response' preparing us for action. The mediators are adrenaline (epinephrine) released from the adrenal glands or noradrenaline (norepinephrine) released at nerve endings. The sympathetic system is activated in the postprandial (after-eating) state to establish homeostasis, i.e. to get the body back to the normal state.

After eating the heart rate and cardiac output increases to propel food to the far reaches of the body (van Baak 2008). Usually not be a problem normally if the meals consumed weren't so massive and if people allowed for a long interval before eating again. However, the overactive sympathetic system after eating can also predispose us to high blood pressure (hypertension), to arrhythmias or abnormal heart rhythms like atrial fibrillation (AF) or ventricular ectopics.

Large numbers of people in the general population suffer from atrial fibrillation (AF) as they age and AF is a stroke risk. Postprandial sympathetic hyperactivity would have to be a major contributor to this risk. Add this postprandial problem to obstructive sleep apnoea or magnesium insufficiency, and you have a recipe for disaster to drive a heart rhythm problem.

The added blood pressure caused by postprandial changes in a 24/7 period, occurs because people just do not stop eating and this causes stress to the heart and in particular the left ventricle of the heart which pumps blood to the body and has to pump blood against an elevated pressure in the arterial system. This heart, as a result, has to work harder to pump blood against a high-pressure barrier. This is analogous to say a garden hose with a kink. You have to increase the pressure at the tap to push water along and overcome this water pressure barrier.

I'm sure you can think of all the problems that can occur by increasing pressure at the tap with holes punched in the hose due to the higher pressure head or the tap head springing an almighty leak. No different to high blood pressure in your arteries with your left ventricle pumping harder and harder to 'punch' through this pressure head. Think strokes instead of leaks in the water hose and think left ventricular hypertrophy (muscle enlargement) and heart failure instead of a tap fitting failing and spraying water all over you.

Diastolic heart failure is caused by the left ventricle becoming stiffer because the muscle has been stressed and damaged and this muscle is thus unable to relax. **You do not have to have high blood pressure to cause the changes in the heart muscle. All it takes is the increased sympathetic/parasympathetic imbalance after eating to cause changes in heart muscle cell growth** (Brook and Julius 2000). The article by Brook and Julius cited is a wonderful article that should be read by every Cardiologist and General Practitioner. Is it any wonder that large numbers of people who undergo an ECHO heart study to assess heart function come back with a report of '**diastolic dysfunction**'.

Here is another 'elephant in the room' as a modifiable cause of heart failure that occurs three or more times every day, year in and year out. Yes, other causes exist but nowhere near the extent of the Western diet as a cause of sympathetic hyperactivity meal-after-meal resulting in prolonged sympathetic activity 24/7, 365 days a year, all because people think will they die if they feel hungry. In fact, they die much younger than they should all because they constantly gorge on food that damages them incrementally and cumulatively over their lifespan. Using the intraday fasting strategy discussed in this book could just be that lifesaver you are looking for especially if you have existing heart disease or other chronic illnesses driven by bad dietary practices.

Stenting and bypass grafting of blocked vessels won't save you long-term

It is interesting that significant blockages in the coronary arteries are discovered through angiography where dye is used to find blocked segments of a blood vessel, and fixed either by stenting or bypass surgery. Stenting is where a metal or plastic tube is inserted into an area of the artery that is critically blocked to allow blood through. Procedures like this can save someone's life in the short-term but in the long-term may have no impact on the risk of an acute vascular event and why? All because diet and lifestyle stay the same.

How can vascular surgery have a long-term impact if those postprandial surges keep on hammering at the blood vessels above and below the stented area? It is naïve to think that the particular blocked segment being stented is the only lesion to worry about, but this is NOT the case. The full length of that particular blocked artery is affected by plaque both soft and hard, and indeed that whole heart vascular bed will be affected as well as other vascular beds like the brain, legs, retina, gastrointestinal tract or the carotid arteries that supply the vulnerable brain with blood. How often would vascular surgery be followed-up by strict control of diet and in particular the strict control of the postprandial (after-eating) factors that lead to vascular damage in the first place?

Dr Michael Ozner is an American Cardiologist and author of 'The Great American Heart Hoax' (Ozner 2008). He indicates that these procedures are just 'Band-Aids' and that 70-90% of these lucrative procedures are 'at best unnecessary'. No doubt this multi-billion dollar industry will tease out as much benefit as possible and obfuscate the issues through massive technically confusing research that will also confuse the regulators.

In fact, at the time the book was published in 2008, the spend on invasive cardiovascular care was 60 billion dollars, and this is just one small corner of medical care!

Ozner goes on to say that: *"...coronary artery angioplasties, stent placements, and coronary bypass surgeries ---are of dubious value, adding little in terms of long-term health outcomes, and sometimes even making things worse than if they hadn't been performed at all."*

Mortality rates for bypass surgery are around 3 – 5% which may not sound like a lot, but that is 3 – 5 people who die out of 100 people undergoing the procedure.

As Dr Ozner points out, that when 500,000 people undergo these procedures the death toll numbers 15,000 to 25,000 people as a result of the surgery. Isn't this an amazing loss of life if the outcomes are of dubious benefit? To make matters worse, 80% of people undergoing these procedures may experience cognitive difficulties after surgery. Cognitive decline may be due to embolic phenomena during the operation where pieces of plaque fly off to smaller vessels in the brain blocking them off and the fact that the cerebral vascular bed is also extensively damaged to the same extent as the coronary arteries undergoing surgery.

It is critical for any individual who has undergone cardiac surgery or is contemplating cardiac surgery to understand that there are short-term benefits but that long-term survival will depend upon absolutely strict dietary management and exercise on a regular basis. Medical practitioners who do not stress this point are simply putting their patients at great risk.

The Lyon Diet Heart Study - The Mediterranean Diet

That dietary measures can prevent or reverse heart disease can be doubted is unbelievable and it should be compulsory for all general practitioners and cardiologists to read this study. The initial study was published in the Lancet in 1994 and examined why mortality was so much lower in countries bordering the Mediterranean in comparison to northern Europe.

It is amazing how incredibly important findings of diet like this vanish into the ether, and we go back to discussing drugs and cardiovascular interventions. This study was supposed to last for five years, was cut short after 27 months because the ethics committee could not allow the placebo group to keep on eating the Standard American Diet (SAD) in the light of the amazing ***70% reduction in all-cause mortality*** (Leaf 1999)

This study marked the beginning of our interest in what is now known as the Mediterranean diet. When we compare the result of dietary management, to say the use of statins that are prescribed to lower cholesterol levels, this quote comes to mind:

> *"Even the best result obtained in a single study with statins in adults reduced CHD by only 40%, and the average reduction achieved in 14 trials was 23%."(McGill, McMahan et al. 2008)*

So the effectiveness of dietary measures far exceed those of medications, and yet the focus is still on relatively ineffective interventionist strategies which as I have stated are all secondary prevention practices as primary prevention occurs lies in optimising dietary factors in pregnancy, development in utero and childhood factors that set the scene for adult atherosclerosis.

That the Mediterranean diet can decrease cardiovascular risk by a margin of 47% **<u>greater than</u>** the average 23% reduction shown with statins that lower cholesterol - is a staggering finding! Can you just imagine the absolute headline-grabbing statements if a drug was found to decrease heart and vascular disease by 70% --- what do you think the headlines would state? 'Staggering reductions in all-cause mortality with Product-X' or 'Stop Press! Unbelievable 70% reductions in heart disease with Product-Y.....' Every doctor's surgery will be flooded with marketing materials and visits regularly by drug representatives time and again in lunchtime meetings or invitations to dinners and conferences to spruik the virtues of Product-X or Y.

So why hasn't this happened with this diet that is thrown in the same basket as other diets when this was amazingly well researched and published in the Lancet no less? The fact is that no one can make a dollar from this apart from governments that could save huge sums of money by aggressively targeting the horrendous Western diets of pregnant women and children and let's not forget the adults who keep on eating the way they did in childhood.

Why is this even debated now? The time to act is now without the 'noise' generated by vested interests including the agricultural and 'Big-Food' industries. It is up to you to look beyond this cacophony and beyond vested interests and marketing and advertising to see food for what it is and to take measures to ensure you stay healthy throughout your life.

The problem with stenting and bypass grafting for established atherosclerosis

If we look at a stent inserted into a blocked (stenotic) area as shown in (A) on the left, this is perhaps how lay people view this and probably many doctors as well. This is seen as a case of – "we have opened up a blockage in the artery, blood is now flowing again, and this has eased the patient's angina, so job well done! see you later."

In graphic (A) we have an isolated blocked area opened up with the stent, but the remainder of the blood vessel looks pristine. Such a scenario in real life is simply not true, and the artery would be more like (B) where you have a diseased blood vessel with both calcified and soft plaque lining the vessel above and below the stented area.

The plaque on either side of the stent is vulnerable to all the metabolic stresses that I have discussed in detail in this chapter. Those after eating metabolic changes in the blood are still adding to the expansion of these existing plaques above (proximal to) the stent, and below (distal to) the stent and are prone to rupture or to form new blocked (stenotic) areas as we can see in (C).

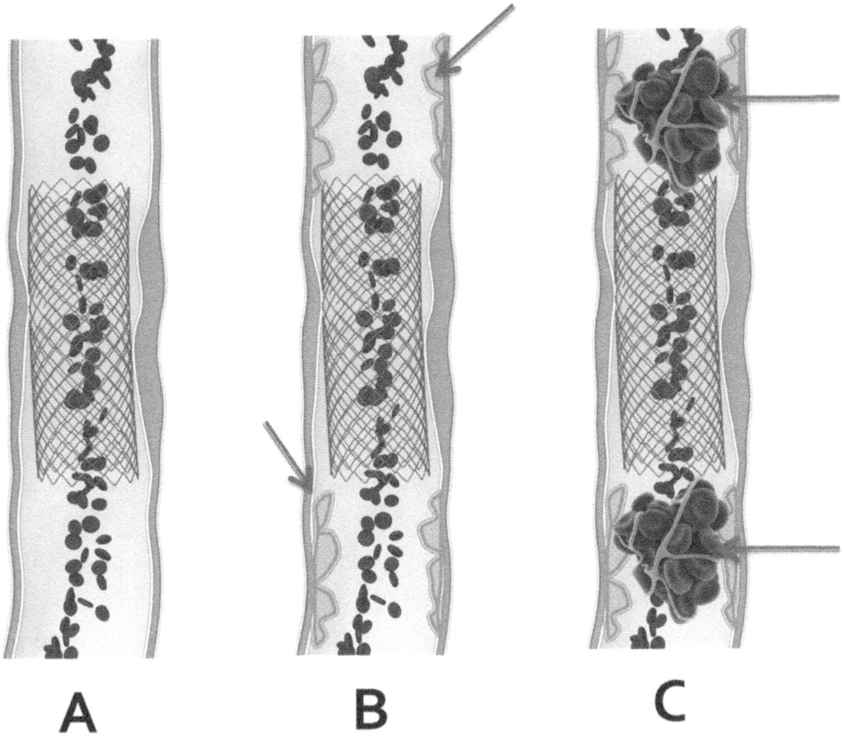

If you are having heart surgery for advanced atherosclerotic disease, it is naïve indeed to think that only one small part of a blood vessel is affected and the rest is absolutely normal.

So if you are unfortunate enough to have to undergo stenting or bypass grafting for advanced arterial disease in the coronary arteries or elsewhere, if you want to live a long life without the risk of a heart attack or stroke after the surgery, you will need to be on a very strict diet using all the tricks outlined in this book to ensure existing plaque not only stabilizes but regresses. All your vascular beds will be affected by plaque to a lesser or greater extent, and it is only a matter of time that an acute event occurs.

The same situation applies if a stent is used to open up a lower leg arterial blockage or if an obstructing area of plaque is being operated on in your carotid arteries.

Meal factors to consider: A Summary

Always think of a meal in the following way:

1. Qualitatively – do you have all the micronutrients, fibre, good fats, phytochemicals present?
2. Quantitatively – Are you eating too much carbohydrate, fats and protein on that plate

The micronutrient content of the meal → Does this meal have a wide variety of vitamins, minerals or trace elements that your body needs to thrive? Low intakes of one or more micronutrients will mean that your body has to decide which organ or organs will receive those micronutrients and which ones will not get their share. The basis of Triage mechanisms that I have discussed.

The phytochemical content of the meal → Is that meal rich in plant chemicals? Does it have a variety of anthocyanins, carotenoids, flavonoids, lignans, glucosinolates and thousands of other phytochemicals that bathe your DNA with signalling compounds commanding your genes to turn on or off (hormesis)? The power of a high intake of phytochemicals is enormous. Hormesis will be discussed in detail. Research has shown consistently that a high intake of vegetables predominantly and fruit modestly, provides you with a huge bang-for-the-buck from a health perspective, decreasing all-cause mortality. Do you have a multicoloured vegetable-rich drink most days? See Appendix-4.

The glycemic effects of the meal → How high will your glucose level climb after that particular meal? Glucose is highly toxic, and for this reason, it is kept in a tight concentration range in your blood.

If you think that because sugar (sucrose or glucose) tastes so nice and seems so innocuous and innocent, that is could not possibly be damaging, just ask any diabetic who has lost their eyesight, lost their limbs, had a stroke or are undergoing kidney dialysis hours every day due to glucose-related kidney damage - if they think that glucose is benign.

How high the glucose levels climb after a meal is a powerful determinant of the devastating complications and short lifespans diabetics experience. If you do not have diabetes and feel reassured, think again. I will show you how glucose damages every cell and organ in your system with every meal you consume whether you have diabetes or not.

Glucose attaches to proteins easily and then damages them (glycation). The protein could be the elastin and collagen in your skin that ages you meal-by-meal or the proteins in your organs that may ultimately become dysfunctional. Glucose glycates the collagen in your bones weakening them as you age and each meal damages not only bone collagen but indeed all collagen and elastin in your body a little at a time. You won't see any immediate difference because the damage is cumulative over your lifespan. You will simply look much older as you age than someone who uses the knowledge supplied in this book to offset a preventable factor in the ageing process.

The inflammatory effect of a meal →The postprandial (after-eating) inflammatory effect of a meal is an independent factor to mark food quality (Margioris, 2009). The food we consume can make up a large part of the inflammatory 'load' the body has to deal with on a daily basis, and this is to a large extent preventable. Inflammation is at the heart of most chronic diseases that affect us, and this includes cardiovascular disease, diabetes, cancer, Alzheimer's, stroke and autoimmune disease. So it pays to keep this diet-induced inflammatory load down as much as possible over your lifetime.

The triglyceride effect of the meal →Triglycerides are a grouping of 3 fatty acids attached to a sugar alcohol backbone (glycerol), and these fats are transported in the blood after a meal. The absorbed and transported triglyceride fats have an independently powerful inflammatory after-eating effect. Researchers often do not make bold statements to describe a research finding, but these researchers stated that triglycerides induce a

"soaring postprandial inflammatory response" (Margioris, 2009).

The amount of inflammation after a meal can trigger off a heart attack or a clot and can lead to ongoing damage of cells and organ systems. High triglycerides in the blood cause a drop in HDL the good cholesterol carrier that removes cholesterol from your arteries and a parallel increase in small dense LDL (sd-LDL) which is a highly atherogenic (arterial plaque forming) form of low-density lipoprotein (LDL). It is interesting that a high triglyceride level and low HDL level were independent risk factors for diabetic kidney disease in a study that involved 15,362 diabetes patients over a four year period (Russo, De Cosmo et al. 2016). Chronic kidney disease is very common in society and so keeping triglyceride levels down with every meal is very good idea.

The diversity of foods consumed in your meals →Individuals in Western populations consume a very small number of foods day-in and day-out. This lack of variety will limit nutrient and phytochemical diversity. Such dietary limitations have a powerful impact on the overall diversity of microorganisms in your bowel known as the Bowel Microbiome. A rich diversity of foods will ensure a rich diversity of organisms in your bowel. The number of organisms in your large intestine is simply staggering. It is estimated, that each gram of faeces has 10^{12} or 1 trillion organisms and remember, this is just in one small gram of faeces (O'Hara & Shanahan, 2006). These organisms have a profound impact on your immune system and long-term health. The diminished diversity of organisms in the bowel in comparison to hunter-gatherer groups may be the basis for a large number of debilitating chronic diseases in Western populations. This concept will be discussed further in this book. Many people have a very small and predictable repertoire of foods they consume on a daily basis, and this is damaging them in ways they have never considered.

The fibre content of your meal →Fibre is food for your bowel organisms. Your good bowel bugs thrive on fibre. Fibre is converted to short-chain fatty acids (SCFA's) such as acetate, butyrate or propionic acid along with many others after fermentation of the fibre by your gut organisms. These SCFA's can produce immunomodulation and anti-inflammatory effects throughout the body and can cross the blood-brain barrier (BBB) through transporters. The effects of these SCFAs are both near and far in the body. As I have mentioned, diversity of the foods consumed that are abundant in fibre will go a long way to increasing diversity of the organisms in your bowels. Because fibre is food for these organisms, you need to aim for a high fibre intake with each meal. Remember, your immune system, and essentially your general health depends on these bowel organisms. The fibre in your food can slow down transit time and alter the biochemical effect of the food eaten, for example, the glycemic effect of the carbohydrate can be diminished by having more fibre in the meal, and the Insulin/IGF-1 response will also be lowered with higher fibre intakes with each meal. We are finding out more and more how vital the daily fibre intake is to your long-term health and survival. A low fibre content of any meal will simply allow all the damaging mechanisms mentioned above such as blood glucose or blood triglyceride spikes to proceed without a braking mechanism in place. The Chia or Basil Seed recipe in this book is packed with fibre and tips on increasing the diversity of fibre you consume.

The insulin response of meal → Insulin is a powerful anabolic hormone that works with its 'evil twin', IGF-1. These hormones have a strong impact on cancer risk and longevity. Insulin and IGF-1 are powerful stimulators of cellular multiplication through mTOR with consistently elevated Insulin/IGF-1 Signalling (IIS) associated with many cancers. Many longevity studies on a large number of organisms including C.elegans a small worm have shown an inverse relationship to insulin and longevity. In essence, the lower your insulin levels are, the longer you will live. As long as insulin levels stay high in the body, your ability to shift fat from your body's fat stores will be severely limited. Constant grazing and the crazy guideline to eat six meals a day ensure insulin levels will stay elevated in the body 24/7, thus trapping the fat in your body. High carbohydrate loads, high protein intakes and dairy are powerful drivers of the Insulin/IGF-1/mTOR pathway.

The antioxidant content of a meal → One of the smartest things you can do with every meal, is to ensure you have a vast array of phytochemical-rich foods in that meal. Eat the rainbow as they say as these colourful foods are rich in thousands of phytochemicals that we have hijacked in an evolutionary sense for our health and cellular benefit over millions of years. Every meal produces trillions of free radicals of various sorts that damage your cells in the process of converting food to energy or in using those nutrient building blocks for synthetic purposes. By not having a huge caloric intake, you will limit the amount of energy extracted and diminish the oxidative stress load of that particular meal, and hence, you will limit the burden of damaging free radicals produced by that specific meal. Remember, each meal damages you, and this is one of the major processes that cause damage at the very heart of your cellular makeup.

By having a high phytochemical and antioxidant intake in that particular meal, you will ensure you have a vast array of antioxidant molecules to neutralise those damaging free radicals produced when your cells chemically process your food, and this will keep the inflammatory effect of that meal low. Ideally, you should have a vegetable-rich, phytochemical diverse drink after eating to limit free radical damage further. Just think of the phytochemical and antioxidant 'wasteland' that is a food court meal or fast food deal. How can anyone in their right mind question the devastating effect of such food being consumed morning, afternoon and night by many people who pay the ultimate price for their health?

Washout periods → Throughout our evolutionary development, we have hijacked the huge numbers of plant chemicals and used them to our advantage. We depend on plant nutrients to survive. We may call these phytochemicals, antioxidants or hormone modulators such as isoflavones or enzyme inducers such as indoles found in cruciferous vegetables. To the plant, these chemicals are ultraviolet (UV) filters, virucides (virus killers) or bacteriocides (bacteria killers) or bitter, toxic compounds that deter either insects or animals from eating them. In the chapter on antioxidants, I mention a term 'hormesis'. If these phytochemical compounds are consumed in the right concentration, they can have hormetic (beneficial) effects if the concentration does not exceed the 'sweet spot'. Going beyond this point can lead to toxic effects.

What the vast majority of people do in Western populations is choose to consume say 10 – 15 foods they like, and this could be the same vegetables, the same fruits or food made by the same grain which is commonly wheat. This is consumed day-in and day-out. The foods harbour not only the thousands of phytochemicals in plants and food but also human-made chemicals that include preservatives, colourings, pesticides, herbicides, flavour enhancers, antifoaming agents, humectants, stabilisers and too many others to name. These add to the mix of human-made and natural toxicities. Humans harbour a vast number of mutated genes, and many of these abnormal genes could be involved in the inactivation of toxic compounds found in plants.

By not consciously avoiding foods on a regular basis, you risk accumulation of toxic compounds in your body. This is why you are asked to eat seasonally and avoid those particular chemicals you have been consuming. Rotate, rotate, rotate foods and constantly try new and exciting foods you have never considered previously. Eat the exotic, strange, new and exciting varieties of foods coming out and exclude these foods every few days. You are now washing out the plant chemicals that may be having adverse effects and providing the diversity in foods that stimulate new populations of bacteria in your bowel to thrive.

Create a Small Wave or Tsunami After-Eating. You decide! → A wonderful way of thinking about the postprandial (after-eating) effects of food is to think about this as a wave. This analogy was used by Professor Antonio Ceriello a renowned diabetes researcher in a paper on the postprandial state and cardiovascular disease (Ceriello, 2000). Your food is simply a combination of carbohydrate, fat, protein and fibre in a complex food matrix with multiple nutrients and phytochemicals in that mix which may be absorbed rapidly if foods in any given meal are highly processed and include high glycemic-index (high-GI) carbohydrates. These components drive up blood glucose spikes significantly. How high your level of blood glucose will climb in your blood and stay elevated will depend on the glycemic index (GI) of the carbohydrate eaten (see Appendix 1) and the amount of carbohydrate consumed. How high your blood triglyceride (blood fat) level will rise and stay elevated will likewise depend on the amount of fat in the meal and the type of fat consumed. The following 'waves' of metabolic change occur in the blood after eating and the extent of these changes as indicated will depend on the composition and quantity of food consumed in any given meal. This postprandial (after-eating) metabolic wave can be one that gently laps on the 'shore' or a 'metabolic tsunami' that wreaks havoc on the body. Let's have a look at these postprandial (after-eating) metabolic effects:

Oxidative stress (Inflammation) → This is where an abundance of free radicals (unpaired electrons) are produced due to the processing of glucose or fats for energy and the subsequent consumption of your body's own intrinsic antioxidants to quench (neutralise) these free radicals. Oxidative stress damages blood vessels and tissues throughout the body after eating. This oxidative stress that occurs meal-after-meal ages all of us. Thus meal composition that limits energy intake but maximises phytochemical and antioxidant intake will limit this oxidative stress and inflammation in the body after eating. Fasting can help make the electron transport chain in the mitochondria (the respiratory chain) much more efficient as I have discussed previously hence reducing free radical production at Complex-I, Complex-III and CoQ10 in the electron transport chain. Having a high phytochemical intake which will increase antioxidant levels in each meal, will offset the damaging effects of that particular meal. Other strategies such as ensuring an optimal intake of the sulphur containing amino acids like cysteine found abundantly in whey protein, will help enhance glutathione levels which is a vital antioxidant in the body. Compounds such as N-Acetyl Cysteine (NAC) can also enhance this glutathione system (see Appendix 7).

Increased Factor VII coagulant activity → Your blood clots due to a cascade of numerous protein factors that are activated in sequence to form a clot designed to stabilise a bleeding point in the body. Clots can also occur pathologically to block off a blood vessel to cause a heart attack or stroke or they may block off the blood supply in a limb. Factor VII activation is directly proportional to high triglyceride levels. Increased coagulation of the blood (increased blood clotting) is a factor in sudden cardiac death after eating. So you can see that what sounded far-fetched that a meal could kill suddenly has a distinct mechanism and a deadly consequence of eating that we just do not think about when we place food in our mouths.

Diminished antioxidant reserves after eating → The surge in glucose, protein, fats and other nutrients into the bloodstream and the subsequent frenetic metabolic response to these nutrients, causes a significant dip in antioxidant levels in the blood (Ceriello 2000). As you now know, antioxidants neutralise (quench or stop) the damaging effects of free radicals (unpaired, reactive electrons). So it stands to reason that your body's level of antioxidants will drop during this time of increased oxidative stress. Without antioxidants, unpaired and highly reactive electrons cause a chain-reaction in cells damaging cellular structures throughout your body with each meal.

Ensure the meals you have, are rich in plant-based antioxidants to at least diminish as much as possible the free radical damage to your body caused by that particular meal you are eating

See if you can guess the metabolic effects now of this common meal.

A burger, fries and soda would have to be a very common type of meal consumed daily by millions of people. You see people in a food court starting their day with such a meal, and this is their first meal of the day! You could easily substitute a pizza in this scenario or a truck-stop meal such as a range of fried meats, sausages, mashed potato or any other fast food you can think of in a food court. Each food type will provide a massive carbohydrate 'hit' from the soft drink (soda), the buns, the fries the sugar in the tomato sauce (ketchup) and sour cream as represented in the graphic. The glycation response of this one meal will be immense, and the effects may last for 6 hours or more in both diabetic and nondiabetic individuals (Ceriello, 2003). There will be a very high blood triglyceride level after eating which comes from the fats in the burger, perhaps butter or margarine on the buns, the oil used to cook the fries and in the meat patty and the oils used in the tomato sauce or mayonnaise. It is important to state that individuals who have prediabetes or Type-2 Diabetes (both caused by insulin resistance), will be impacted far greater by the metabolic effects of this one meal and the blood glucose and triglycerides may never come back to normal in a 24 hour period in these individuals. The sugar and triglyceride levels in the blood stay elevated and to add insult to injury, they have other meals like this at lunchtime and dinner, perhaps replacing the burger with a large pizza, garlic bread and cheesecake. That this happens on a daily basis shows you why people are dying prematurely, why the medical system is being burdened and why we pay such a tremendous bill for the medical care of disease states that are highly preventable.

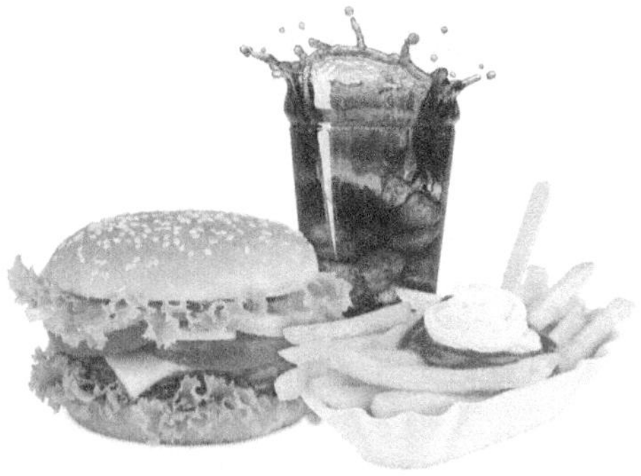

What are the downfalls of this meal?

- **Fibre – minimal at best.** Your bowel microbiome is not something distinctly separate to you as an individual; it is a part of you. Fibre is the food of bowel microorganisms. Feed them fibre, and you live a longer life

- **Nutrient density – very poor.** Easy enough to see why micronutrient deficiencies abound. Eat an optimal diet is what some nutrition experts say. For those who do not know better and this is 6 out of 10 people in society who are overweight or obese, meals like this are an optimal diet to them
- **High carbohydrate load** – increasing glycation, Insulin/IGF-1 blood levels. Keep in mind the sugar in the tomato sauce (ketchup) or mayonnaise as well as possible fructose which is far more glycating than glucose
- **High fat load** – It is interesting that even one fatty meal can increase a dangerous compound that floats around in your bloodstream after eating called lipopolysaccharide (LPS) from certain bowel bacteria. This is a powerful trigger for inflammation in the body, and this is discussed further in the chapter on the gut microbiome. It is of great concern that there is a high-fat intake movement in dietary circles as this is a known problem in nutritional research. For many people, it is one high-fat meal after another putting anyone who has these high-fat meals regularly at grave risk long-term. Do not allow your children to become used to these types of meals as cardiovascular disease begins in childhood. We simply add to the fatty streaks formed in childhood as we grow older into our adult lives.
- **High animal protein load** – You are now well aware of the AMPK/mTOR mechanisms for cellular multiplication. Some fast foods can provide large portions of animal-based protein. We know from recent studies the dangers of red meat and cancer from the heme component, and this is now fact through a large research base.
- **Advanced Glycation Endproducts (AGEs)** – these are glycated proteins and occur when glucose has attached to and then damaged proteins irreversibly. These can be created when food is cooked and absorbed from food or AGEs can be created in the body from high glucose levels after eating attaching to proteins. AGEs, in turn, can damage the proteins in your body and often this is collateral damage. Why? Because your body will see damaged proteins (AGEs) as foreign stimulating an immune system attack on them. Proteins nearby will suffer collateral damage and in turn also become foreign and stimulate the immune system. A domino effect. Even if you avoid this type of meal, you may suffer from all these pitfalls. AGEs are created in the body with each meal and especially so if you have insulin resistance (prediabetes) or diabetes which drives glucose even higher in the blood after eating. The glycemic index (GI) of the carbohydrate and the quantity consumed will determine how high glucose rises in the blood and for how long. The higher the blood glucose level and the longer it stays elevated after a meal will determine how damaging it will be to all the proteins in the body. More on this later.
- **Bowel bacteria adaptations** - your bowel organisms adapt to the type of food you consume. Changes in your bowel bacterial composition (the bowel microbiota) will change to a population of organisms that thrive on high energy foods like these. The sobering thought is that once these abnormal organisms are established, they seem to alter cell signalling through various mechanisms so that you crave these kinds of foods. In other words, your bowel organisms are calling the shots and telling you what to eat to ensure their survival at the cost of your health and your survival (Spector 2015). Remember these bacterial cells outnumber your human cells many times over. What a strange concept that our non-human partners in life manipulate us in ways we are only just becoming aware of. I suppose these organisms have had millions of years to work it all out.
- **Phytochemicals** – minimal at best yet vital to good health.
- **Omega-3's** – very limited if any. Important to dampen down inflammatory processes.

- **High Omega-6 levels** – often vegetable oils will be used in the cooking process, and these are high in pro-inflammatory omega-6 fats. This will add to the overall inflammatory effect of the meal. See Appendix 2 for more information on Omega-6's and Omega-3's
- **Minerals and trace elements** – these types of meals are calorie-dense and nutrient-poor. Micronutrients like selenium or iodine will be very deficient in such as meal leading to thyroid problems and ultimately systemic effects. Your bones and organ systems will suffer from micronutrient deficiencies, and your enzyme systems will malfunction.
- **High acid load**. Large intakes of carbohydrate and protein lead to high acid loads that need to be neutralised at the kidney. Your body draws compounds from the muscle and bone to neutralise these acids leading to gradual sarcopenia and osteoporosis. See Appendix 9
- **High Phthalate levels** – phthalates are hormone disruptors. In other words, they interfere with the hormone system of your body. Think breast, prostate, thyroid gland problems. Those individuals, who derive 35% or more of their calories from fast-food, had 23.8% and 39% higher levels of two phthalates: DEHP and DiNP in their urine respectively. Even modest consumers of fast foods had high phthalate levels in their urine (Zota, Phillips et al. 2016)
- **Acrylamide** – this is considered a potential carcinogen with ongoing research being carried out about its carcinogenicity. It is found in foods such as chips that have been cooked at high temperatures. Another good reason to avoid fast foods.
- **Trans fats** – from deep-frying in vegetable oils and animal products. There is no safe lower limit, and the consumption of fast foods on a regular basis in large amounts means a significant risk of premature cardiovascular disease, Alzheimer's Disease, cancer, depression, decreased fertility, diabetes and declining cognitive functioning. Many good reasons to avoid fast-foods.

Thinking about meal composition is one of the most important things you can do if you want to live a long and healthy life. This example of a meal combo is not a meal; it is a slow and inexorable death-trap if you regularly consume these types of meals on a daily basis.

Postprandial blood glucose - Highly individual responses to the same food

A groundbreaking Israeli study is looking at how to personalise diets highly and in particular, how to modify the postprandial glucose responses in individuals by looking at the gut microbiome and matching them to the blood glucose responses produced in the cohort of people studied.

The findings were that there is a great deal of variability among people consuming the same food and that this response was not just due to the glycemic index (GI), but due to variability in the gut microbiome that determined the glycemic(glucose) response after eating.

The study involved 800 people's blood glucose responses monitored for one week by the Israeli team. They chose blood glucose responses to food as the parameter to study because of the ever-increasing numbers of people with prediabetes and diabetes and the higher glucose levels in the population due to the obesity epidemic. This study was published in the journal Cell (Zeevi, Korem et al. 2015). The researchers state that to control blood glucose levels, individuals need to make the right choices of food to consume. So by comparing the groupings of bacteria in individuals using the 16s RNA marker that I have explained in this book and then looking at the blood glucose responses in individuals to certain foods, assumptions can be made and thus what is emerging is a powerful new tool to ascertain personal responses to food. At this stage, we have data on glucose but no doubt, many individualised responses will be mapped in future to predict adverse outcomes with food consumption. The tools that will be used to personalise your blood glucose responses will be:

- Analysing your gut microbiome
- Analysing your diet (See Appendix-17)
- Baseline blood testing and follow-up
- Baseline body composition measurements such as DEXA scanning, scales, waist circumference
- Possible continuous blood glucose monitoring through patches or surgically inserted probes under the skin that can be paired with a smartphone for monitoring and assessing blood glucose spikes after eating certain foods

Blood glucose monitoring

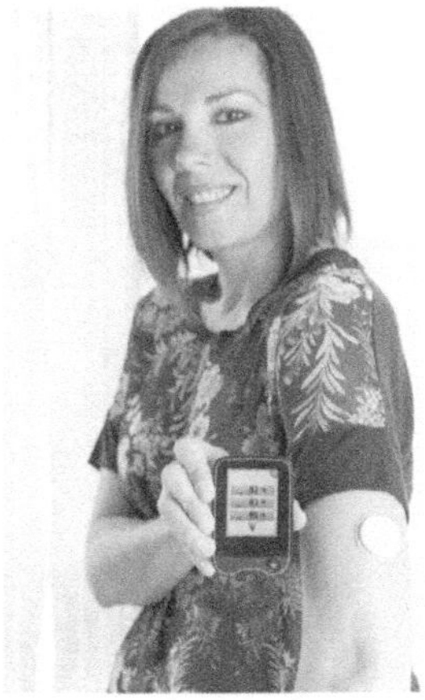

Technology is moving rapidly, but even now, patches are available that can monitor blood glucose levels either paired to a dedicated device that can record the readings or to your smartphone.

This glucose monitoring system would have to be one of the best investments for anyone who has existing heart disease, peripheral vascular disease, a history of TIA or strokes, prediabetes, diabetes, early onset dementia like Alzheimer's and anyone wanting to prevent Alzheimer's or vascular dementia and those with cancer or pre-cancerous conditions.

Such an electronic system will scare the living daylights out of people who see food as benign and will realise how high their blood glucose levels will rise after eating a meal. Let's see how many times a year people who monitor their blood glucose levels will ever sit down to waffles smothered in chocolate, ice-cream with sweet chocolate bars sticking out of them with a topping of some creamy and sugar-sweet syrup. You get the picture. This scenario of eating such meals is a regular occurrence no matter where you go in the Western world. It is important also to remember that it is not only the consumption of meals like this that will spike blood glucose levels but many foods regarded as healthy.

Such emerging technology is truly going to move humanity forward, and future generations will have a far more enlightened view of the effects of food than this one.

CHAPTER 6

Blood Glucose Dangers

To many people, this sweet white substance called glucose seems harmless enough. It is found in confectionery and many processed foods and sodas and makes up 50% of table sugar. Any carbohydrate you have such as bread, pasta, pastries, potatoes or French fries, rice and other grain products, are all essentially broken down into glucose in your body. Have a large serving of mashed potato or fries for example, or a large serving of rice and essentially what you are doing, is having a massive hit of glucose.

Why is this important to you? The reason is that with each surge in blood glucose level, you are significantly damaging a vast array of proteins in your body. Glucose also greatly increases insulin and IGF-1, and these are powerful hormones that drive protein synthesis and cellular multiplication. Every organ is affected by the high spikes in glucose after you eat, and these damaging effects are cumulative over your lifespan as I have pointed out earlier. It is important to note that I am not talking about glucose in the context of a pre-diabetic or diabetic state, although these groups are at higher risk for after-eating spikes in glucose. I am talking about blood glucose levels that occur after eating in the healthiest of individuals consuming everyday foods they consider healthy, that slowly damage and age them.

A high starting point for glucose with a fasting glucose level even in the high 'normal' range, will result in a greater glucose spike after eating and all because your glucose 'springboard' is set at a higher level.

If you want to age well, then this is a crucial modifiable factor that is well within your control. Proteins like collagen and elastin in your skin, soft tissues and organs provide strength and elasticity and these are damaged through glycation after eating, and this protein damage hastens the ageing process. Sun damage is not the only cause of wrinkles in your skin. You need to protect your skin from the inside out by limiting these after-eating glucose surges or spikes that ripple through your blood vessels to the tissues and organs including your brain which is damaged by high glucose spikes after you eat.

Vegetarians or Vegans consuming a lot of grains and legumes are putting themselves at risk for large and prolonged glucose spikes after eating, and these groups may be deficient in numerous essential nutrients (Cordain 1999).

The 'Normal Range' of blood tests: How this can be deceiving?

It is interesting that when a doctor gives you a result, there seems to be a blatant acceptance that if the level falls anywhere between two goal posts of the 'normal' or reference range, the result must be perfect no matter where in that range that level falls. A simplistic interpretation of test results is naïve indeed!

This seemingly normal result is deceptive and puts you at significant cardiovascular risk. The fasting blood glucose level regarded as normal in my practice is 3.5 mmol/L – 5.4 mmol/L (63 mg/dl to 97 mg/dl) and this range can be divided into four (x4) parts called quartiles, which are labelled the 1st, 2nd, 3rd and 4th quartile.

A study published in the journal Diabetes Care followed 1,998 seeming healthy nondiabetic men for 22 years and what they found was worrying - 483 men out of the 1,998 in the study with fasting blood glucose levels at just 4.72 mmol/L (85 mg/dl), died of cardiovascular disease making up 53% of that group.
Keep in mind this level of 4.72 mmol/L was well within the upper limit of the 'normal range'. These men simply had levels in the upper (3rd) quartile of the normal (reference) range.

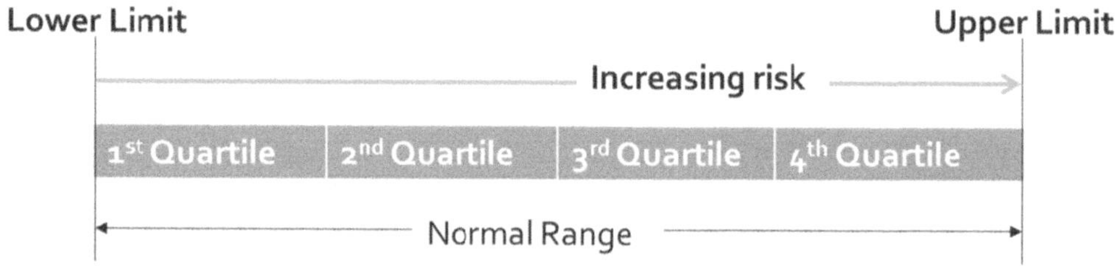

Knowing your fasting blood glucose result

Many people in the Western world will have had a fasting blood glucose test done especially in their middle years, as prediabetes and diabetes are so common in these Western countries but also rapidly increasing in Third World countries. It is important to know your fasting blood glucose figure because so many diseases are associated with higher levels of glucose **within** the normal or reference range which has relevance to meal composition as you will soon see. To understand how much of a risk a high-normal fasting glucose is or even a level just beyond the upper goal post, just look at the following graphic.

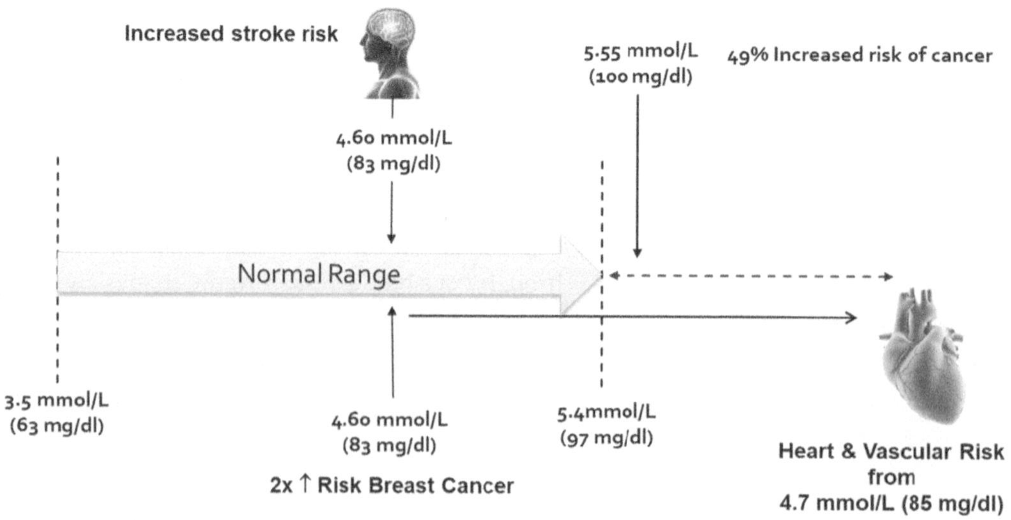

The important points to note in the graphic above are:

1. That at a level of just 4.60 mmol/L (83 mg/dl), you have an increased risk of stroke. For every 1 mmol/L beyond 4.60 mmol/L, there was a 27% increased risk of dying from stroke (Batty, Kivimäki, Smith, Marmot, & Shipley, 2008).
2. That there is a two to three-fold risk of breast cancer at this 4.60 mmol/L (83 mg/dl) level and above (Muti et al., 2002)
3. At a level of only 4.7 mmol/L (85 mg/dl), you now have a significant risk of developing heart and vascular disease (Bjørnholt et al., 1999).
4. That you have a 49% increased risk of cancer at 5.55 mmol/L (100 mg/dl) which is just beyond the normal range (Hirakawa et al., 2012)

These seemingly normal fasting blood glucose levels lead to deadly outcomes and all well within, or just beyond the range that doctors use as a guide in clinical practice to classify someone as 'normal' or having overt disease. These ranges, however, are interpreted simplistically. The rule, not the exception is that the general practitioner will pat a patient on the back often saying; *'well done, your results are perfect. You are well within the normal range.'* Such simple interpretation of results seals the fate of the individual and condemns them to be cardiovascular, dementia or cancer risks.

Too often in medicine, nothing is seen as important unless there are overt blood markers, signs or symptoms. Nothing could be further from the truth. Molecular changes at the cellular level begin long before overt signs develop and this recognition along with developing technologies to test and map these early markers of disease will revolutionise medicine. Remember, the higher you set the bar, i.e. the higher you set a test result to define a disease, means that you have a smaller number of people needing treatment and this saves money for governments.

It is important to know that these levels are commonplace findings in general practice, and yet little attention is drawn to the higher risk of cancer, dementia or higher cardiovascular risk. These are utterly commonplace problems seen in medical practice. Cancer, Alzheimer's, heart and vascular disease are common killers in society, and your diet and meal composition is the number one contributor to a large number of chronic disease states.

So why does your fasting blood glucose creep higher?

1. **The higher the glycemic load of a meal** (high carb intakes), the higher the likelihood of insulin resistance (IR) (O'Sullivan, Bremner et al. 2010). See Appendix-1
2. **The higher the blood insulin levels after eating**, the higher the risk of insulin resistance (Hoyt, Hickey et al. 2005).
3. **Sarcopenia** (muscle loss with ageing). As we age, we have a gradual and inexorable loss of muscle from our mid to late 20's onwards. Hormones, ageing, sedentary lifestyles and poor diets all have a part in sarcopenia. Losing such highly active tissue from the body will be the catalyst that ensures fasting blood glucose levels will creep higher. In fact, we lose our most powerful Type-IIX muscle fibres as we age (Doherty 2003), making us progressively weaker. Losing these powerful Type-IIX muscle fibres means that we are losing highly active tissue that would if they were maintained by regular resistance training over our lives, burn off any excess glucose for energy keeping fasting levels down. Our sedentary lifestyles hasten muscle loss. Never perform just aerobic exercises at the expense of resistance training.

4. **Lower NAD$^+$ levels** as we age. NAD is a Vitamin-B3 derivative and vital for oxidation-reduction reactions in cells. We discussed NAD$^+$ as the molecular master of the Sirtuins. Suffice it to say that lowered NAD$^+$ levels due to ageing results in decreased energy-producing efficiency in the respiratory (electron) chain within mitochondria. Creating energy (ATP) from food becomes less efficient. You won't burn off glucose as effectively as when your NAD$^+$ levels are optimal.
5. **Glucose-6-Phosphatase** is an enzyme that is involved primarily in the liver and catalyses the final step in gluconeogenesis and glycogenolysis processes (Henry-Vitrac, Ibarra et al. 2010).
Both of these processes are geared to increase glucose availability. Gluconeogenesis is where compounds such as glycerol or amino acids, are converted to glucose in the liver and glycogenolysis is where the complex glucose compound, glycogen is broken down into glucose.
Glycogen is found in liver and muscle. Diabetics can have a 2 – 3 fold (2x-3x) increase in Glucose-6-Phosphatase activity. Likewise, ageing seems to produce an insulin resistant state due to the mechanisms discussed in the points above, and thus we do not just have to contend with decreased glucose clearance from the blood we now have to worry about increased glucose production in the liver by the action of Glucose-6-Phosphatase. Chlorogenic acid from green coffee has been known to suppress this activity (Henry-Vitrac, Ibarra et al. 2010).

How can meal composition make things worse?

This book is all about meal composition and the consequential metabolic impacts each component has in your blood and indeed the whole body. It is important to see each meal as either causing great harm or the least harm. By 'least harm' I mean that we can't stop the damaging effect of food entirely but what we want to do is dampen significantly the detrimental metabolic effects that occur after eating.

So knowing your fasting blood glucose level is highly recommended for anyone from early adulthood onwards. What is important to know is how does a spike in blood glucose add to this risk? The fasting blood test is a baseline level that signals risk outcomes (O'Keefe and Bell 2007). The after-eating spikes in blood glucose amplify this baseline risk.

As discussed above, the baseline is like a springboard where the higher the foundation (fasting) glucose level rests, will determine how high after eating glucose spikes reach. How far your glucose level rises and stays elevated after eating is a powerful determinant of vascular disease.

The Glucose Tolerance Test (GTT)

The research tool used is glucose load (GL). A glucose tolerance test (GTT) can be used to work out after eating (postprandial) levels and what these levels mean regarding medical outcomes such as heart disease, dementia, progression to diabetes etc. The blood glucose is measured at fasting, and then the individual is given a 75-gram glucose load. Blood glucose is then measured again at 1 hour and 2 hours after this glucose load. Someone whose level stays below 4.83 mmol/L (87 mg/dl) 2 hours after eating has been shown to have the blockages in their heart vessels regress (become less of an obstruction) (O'Keefe, Gheewala, & O'Keefe, 2008).

A known factor is that a minor jump of just 1.05 mmol/L (19 mg/dl), beyond 4.83 mmol/L (87 mg/dl), at 2 hours post-glucose load or post-eating causes progression of blockages in the coronary arteries (O'Keefe, Gheewala, & O'Keefe, 2008).

How many deaths can be avoided just by strict control of after-eating blood glucose spikes? These spikes in blood glucose can actually be controlled through strategies I will shortly describe. It is important though to know that these damaging effects on your blood vessels occur whether you have an underlying cardiovascular disease or not. You develop cardiovascular disease only because of a lifetime of constant and cumulative damage caused by poor dietary habits and sedentary lifestyles and you damage every artery and organ in your body meal-by-meal! This was discussed in detail in the chapter on postprandial effects.

That heart artery blockages can regress is a staggering outcome when you take into consideration statistics provided by the Australian Heart Foundation

- **Over 43,000 deaths in Australia are attributed to cardiovascular disease per year**
- **Cardiovascular disease kills one Australian every 12 minutes**
- **Cardiovascular disease affects 1 in 6 Australians; this is a whopping 3.72 million people**

Think of the lives that could be saved. That these dramatic outcomes could so easily be prevented through dietary and exercise measures is a great indictment on Western governments.

Having large carbohydrate loads, piling on the rice, potatoes, fries, bread, pasta, sweets, pastries will ensure large and prolonged glucose levels in your blood that will result in widespread tissue damage to your body as a whole with every meal consumed having these kinds of carbohydrate loads. Grazing on snacks constantly will mean a constant topping up of blood glucose, Insulin/IGF-1 levels.

Advanced Glycation Endproducts - AGEs

AGEs are damaged proteins caused by glucose binding to the protein in a process termed glycation. Once glucose attaches to proteins (or lipids), it changes the characteristics of that biomolecule as the protein becomes distorted.

With wave after wave of glucose spikes after eating, more and more glycation damage is occurring to a variety of proteins throughout the body. Early and reversible changes to a protein are called Schiff Bases, and these are fully reversible. However, with further glucose insults, we now progress to Amadori Products, and these are partially reversible. Further glycation results in Advanced Glycation Endproducts (AGEs) an aptly named irreversible product of damage.

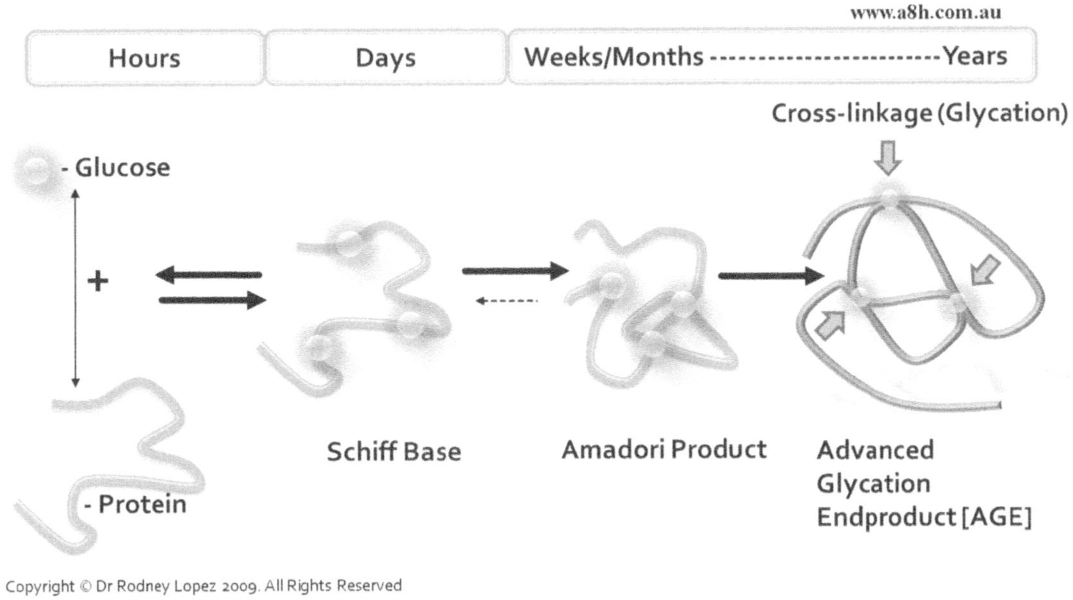

AGEs are a part of the destructive process of diabetes, and the complications that ensue like chronic kidney disease or blindness or vascular disease and AGEs occur after eating due to glucose interacting with proteins. You can also consume AGEs through your diet. That someone can produce these destructive AGEs is easy enough to understand when you see what people eat and have a look at the carbohydrate content of that food. It matters not whether these are simple or complex carbohydrates, they all get broken down to glucose in the body.

When vast quantities of carbs are consumed throughout the day with 3 main meals and snacks consumed in-between, you can easily see that significant elevations in glucose can occur on a daily basis. These clucose levels stay elevated for 6 hours or more after a single meal in both diabetic and nondiabetic individuals (Ceriello, 2003).

Because glucose stays elevated so long after eating, it gives it plenty of time to attack and damage proteins or lipids keeping in mind that glucose levels may never come down in a 24 hour period but stay permanently elevated in someone with insulin resistance. This glycation process and AGE formation are occurring 24/7, 365 days a week so is it any wonder why those with insulin resistance or diabetes die younger, develop Alzheimer's Disease or cancer at much younger ages. The important point to make is that you do not have to be insulin resistant for this process to happen! It is happening in so-called normal people and all because of the food choices they make.

Thus if you eat a carbohydrate-rich breakfast (toxic breakfast in a box), blood glucose levels will still be elevated at lunch time especially if you have also eaten a mid-morning snack. At midday when you have your lunch you are adding to the glucose and triglyceride elevations produced by your breakfast. The lunchtime meal may produce glucose and triglyceride elevations that extend to your dinner especially if you have had a snack between lunch and dinner. If your dinner includes a large meal made up of a high carbohydrate load and why not throw in that much-loved dessert that is the norm for so many people, and you now have glucose and triglyceride elevations that extend throughout your sleep and guess what? Breakfast waits!

The Activ8Health Plan-A diet that hopefully, you will have personalised through a Dietitian at www.a8h.com.au to ensure it meets your individual needs will be of great help to decrease these after-eating damaging effects of foods on your body. Do not start your day with breakfast in a box as these cereal breakfasts are toxic. An Activ8Health Plan-A blended meal will be a brilliant start to your day and will have all those highly desirable components in a meal to help your body thrive. Nothing in a box can match this! Stay away from toxic fast foods and food in food malls as these are huge killers in society providing the type of calorie-rich, nutrient-poor foods that are indeed killing millions of people every year and making people fatter and sicker worldwide. Try to understand what real food is!

Arterial stiffness, elevated central blood pressure and heart disease. Future risk for you

The large elastic arteries such as the wide aorta and its main branches have a thick tunica media component of the arterial wall which is rich in elastin and collagen fibres. See graphic-Blausen.com staff (2014). The smaller arteries do not have as much elastin or collagen (Soldatos & Cooper, 2006).

Elastin enables the artery to stretch with a blood pressure wave caused by the heart contraction to eject oxygenated blood into the body and then return to normal whereas collagen helps provide the structure of the artery. If either the elastin or collagen or both are affected by glycation (glucose damage), stiffness of the arteries will ensue. As a result, these large arteries are prime targets for glucose damage where glucose binds to these vascular elastin and collagen fibres, glycating and damaging them in the process of creating advanced glycation endproducts (AGEs) (Soldatos & Cooper, 2006). Remember, this occurs with every large carbohydrate meal you consume).

Glycation damage to large blood vessel elastin and collagen will lead to gradual arterial stiffness and because of this stiffness, there is a back-pressure that your heart will need to overcome with each beat of the heart. In other words, your heart has to pump even harder to overcome this backwards pressure to supply your body with oxygenated blood. Anything overworked will fail much sooner.

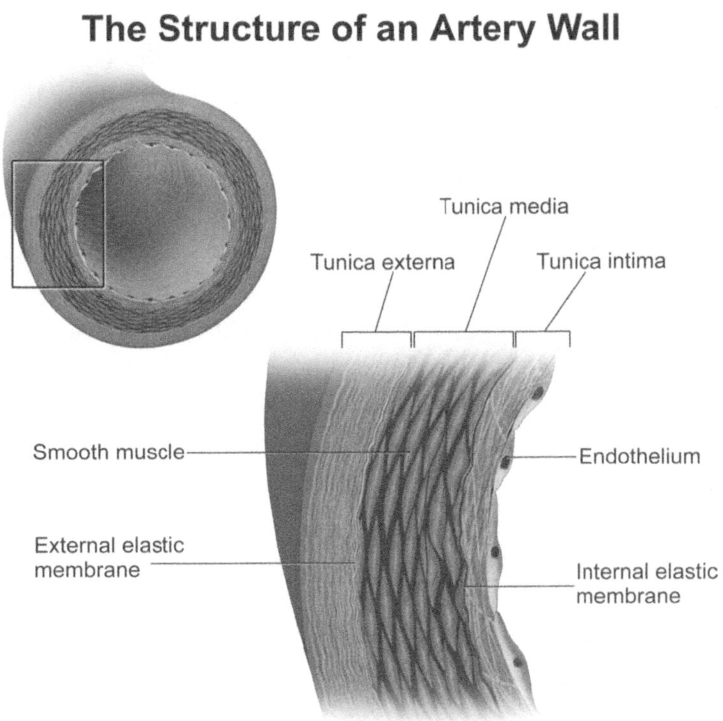

With the heart having to work harder and harder over your lifetime, the walls of the left ventricle which is the heart chamber that forces blood out of the heart into the aorta and then to the other arteries that branch off this major vessel becomes stiffer and thicker. This ventricular wall stiffness and thickness can lead to diastolic heart failure over time as less oxygenated blood can be pumped out of the heart with every stroke.

Heart failure is common, and people hasten heart disease just by the meals they have and the starchy carbohydrate content of those meals. This risk is undeniable and well-researched. There is a wealth of scientific papers to back this scenario of progressive food-related (glycation) damage. Remember, a lack of the blood vessel-dilating compound, Nitric Oxide (NO) contributes to this effect because the vast majority of people in Western societies do not consume the requisite number of fruit and especially vegetable servings, decreasing the intake of valuable nitrates consumed in the diet. A lack of nitrates results in lowered nitric oxide (NO) availability making worse the blood vessel stiffness which then impacts on the function of the heart.

So you can see that overloading on carbohydrates over time is not a great idea if you want your arteries to be flexible and if you want your heart to be strong for as long as possible. With over 43,000 cardiovascular deaths in Australia per year and similar numbers in other Western populations pro rata to their population size, what you put in your mouth, meal-by-meal, will determine whether you become one of these statistics. Do not forget the sympathetic hyperactivity that occurs after eating which can cause blood vessels to clamp down (vasoconstriction) and thus increase blood pressure as well and even change the nature of your heart cells and increase the risk of arrhythmias of the heart which are either missed beats or atrial fibrillation. Does a doctor or Cardiologist ever thing of food composition as a contributor to atrial fibrillation (AF), other abnormal rhythms of the heart or poor heart function?

Prediabetes

The numbers of people in Australia who are in the pre-diabetic state is simply staggering. It is estimated that in Australia alone, 16.4% have prediabetes and this is close to 4 million people and in the USA 86 million people have this problem, almost 1 in 3 individuals there. Most of these people will progress to full-blown type-2 diabetes mellitus (T2DM) but of great concern is the risk of cardiovascular disease which matches true diabetes at 2x the risk and this risk effect may be greater in women (Ford, Zhao et al. 2010).

What brings home the importance of this pre-diabetic state is that even in individuals with fasting blood glucose levels in the 'normal' range, in the upper quartile of this range , that they will have lost 30% of their pancreatic beta-cell mass before their pre-diabetic diagnosis, and by the time they have been diagnosed as having full-blown type-2 diabetes, they will have lost 80% of their pancreatic beta-cell mass (Rea and Tien 2017). Beta cells in the pancreas produce insulin. Keep blood glucose levels in the low normal range through the dietary and exercise programs outlined in this book.

A study of 1800 individuals with prediabetes and diabetes in comparison to individuals with normal blood glucose levels were followed-up for ten years and assessed for coronary (heart) artery disease (CAD). What this study found was that those with prediabetes and diabetes had essentially identical risk for heart disease at ten years (Li, Chen et al. 2010). This study indicates that the distinction between the pre-diabetic and diabetic state is clinically irrelevant and creates a false sense of security in both doctors and patients. This study shows that prediabetes cannot be ignored and by doing so, it condemns an extremely large number of people in Western populations to an early cardiovascular event or death. We need to find a different name for pre-diabetes as this seems to confer a benign state in the minds of both the public and doctors alike. A deadly assumption.

It is important to remember that intermittent fasting which includes intraday fasting mentioned in this book, can lower fasting glucose by 3% to 6% especially so in pre-diabetics (St-Onge, Ard et al. 2017). These are significant percentage reductions.

Metformin

I find it truly amazing that a highly effective medication like Metformin a first line drug for diabetes and amazingly cheap in comparison to many medications, is not being used in prediabetes. This medication has a fabulous track record in terms of safety, but is just not being used in the pre-diabetic state to delay or prevent the onset of diabetes or to improve insulin receptor sensitivity and improve blood glucose clearance.

Why use Metformin? Where is the research to support this? Well, this comes from none other than the 15-year Diabetes Prevention Program Outcomes Study (DPPOS) funded by the National Institutes of Health (NIH) in the USA. What this study shows in an incontrovertible way is that in a diverse group of people with a high risk of developing diabetes, that lifestyle modification such as increased activity and weight loss or Metformin reduced the risk of developing diabetes by a highly impressive 58% and 31% respectively. If you just think about the vast numbers of people with prediabetes and diabetes with 4 million people in Australia and 86 million people in the USA having prediabetes alone, then these percentages will staggeringly decrease the burden of diabetes.

So why hasn't Metformin been used more in this setting? In my opinion, medical practitioners including specialists have truly underestimated the damaging effect of the pre-diabetic state and the long-term complications caused by the dysregulation of blood glucose and the after-eating surges in glucose that occur due to the underlying abnormal glucose regulation processes. Using short-term studies to work out long-term problems is a recipe for disaster, and this is why the DPPOS study is so important in that this has been a very long ongoing study.

You can see by the tremendous amount of research that already exists that lowering fasting glucose or lowering those after eating surges in glucose by improving glucose clearance, produces positive clinical outcomes in cardiovascular disease.

Will the long-term use of Metformin improve heart diseases like heart attacks or prevent cancer? It has yet to be established in the DPPOS study. I hope they look at the **timing of treatment** much more closely than research projects of the past i.e. looking at the outcomes if someone commences Metformin early in the prediabetes phase rather than later. Once cardiovascular disease is well established and entrenched, then throwing medications or nutraceuticals at an individual with advanced disease may simply be futile.

Not taking timing into consideration has been the real failure of research in the past in that short-term thinking has created erroneous results. We might have truly progressed in the treatment of so many chronic disease states if long-term treatment approaches were studied and then implemented in much younger age groups. Heart attacks and cancer are not the only endpoints we need to worry about high glucose surges which damage every organ in the body including the brain.

Lactic acidosis with Metformin use is another reason that may have tainted the thoughts of medical practitioners in the treatment of prediabetes. Lactic acidosis as a complication of treatement is rare, but an individual with prediabetes should **not** be discouraged from using Metformin for this reason. Most medications have some horrendous yet unlikely side-effects, so what is so different about Metformin and lactic acidosis? If an individual has normal liver and kidney function, is not a heavy alcohol drinker, then their risk is extremely small. Patients should be instructed to cease Metformin if there is a chance of dehydration which may occur on extremely hot days or if that individual is suffering from significant gastroenteritis or an acute medical or surgical condition. As one of the lead authors of the DPPOS study stated:

> *"Other than a small increase in vitamin B-12 deficiency, which is a recognized consequence of metformin therapy, it has been extremely safe and well-tolerated over the 15 years of our study,"*

This quote was from Professor Jill Crandall, Professor of Medicine at the Albert Einstein College of Medicine and stated on the American Diabetes Association website. Vitamin-B12 should also be checked and a simple Multivitamin most days or B12 injection once or twice a year may be all that is needed to prevent this vitamin becoming depleted. Micronutrient or mineral depletions by medications are commonplace.

Thus anyone with prediabetes should consider Metformin based on the strong evidence as it now stands. A great advantage of using Metformin is that it increases AMPK which represents a fasting signal or a just exercised signal – i.e. an energy-depleted state. Metformin is thus calorie-restriction and exercise in a pill! High AMPK indicates that the cells do not have a lot of energy available to build things like cells and you may remember high AMPK levels dampens mTOR which in turn will dampen cell multiplication.

Using Metformin in pre-diabetics can prevent the onset diabetes by a huge margin. In my opinion, it is irresponsible for the medical profession not to recommend such a cheap and safe medication in the face of an epidemic of prediabetes/diabetes and the burden of disease these conditions cause that they then require complex and extremely costly interventionist modalities of treatment just to keep people alive. How logical is this?

A heart attack or stroke is a common complication of prediabetes, and this can change a person's life irrevocably. Do not be conned into thinking this is the 'mild' end of the diabetes spectrum as time-after-time research has shown an equivalent rate of cardiovascular disease with the full-blown diabetic state. Studies using fasting glucose levels may have underestimated the risk and HbA1c a glucose-damaged (glycated) protein is a far more reliable and reproducible marker of long-term risk in non-diabetic individuals (Selvin, Steffes et al. 2010). The American Diabetes Association states that a person is pre-diabetic if their HbA1c is between 5.7-6.4% and recommends Metformin in this group. There is a high risk for progression to diabetes with an HbA1c of 6% and the HbA1c is a better marker for cardiovascular risk than fasting glucose (Selvin, Steffes et al. 2010). Once again research has used the wrong tool (fasting glucose) and put lives at risk.

CHAPTER 7

The Telomere Story

What are telomeres? Why are they so important?

Telomeres are non-coding areas on the tips of chromosomes. They are composed of constantly repeating base pairs of nucleotides that are not genes – i.e. they do not code for proteins. Telomeres are there to protect the ends of the chromosomes from damage and to prevent fusion to other chromosomes. Chromosomes, as you are aware, contain your DNA and its precious gene cargo. The genes are essentially the blueprint of life that created you and how you look the colour of your hair and eyes, but beyond your creation and appearance, the DNA keeps on instructing cells throughout your life in a molecular sense, orchestrating an array of biochemical processes necessary to sustain life.

Elizabeth Blackburn is an Australian researcher who co-discovered Telomerase and awarded the Nobel Prize for this discovery in 2009. Blackburn likens telomeres to the aglets on shoelaces which are the plastic or metal tips at the ends, placed there to help prevent fraying of the shoelaces at the tips. Telomeres shorten with each cell division and how fast these shorten will determine how you age, how long you will stay in the healthspan (your healthy time on the planet), your diseasespan (how early you develop a chronic illness and stay ill on the planet) and how long you essentially live. So telomeres are an important marker of ageing and the health of your cells. Some lucky people are born with long telomeres, and these individuals often live past the age of the highest mortality rate, and this is 75 years of age.

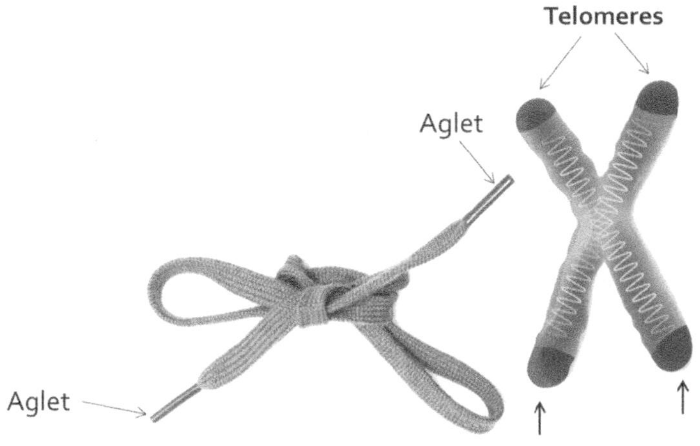

The Hayflick Limit

It was in 1961 that Leonard Hayflick, a biologist discovered that human cells have a limit to the number of times they can divide. This number is around 50 times, and each time a cell divides, the telomeres shorten to a critical point where cell division just cannot occur anymore. Another Australian, Sir Frank McFarlane Burnett who received a Nobel Prize for his critical work on the immune system, coined the term 'Hayflick Limit' for this restriction in cell division. Until this point, they thought that human cells were immortal.

Are all cells restricted by the Hayflick Limit?

Some cells are immortal. Henrietta Lacks was an African-American woman, born a descendant of slaves in 1920. In 1951 she was initially but incorrectly diagnosed as having a particular form of cervical cancer which was later found to be an adenocarcinoma a malignancy of particular cells in epithelial tissues which line certain parts of the body. These cells can be highly malignant with a great potential to spread. Henrietta Lacks cells survive today in culture medium and are known as the **HeLa Immortal Cell Line** which has been used extensively for biomedical research.

So why can cancerous cells divide indefinitely? One of the answers is telomerase, an enzyme that helps keep the telomeres long and functional allowing chromosomes to divide without a Hayflick Limit. Other cells like stem cells are also immortal as long as they are healthy cells and not damaged by dreadful diets, poor lifestyles like smoking or a lack of exercise or perhaps living in a toxic or stressful environment.

What is Telomerase?

Telomerase is an enzyme that helps keep the 'aglets' of the chromosomes, the telomeres, healthy and long to enable cells to keep on multiplying. Having too much telomerase in damaged cells like the HeLa cell line is not a good idea. The concern with repeated cell divisions over generations is that DNA mutations can occur with each division of any cell line. Over time the cumulative effect of a number of these DNA mutations can lead to cancerous change. So telomerase is a double-edged sword. This advice in this book will help to optimise telomerase in a natural, safe way.

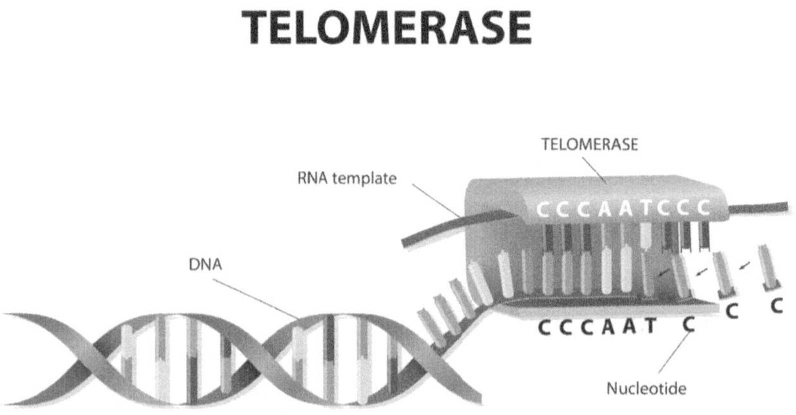

Learning how to harvest the good part of telomerase's personality, that keeps healthy cells dividing longer versus allowing a damaged cell to keep on dividing and becoming malignant, is key to a long healthspan and to delay chronic disease.

Cell senescence (ageing) and apoptosis (cell death) is a way of getting rid of damaged and perhaps dangerous cells in your body, and we do not want to hamper this process through artificial ways of increasing telomerase until the research shows that this is a safe thing to do.

Western diets are driving cell multiplication and telomere shortening

With large caloric intakes devoid of many micronutrients, we have a perfect storm for ageing our cells rapidly. A high carbohydrate, protein and dairy intake drive the AMPK/mTOR pathway to drive cell multiplication, and with each cell division, you are shortening the telomeres and ageing yourself.

Just one large hamburger can provide nearly 600 calories (2508 kJ) and 25 grams of protein. Many restaurants will provide 300 to 500-gram steaks which will have 75 – 125 grams of protein in just one meal which is a whole day's worth for the majority of people in one hit! We have discussed how people start their day with a fast food feast such as a hamburger, sugary soda, milkshake and fries and then have another similar meal for lunch and dinner. Look at what people have in front of them in any food court or fast food outlet.

Eating this way is the reality of life, and many individuals have had this eating behaviour instilled in them from a young age. How many times have you seen people pile on the food on a plate in a buffet setting and then go back for seconds or thirds and let's not forget that large calorie-rich dessert at the end of it all?

The sad part is that people, including medical professionals, do not see food as truly damaging to the body and see food as something quite benign. What is emerging scientifically, and at a molecular level is how food ages us and how food drives so many of the chronic illnesses we see in society

The feast signal driving the AMPK/mTOR pathway towards rampant cell multiplication is also causing us to push our cells headlong into senescence and then cell death or cancerous change. Cell multiplication driven by the calorie-laden Western diet reaches a point where this telomere shortening stops cells dividing any more. These are the cells at the end of their lifecycle and thus are aged, senescent cells no longer capable of youthful cell division.

As we push more and more cells into senescence (ageing), we are creating a situation of ongoing inflammation in the body as these damaged senescent cells cry out for help by sending chemical messengers to other cells for assistance in a process called SASP (Senescence-Associated Secretory Phenotype), which I will now discuss.

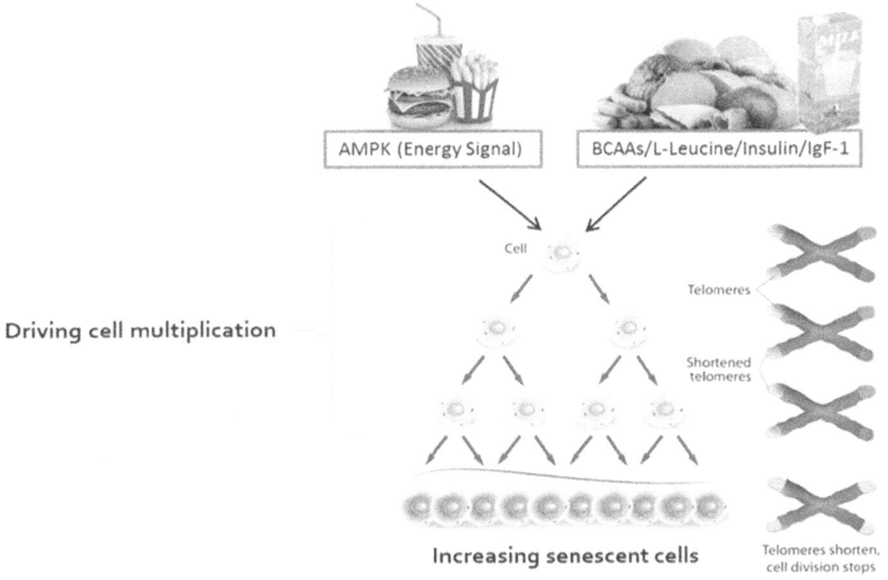

SASP - a cry for help that damages the whole body

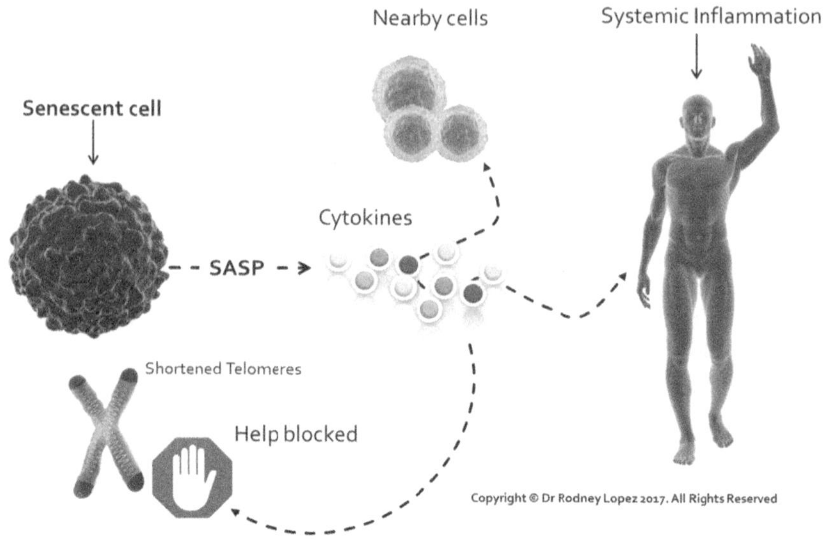

Senescence-Associated Secretory Phenotype (SASP) is a process described in an excellent book on the subject by the absolute expert on this topic, Dr Elizabeth Blackburn. The book is titled 'The Telomere Effect'. Consider purchasing this book to read about this important topic which covers far more than I can in this chapter on telomeres. It is interesting that an ageing (senescent) cell with DNA damage and telomere shortening will send out help signals in the form of chemical messengers called cytokines. SASP is a DNA damage response for self-preservation. These injured cell signals are crying out for repair mechanisms to spring to action, but the interesting thing is that when telomeres are damaged, they seem to hamper the repair mechanisms sought after by the cell itself. As Dr Blackburn states, these shortened telomeres (essentially damaged DNA), can linger on in the cells for months allowing the cell to constantly send out distress signals and yet paradoxically not accept help when it arrives. Such is the power of the telomeres on the overall health of the cell as they call the shots issuing commands yet preventing their execution!

We need to consider then that these chemical signals and many of them are pro-inflammatory cytokines, keep pouring out of the old damaged cell causing near and far inflammatory changes. This systemic inflammation will ultimately lead to organ systems failing, clumping of protein in organs like the brain as is seen in Alzheimer's disease with ongoing dysfunctional signalling in a multitude of cells leading to progressive deterioration of the whole body as you age.

Blackburn uses the analogy of one rotten apple floating in a barrel-full of good apples. After a short period, the toxic elements from this rotting apple will permeate throughout all the apples in that barrel, speeding up the deterioration of all of them. Another analogy of this mechanism occurs in the fruit and vegetable drawer of your refrigerator where gasses released by rotting fruit and vegetables affect all the other fruit and vegetables in the same fridge drawer speeding up their deterioration.

Inflammatory processes and ageing (termed inflamm-ageing)

Inflammation is shaping up to be a critical component driving many common disease states such as cardiovascular disease, diabetes, cancers, Alzheimer's and a range of other medical conditions.

Many factors contribute to inflammatory processes, and these include, but are not limited to the following:

- Central abdominal adiposity (deep visceral fat) – generates numerous inflammatory cytokines

- Postprandial (after-eating) effects such as raised glucose and triglycerides caused by poor dietary choices can cause significant body-wide inflammatory changes.
- Sedentary lifestyles – exercise can help decrease inflammatory processes in the body through myokines (muscle cytokines) produced after exercise that dampen down inflammation.
- Advanced Glycation Endproducts (AGEs) caused by raised fasting glucose, raised postprandial glucose or consuming AGEs from charred foods or from processed foods that have high AGE levels. These stimulate inflammatory responses.
- Senescence-Associated Secretory Phenotype (SASP) – as I have just described. As we drive more and more cells into the senescent phase from relentless cell multiplication caused by consuming an abundance of food - we are driving inflammatory processes in the body from these ageing cells.
- High protein intakes in particular high animal protein intakes driving the mTOR pathway and stimulate cell proliferation and early cell senescence with subsequent SASP mechanisms for inflammation. Animal protein may also contain a high level of inflammatory omega-6's and arachidonic acid which is the precursor to inflammatory eicosanoids.
- High omega-6 intakes – vegetable oils, fast foods, processed foods. The Omega-6 essential fatty acid linoleic acid is the precursors for arachidonic acid which then results in the production of all the inflammatory eicosanoids.
- Low omega-3 levels – low intakes of alpha-linolenic acid (ALA) and oily fish. Omega-3's are necessary to offset the effect of the Omega-6's
- High arachidonic acid intakes from various sources like meats, egg yolk, dairy, processed foods
- Micronutrient deficiencies leading to impaired cell and damaged protein repair damaged DNA and impaired cell renewal processes
- Low micronutrient intakes impairing enzyme function, and innate antioxidant production processes
- Poor antioxidant status – poor intakes of phytochemicals and low intakes of sulphur containing amino acids like cysteine can lead to impaired antioxidant production (see Appendix 7 – NAC)
- Genetic mutations like single nucleotide polymorphisms (SNPs) could be present and impair antioxidant systems in the body
- Exposure to environmental toxins through our air, food, water

These are just some of the mechanisms that lead to ongoing and progressive low-grade inflammation that affects us as we age. To this list, we can now add telomere shortening. Controlling our inflammatory processes through our diet, intraday fasting and effective exercise is vital if we want to enjoy health long into our senior years.

The Omega-6 to Omega-3 Ratio

The metabolic pathways for the omega-6 and omega-3 essential fatty acids are complex. View these pathways in Appendix 2. These pathways, are complex, and the discoverers of the compounds called eicosanoids derived from omega-6 and omega-3 essential fatty acids received the Nobel Prize in 1982. Since then, this complexity has increased greatly as our understanding of eicosanoid production and molecular action has increased.

Of concern is an increased intake of omega-6 essential fatty acids through vegetable oils such as palm, sunflower, safflower, canola and soybean oil. These are metabolised to arachidonic acid (AA) the parent compound for the inflammatory eicosanoids. Whenever you purchase an anti-inflammatory product from the chemist for pain or fever, what you are doing is buying a compound that blocks the effects of these inflammatory compounds (eicosanoids) derived from AA - the series 2 and 4 eicosanoids.

The ratio of omega-6 to omega-3 in Western societies may be as high as 15:1 meaning 15 times more omega-6 consumed than omega-3's. Processed foods will use the most economical oils, and this is not going to be a high-quality extra virgin olive oil so beware of processed foods, fast foods and food halls that have foods riddled with these cheap omega-6 oils.

Omega-3's have a parent compound for anti-inflammatory eicosanoids, and this is eicosapentaenoic acid (EPA). This EPA long-chain omega-3 produces the series 3 and 5 eicosanoids. Ideally, for every omega-6 essential fatty acid consumed, one omega-3 essential fatty acid should also be consumed to make the ratio 1:1 or at the most 4:1. This ratio is important because if you view the diagram in Appendix-2, you will see that the enzymes that work on each stage of the pathway are the same. Sharing the same enzymes makes the two pathways competitive and so, if you are consuming predominantly omega-6 fats then logically, more arachidonic acid (AA) will be produced and more inflammatory series 2 and 4 eicosanoids are created. You are shifting your body into an inflammatory state just by consuming the wrong oil!

Of great value are the **resolvins** derived from EPA and DHA and these compounds are also known as **specialised pro-resolving mediators (SPMs)** vital to your body helping it put an end to inflammatory processes as they are potent anti-inflammatory compounds that put out the 'fire' caused by your immune system. Even everyday stress and the release of noradrenaline can trigger inflammatory responses. By limiting intake of omega-3's, you are putting your body in harm's way and increasing the inflammatory load on your body thus increasing the risk of a huge variety of chronic diseases including cancer and dementia.

The AA and EPA embed themselves in cell membranes, and these include the membranes of all the immune system cells. The inflammatory eicosanoids and resolvins are a part of the immune defence mechanism, but you do not want your cells primed for inflammation all the time.

People in most Western societies rarely consume the omega-3 rich small cold water fish like sardines, herring, mackerel, salmon and trout. They often mistakenly consume white-fleshed fish like perch or barramundi thinking these are good sources of omega-3's which they are not. Also rarely do people ensure they have an adequate intake of alpha-linolenic acid (ALA) which is the parent compound for the omega-3's including EPA and DHA so important for health.

Gamma Linolenic Acid (GLA) although derived from the omega-6 pathway, is also a powerful anti-inflammatory compound from Borage and Evening Primrose Oil. GLA results in the series-1 anti-inflammatory compounds.

Human beings do not convert ALA easily to EPA or DHA with only a 5% efficiency rate at most for conversion, but marine algae are excellent at converting ALA to EPA and DHA and fish that eat the marine algae, accumulate the EPA/DHA in high concentrations in their flesh and blood. The EPA/DHA act like anti-freeze for these fish in those extremely cold waters, and we then benefit from the omega-3's when we consume those types of cold water fish.

ALA can be found in high concentrations in seeds like flaxseed and chia. Getting that ideal meal composition on your plate is vital to ensure you do not add to the inflammatory burden of your body.

Ensure you get the whole raft of anti-inflammatory compounds EPA/DHA/ALA/GLA (See Appendix-2 & 18).

The wrong level of intake of omega-6's does add to the inflamm-ageing process.

Testing Omega-6 and Omega-3 Ratios

You can take away the guesswork out of your omega-6 to omega-3 ratios by having this analysed. Go to Appendix-18 to see how. You can have your arachidonic acid (AA) and EPA ratio assessed as this is important. Your AA level may be in the reference range or even lower but if your EPA level is also low then the ratio of AA/EPA is affected meaning that the AA series 2 and 4 inflammatory eicosanoids will predominate because of that competitive nature of the enzyme system discussed above.

Testing your omega-3 to omega-6 ratios will give you a great idea of how you are tracking regarding these important essential fatty acids and whether you are primed for inflammation and are at risk for so many diseases of inflammation from Alzheimer's Disease to cancer. You can target treatment more effectively as a result. Like any test, service or product, it is important not to take any action until you have discussed this with the doctors that are caring for you especially if you have a chronic illness or are on one or more medications.

Find a practitioner at www.a8h.com.au to help you with this important test.

CHAPTER 8

Weight Loss Principles

For the first time in the history of humanity obese individuals far outnumbers those starving on this planet with around 1.5 billion people overweight (Popkin, Adair et al. 2012), versus around 800 million people underweight (Mirsky 2007). For the first time in our evolution, we as a species are not laboriously hunting for calories; we are now actively trying to avoid them. Many overweight or obese individuals may try to avoid calories but paradoxically, these same individuals, seem to struggle with weight gain as they get older. People have a honeymoon period up to 25 years of age, and the battle then gets harder to keep weight off. Even those that appear slim may have an abundance of intra-abdominal fat called visceral fat deep in the abdomen that surrounds the internal organs, and these individuals are the so-called TOFI's (thin on the outside, fat on the inside). These individuals are at high risk for metabolic diseases such as prediabetes or diabetes and the Metabolic Syndrome and all because this toxic deep visceral fat pours out chemical compounds called **adipokines** that are highly inflammatory and damaging to the body even inducing insulin resistance which adds not only to cardiovascular risk but cancer and dementia risk. Losing weight is obviously a difficult task.

The number of health books about this topic abounds. Some people just love food, and the thought of not indulging is anathema to them. In this instance, these individuals know there is a price to pay regarding weight gain or poor health or both with indulgence.

Can you be 'fat but fit'? Politically Incorrect Madness!

A lot of dangerous comments are made in the press or in social media and all in the name of political correctness that ensures inclusiveness to the detriment of a huge number of individuals in society. By stating that you can be obese and yet still enjoy a long healthspan and be fit irrespective of being obese is a fallacy putting millions of people at great medical risk. This notion was shattered by a huge Swedish study of 1.3 million Swedish men carried out by Peter Nordström et al. The research found that aerobic fitness reduced the risk of death from **'any cause'**. However, and this is the important point, the benefit of aerobic fitness was reduced in obese individuals. Further, it was found that even **unfit normal weight** individuals had a **30% lower risk of death** from any cause in comparison to obese individuals (Högström, Nordström et al. 2015)

How aerobically fit an individual is in late adolescence is a determinant of early death. Our sedentary children may not enjoy long lives based on this research. So no matter how many factors you throw into the mix whether these are genetics or overconsumption, a sedentary lifestyle is a major determinant of mortality risk.

Why are we trying to embrace obesity as if this is an accepted norm? With increasing weight comes an increased risk of knee and hip osteoarthritis. There is a distinct loading pattern on the joints with a 1 to 4 ratio (1:4) between excessive weight and loading on the knees. So what this means is that for every kilogram you carry as excess weight, there will be a 4 kg effect on the knees per 1.6 kilometres walked (Messier, Gutekunst et al. 2005). So let's look at this a little further and let's say an individual is carrying a modest excess weight of 20 kg beyond their ideal weight. So this 1:4 loading will mean that each knee is now taking the brunt of 80kg of loading on each knee per 1.6 km. So if we walked say 10,000 steps a day, this would mean a massive cumulative loading of 381 kg (840 lbs.) on these joints per day (assuming a stride length of 0.762 metres). So is it any wonder that knee and hip replacements are some of the most common Orthopaedic procedures in medical practice? What about the lower back? Similar stresses would also apply increasing the risk of disc herniation and progressive osteoarthritis of the vertebral joints and degeneration of the intervertebral discs.

As joint pain worsens, so too will be the ability for that individual to exercise producing a progressive deterioration of aerobic fitness associated with diminishing lung function caused by a multitude of complex pulmonary factors associated with obesity.

Let's not forget the increased risk of insulin resistance, hypertension, cardiovascular disease, increased risk of gallstones and gallbladder disease, the risk of many obesity-related cancers, significant risk in childbirth and great surgical risk if anything goes wrong that needs immediate surgical correction like traumatic injuries. Complications such as gallstones in the obese state can prove fatal. There are many other complications. Let's not forget that someone obese will cause epigenetic changes in their eggs or sperm with the female affecting the next three generations and the male affecting the next two generations condemning the offspring of future generations to ill health and perhaps early death all because of obesity. So keeping your weight down to an ideal weight is the best insurance policy to protect against a myriad number of chronic disease states that will diminish your healthspan and truly diminish your lifespan.

'Large waist raises cancer risk.'

Was the title of an article published in Medscape (http://www.medscape.com/viewarticle/880719), the peer-reviewed website for health professionals. This article pointed out that:

> *"An analysis of data on more than 43,000 individuals revealed that, while increases in BMI raised the risk of developing a group of 10 obesity-related cancers by 11%, similar increases in waist circumference and waist-to-hip ratio (WHR) raised the risk by 13% and 15%, respectively."*

So you can see, that being overweight irrespective of whether you use BMI, waist circumference or waist-to-hip ratio is a statement that if you are fatter, you are at significant risk of a devastating disease. This generation is certainly fatter than generations that have gone before. The problem is perception. Many people walk around with BMI's of 30 or more and still see themselves as normal and all because they view people around them that are so much fatter when a BMI of 30 or more in them means they are obese!

Cancer is so rife in the community, with a range of coloured ribbons around to signify a particular cancer cause, and yet, little public attention is drawn to this devastating problem in the community where 60% of people, i.e. 6 out of 10 people are overweight or obese, and these individuals keep on eating foods that ensure they become bigger over time with ever-expanding waistlines. Regarding obesity-related cancer, one study stated:

> *"Results from epidemiological studies that largely began in the 1970s indicate that adiposity contributes to the increased incidence and/or death from cancers of the colon, breast (in postmenopausal women), endometrium, kidney (renal cell), oesophagus (adenocarcinoma), gastric cardia, pancreas, gallbladder and liver, and possibly other cancers. It has been estimated that 15–20% of all cancer deaths in the United States can be attributed to overweight and obesity" (Calle and Kaaks 2004)*

So many of these cancers such as breast cancer and bowel cancer are occurring at much younger ages and for experts to scratch their heads, wondering why strikes me as insane when obesity as a cause is the elephant in the room. Sure other factors will be involved such as genetics and the environment, but obesity would have to be a huge trigger. There is a tremendous loss of time, effort and huge sums of money in treating these cancers rather than trying to prevent them.

The money lost could be used for so many other causes in society and let's not forget the human cost and unbelievable sadness at the preventable premature loss of life that can be avoided.

That governments are complicit in this ignorance is truly shocking. A concerted educational push is the only way forward with fresh food prices driven down by subsidies and taxes on all the damaging foods sold in supermarkets, food malls and fast food outlets. Allowing Big-Food to keep on killing people just to ensure job numbers are maintained or to derive tax benefits from the sale of those foods is sheer madness when you consider the enormous health bill and the loss of life at the end of all of this. Governments need the courage to effect change.

So let us get away from that myth of being fat and fit and that you can be fat and healthy. It is simply not true!

Why is weight loss so difficult for some?

The problem with weight loss attempts is that one of two strategies will be used:

1. **Decrease caloric (energy) intake (avoid calories)**
2. **Increase energy expenditure (exercise more)**

However, both strategies are doomed to failure. In the first instance, if calories are reduced, there is a corresponding reduction in **basal metabolic rate (BMR),** also known as **resting metabolic rate (RMR)** which is the energy used by the body at rest to drive breathing, your heart action, brain function, excretory functions, metabolic and hormonal processes, all in the resting state for the body. This RMR consumes 60%-70% of the total energy expenditure (TEE) in the body (Martin et al., 2007).

Numerous studies have shown that lowering calories results in a massive 30%-40% drop in basal metabolic rate (Song & Thomas, 2007). This is the body shifting to energy conservation as the signal you are giving your body by dropping calorie intake for weight loss, is a famine signal. Your body will want to conserve precious energy, and so it will start to shut off many metabolic systems that 'chew-up' energy. You will feel the cold as your body temperature will drop to conserve energy, and your activity will also decrease as your body's energy levels drop, and you feel too fatigued to move.

You may be hoping that by decreasing calories you are sending a starvation signal to your body in a bid to mobilise your fat stores. However, this drop in RMR may persist long after you have resumed normal feeding to pre-caloric restriction levels. Your body fat may rebound, and fat stores may grow larger than pre-dieting levels. It is unfortunate that with a significant reduction in calories, you will also lose lean mass from muscles and organs and even lose protein from your bone. You can see in the graphic on Total Energy Expenditure (TEE), that RMR accounts for a large part of total energy expenditure per day and that lean muscle mass accounts for 18% of this RMR (Durnin, 1981).

If you lose muscle in the process, you will significantly decrease metabolic rate and to try and get back this lost muscle tissue will take a great deal of effort and dedication. Muscle loss is an important reason why the effect of calorie restriction may persist long after you stop this dietary weight loss strategy because of the great impact muscle loss has on the resting metabolic rate (RMR). This effect ensures that when you go back to your regular diet that those calories now cannot be burnt off as energy as you have less active lean muscle mass to devour those calories. You now pack on the fat where before the calorie restriction, these same calories may have maintained a steady weight; they are now conserved as fat due to the metabolic changes induced by calorie restriction. Not a good strategy for weight loss! Your weight setpoint moves higher.

You may be thinking that this low energy signal and low protein sufficiency signal caused by a significant drop in calories will be decreasing the cellular proliferating mTOR signalling pathway as a result. This is all true and does happen because your body is conserving energy and resources. However, persistent lowering of calories and a prolonged scarcity of precious nutrient resources will induce a deleterious effect on the body resulting in loss of lean muscle mass which is never a good thing. Semi-starvation diets will cause your bones to lose protein and minerals putting you at risk of lower bone mineral density and lower bone protein concentration resulting in osteopenia or osteoporosis (bone weakening). Your body will start to cannibalise itself because of the Triage mechanism we discussed before, where critical nutrients are shunted from less immediately important tissues like muscle and bone to critical organs like the heart, kidneys, lungs and brain. Lowering calories long-term is not sustainable, and organ systems will start to crumble and fail.

If you try to increase exercise, all you will do is create an energy deficit, and your body will try to get you back to the setpoint you started by increasing hunger signals. Give in to your hunger signals, and all is lost!

Many diet combinations have failed and these include:

- **Low-fat diets** – like the Ornish diet have been a huge disappointment. The Ornish diet was favoured by the American Heart Association and the medical profession for the past few decades. The obesity epidemic has thrived on this type of diet. Low-fat diets according to Harvard professor David Ludwig, lowered metabolic rate the most (Ebbeling et al., 2012).
- **Low-carb diets** - like the Atkins Diet (short-term weight loss only). If you decrease carbs, you increase protein and fat to compensate.
- **High-carb diets** can increase net fat (triglyceride) production by **296%** (Minehira et al., 2003). High carbohydrate intakes can produce high triglyceride levels in the blood both in the fasting state and the after eating (postprandial) state (Minehira et al., 2003). Modern Western diets are tremendously carbohydrate-heavy, and the high rates of so many diseases are a result of the skewed intake of this one macronutrient. This is a disaster for anyone with existing heart disease or blood vessels starting to become blocked due to atherosclerotic plaques.
- **High-protein diets** - Also a failure and a high-risk with the new findings on protein intake and cancer risk and mTOR signalling (Levine, Suarez et al. 2014). For those who like to think that protein cannot be converted to fat, expert biochemists would love to argue the point – you cannot argue and win when the issue is an incontrovertible fact! This following quote should put an end to this way of thinking:

"In spite of the exhortation by some popular weight-reducing diets to eat large quantities of protein, it should be remembered that surplus dietary protein can be converted to fat. For protein to be converted to fatty acids and triacylglycerols, the essential precursors for fatty acid synthesis, namely a carbon source, acetyl CoA, and biosynthetic reducing power as NADPH, must be formed." (Salway 2006). The other name for triacylglycerols is triglycerides.

- **High-Fat Diets** – the latest craze that will backfire. It is a well-known fact that a high-fat diet will lead to obesity and that high-fat intakes (around 30% of energy) can readily induce obesity in both Humans and in mice and rat models (Hariri & Thibault, 2010). Studies are emerging that even one fat-laden meal can increase **systemic lipopolysaccharide (LPS or endotoxin)** that can **trigger marked inflammatory responses** in the body and can damage the endothelial lining of blood vessels (Erridge, Attina et al. 2007). This occurs in healthy individuals even with just one fatty meal. I will discuss LPS (Endotoxin) in more detail later. Another disaster that awaits anyone with existing heart and vascular disease as chronic inflammation in the body drives a myriad number of diseases seen in society.

If you look at these common types of diets, you will notice that we are looking for a magic-bullet solution by focusing on one of the macronutrients (fat, carbs or protein) and increasing one of them while decreasing one or more of the others. The problem with this reductionist thinking about diet is that it is doomed to failure as human beings have always had a varied diet based on availability and seasonality. Such restrictions can result in malnutrition.

Pushing people towards starchy grains is absolute folly as there is nothing essential about having a grain or cereal product. These grains are rich in energy, nutrient poor and have inherent problems such as gluten-sensitivity, non-coeliac gluten sensitivity (NCGS) and also have FODMAP (Fermentable carbohydrate) concerns that could make anyone with irritable bowel syndrome (IBS) suffer. These problems affect a vast number of people. Grains and cereals are far from wonder foods! See Appendix-28.

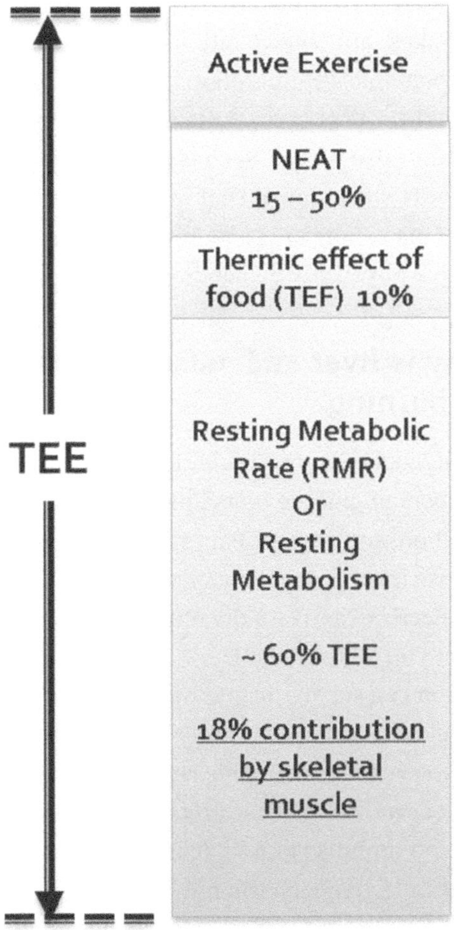

Total Energy Expenditure: Let's have a look at how you burn energy

Most of the calories that you burn in a day for energy is known as the **Resting Metabolic Rate (RMR)** sometimes called Basal Metabolic Rate (BMR). Thus 60-70% of the energy you consume in a day is taken up by the RMR which includes the energy needed by your body while at rest and 12 hours after any exercise. RMR includes the energy used for breathing, your heart beating, your kidneys functioning, the energy consumed by the brain during rest and all the cellular functions that require energy in the rested state.

Energy is also consumed by the very process of eating food and this is called the **Thermogenic Effect of Food (TEF).** We also have **Non-Exercise Activity Thermogenesis (NEAT)** which is activity other than formal exercise, and this will include how much you walk in a day, how many stairs you take, how much you fidget, and then there is the energy expenditure of formal exercise. All the energy consumed by your body in a day is called **Total Energy Expenditure (TEE).**

You will see that NEAT can vary from 15 – 50% respectively in sedentary and active individuals (Levine, 2004). NEAT is so easily targeted by an individual as it is in their control to walk faster or longer in a day, take stairs as often as possible, go for a brisk walk for a few blocks during lunchtime, and do short bursts of high intensity training lasting just seconds throughout the day. NEAT is an easy exercise alternative for those that hate exercising providing a huge 'bang-for-the-buck'.

A simple act such as walking fast as if you are rushing to catch a bus or train can *"triple ones metabolic rate above the basal level"* (McCrady-Spitzer & Levine, 2012)

NEAT activity is a highly effective way to increase metabolic rate above the resting level and significantly so. However, for this to be an effective way of shifting fat you need to have the following in place:

1. A low blood insulin level that will allow mobilisation of fat --- **Intraday Fasting (IDF) using IDF2M or IDF3M strategies (**discussed soon)

2. Eating just 2 - 3 meals a day spaced apart without snacking to allow prolonged blood insulin dips

A diet predominantly based on whole vegetables and low carb fruit along with the right amount of protein that takes into consideration hidden protein sources (see the section on protein), with optimal phytochemical & micronutrient intake and no starchy carbohydrates in the Plan-A diet can provide the basis for fat loss. You replace starchy carbs by plenty of low-glycemic-index vegetables (Low-GI carbs) and low-GI fruit (also carbs). Such is the **Activ8Health Plan-A Diet designed for fat loss or weight maintenance.** My **Activ8Health Plan-B Diet** includes meaningful starchy carbs, i.e. ones that have a lot of fibre or minerals, and other micronutrients and not just empty carbs. The Plan-B diet is designed for those who exercise intensely or have physically demanding jobs.

Why is liver and muscle glycogen important in fat burning?

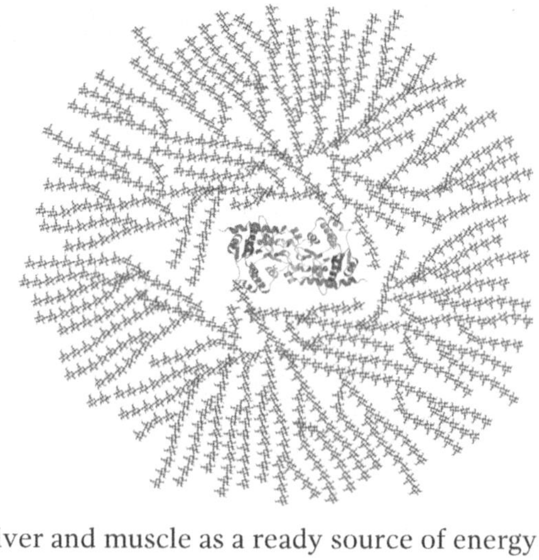

Glycogen is a molecule rich in glucose tightly bound in vast numbers of glucose units linked together. Glycogen is a storehouse of glucose energy for times of emergency, when the glucose level is dropping or when there is a fight-flight response that needs to activate the most powerful Type-IIX muscle fibres to get you out of trouble.

You can see in the graphic by Mikael Häggström, (2014), that glucose units are tightly bound in the glycogen, and each dot you see in the graphic represents a glucose molecule. Tens of thousands of glucose units are thus bound in glycogen within liver and muscle as a ready source of energy that can mobilise rapidly in an emergency with the aid of adrenaline.

Muscle glycogen can only be used for local muscle needs whereas liver glycogen can be used to provide the whole body and brain with glucose energy as required. Adrenaline is the principal molecule that mobilises muscle glycogen, and glucagon is the principal molecule for liver glycogen mobilisation (Berg, Tymoczko et al.).

The key to fat loss

What I am describing here is the absolute key to fat loss. You will find out why glycogen is so important in an evolutionary sense and how you can take advantage of this evolutionary imperative. Please read this time and again if you have to. This understanding is vital to you shifting fat and to stimulate fat loss in the body. The strategy all hinges on you also ensuring low blood insulin levels which will enable fat (triglycerides) to be released from fat cells and to stimulate adrenaline release to release glucose from glycogen and triglycerides from fat.

For fat loss, it is important to use the Activ8Health Plan-A diet that has been designed to support exercise and the mobilisation of your fat stores and to use intraday fasting as an aid to diminishing blood insulin and glycogen levels. The whole idea is to ensure you have all the nutrients you need and that you consume a protein intake based on that recommended in this book or through your Dietitian.

HIIT Simulates the Fight-Flight Response

Short bursts of high intensity exercise or high intensity interval training (HIIT) in essence produces a fight-flight response as far as the body is concerned. Consider yourself on a stationary bike, and you peddle as fast as you can for 20 – 30 seconds and then at a very slow pace for a few minutes. That rapid burst of activity which will leave you breathless if you do it well, is essentially perceived by the body as you trying to escape something threatening stimulating adrenaline to increase significantly in your body and adrenaline has the following effect:

1. It rapidly releases glucose from glycogen in the liver for use by the body's muscles, organs and brain

2. It rapidly releases glucose from glycogen in the muscle for use by the muscle only. Muscle lacks a particular enzyme, and thus muscle glycogen can only be used locally in actively contracting muscles during a fight-flight response.

If you can ensure your blood is not flooded with glucose constantly through nonstop grazing on starchy carbs, then insulin levels should be low enough in your body allowing fat stores to be plundered and the stored triglycerides in those fat cells to be used for energy and to replace the glycogen lost through the glycerol in those released triglycerides.

Adrenaline's Cascade Amplification

The body has produced an exquisite system to rapidly release glucose units from this tightly coiled glycogen structure when glucose is required. There is an amplification process where just one (x1) molecule of adrenaline (or glucagon), can lead to multiple secondary then tertiary molecules and so on to the last step that then converges on the glycogen at multiple sites to release vast quantities of glucose units simultaneously in times of crisis – the fight-flight response. These amplification steps can be seen in biochemistry books like Berg & Stryers Biochemistry 5th Edition for those who want to see this action in detail (Berg, Tymoczko et al.).

The graphic below has been created by me to give you a visual understanding of this process, and this will help you understand what is happening with HIIT and how glycogen in muscle will be depleted with exercise. One molecule of adrenaline (or glucagon) can result in the release of 10,000 glucose molecules from glycogen (Heilmeyer 2012).

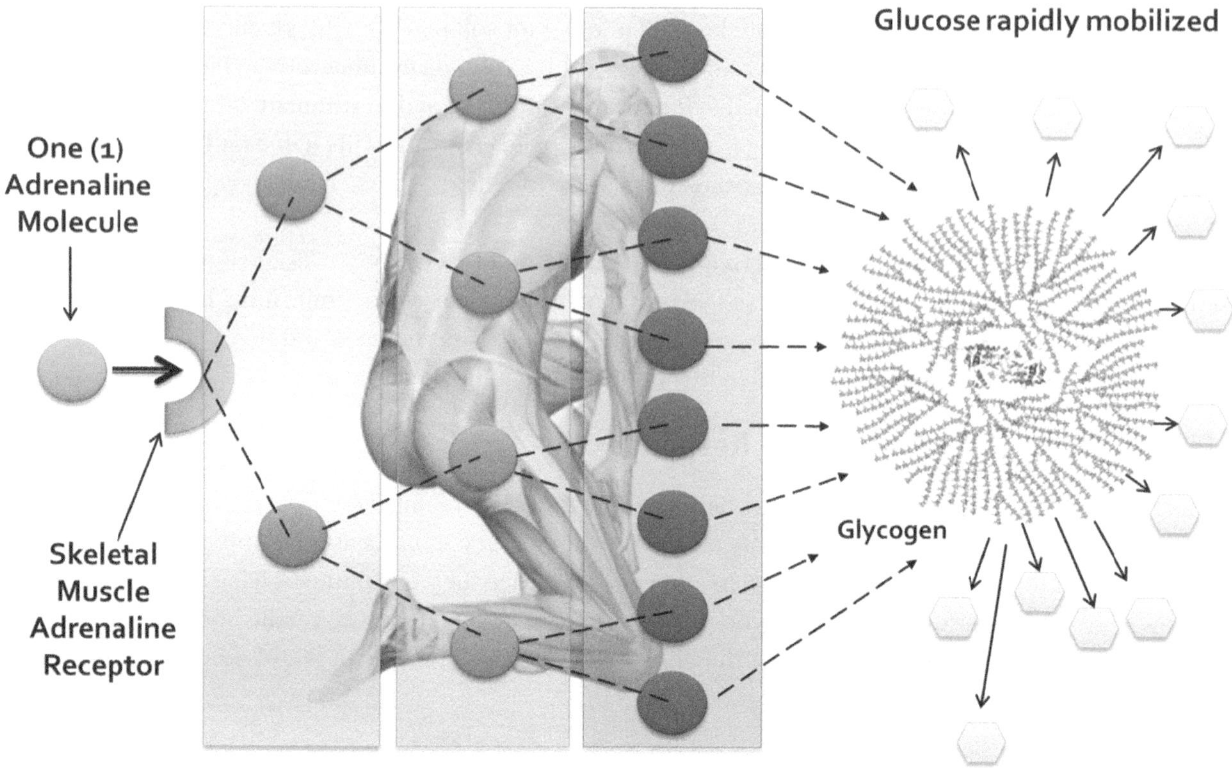

A NutriDesk presentation. Graphic © Dr Rodney Lopez 2013 .All Rights Reserved

Why is glycogen so important? Let's discuss the evolutionary imperative

Glycogen is your ticket out of trouble in times of danger. You will gear yourself to fight or flee the scene, and you need energy that can be used immediately in this time of danger. Fats cannot be burnt off fast enough in this emergency state, but glucose can be rapidly utilised and used as energy by the muscles and in particular, by the powerful Type-IIX muscle fibres to help spring you away from trouble.

Type-IIX muscle fibres are glucose and energy 'guzzlers' that are inefficient energy producers, but they serve a purpose in times of trouble because of their power and hence the Type-IIX muscle fibres need to have full glycogen stores at all times as an energy reserve for times of crisis.

Thus glycogen replacement is an **EVOLUTIONARY IMPERATIVE --- your body is programmed to replace these stores rapidly to ensure you are ready for the next threat.** According to the wonderful biochemistry text 'Metabolism at a Glance' (Salway & Granner, 2004), the author states:

> *"Next, after a strenuous chase, the prey (assuming it has survived) must quickly replenish its glycogen reserves for the next emergency, whether food is available or not."* The operative words are, *"whether food is available or not"*.

When food is not available, you mobilise body fat stores as this is a large energy reserve waiting to be plundered to help replace depleted glycogen stores. This understanding is vital to shifting troublesome fat in your body. Let's use this evolutionary survival loophole to our advantage and chip away at these fat reserves.

Using glycerol from fat to our advantage

Your fat cells pack in vast numbers of fat molecules called **triglycerides**. As you have cleverly guessed by the name, this molecule has 3 of something, and these three things are fatty acids.

The three fatty acids are attached to a glycerol backbone, and by that name, you may also guess that glycerol sounds like glucose and it is indeed a sugar alcohol.

The important thing to understand, is that when fat is mobilised for energy, the 3 fatty acids are split from the glycerol backbone, and these fatty acids can provide a lot of energy for cellular functions and the glycerol can also be used after it has been converted to glucose in the liver through a process called gluconeogenesis, to fill up all that lost muscle and liver glycogen.

Depletion of muscle glycogen can occur through intraday fasting (IF), increasing NEAT exercise and through high intensity interval training (HIIT) and other forms of formal exercise.

Your most powerful Type-IIX muscle fibres are rich with muscle glycogen, and you need to target these fibres effectively to release as much stored muscle glycogen as possible thus leaving this glycogen 'hole' that will need to be filled in from tapping into your fat stores.

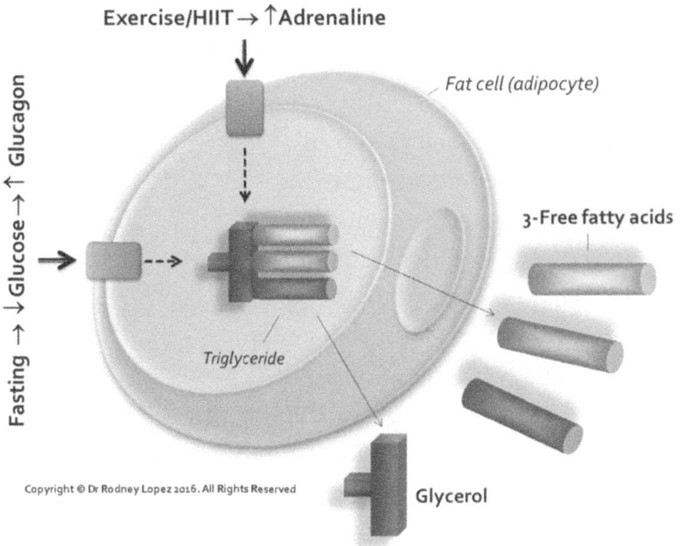

Just understanding the importance of glycogen in the scheme of things and then knowing that if you do NOT supply your body with a ready source of glucose from starchy carbohydrates whether whole-grain or not, means your body has to find a way to replenish the vital glycogen stores and this will be from the huge reservoir of fat that exists in 60-70% of people in Western countries.

Using fat in your body to replace the glycogen loss in muscle and liver

It is preferable that you have not eaten for at least 2 hours before exercise so that readily available glucose will be low. Limiting glucose availability will force your body to tap into your fat reserves and draw from the wealth of glycerol in this fat. The graphic highlights how glycogen stores will trigger fat use as long as you do not provide a readily available glucose source through starchy carbs throughout the day or around exercise by sipping on glucose-rich sports drinks!

Remember, glucose from any source will raise insulin levels and this is true of dairy and high intakes of protein. All of these raise insulin, and this hormone then traps fat in the cells. If glucose and insulin levels are low, it will force your body to break down the fat (triglycerides) in your adipocytes (fat cells) to release 3 fatty acids and 1 glycerol molecule from each triglyceride molecule.

There are thousands of these triglyceride molecules in just in one fat cell. The free fatty acids will be used to drive energy utilising processes and can provide the energy for the homeostatic adjustments of EPOC after exercise, and the glycerol will undergo gluconeogenesis in the liver to glucose. Use your fat to replenish these depleted glycogen stores and not sugar in a sports drink or a carb.

What you are aiming for is a cycle of glycogen depletion followed by the use of fat (triglycerides) to replace the lost glycogen. By doing this daily, you will constantly tap into fat stores that are seemingly difficult to rid. Remember, the Activ8Health Plan-A Diet is highly supportive of this fat loss process.

Essential Amino Acids (EAAs) before exercise, during exercise and after is worthwhile as the energy content of EAAs is extremely low, they provide all the amino acids your body needs for protein synthesis keeping in mind the body can create any non-essential amino acid.

EAAs will limit the amount of insulin produced, and these free-form amino acids are rapidly absorbed, unlike whole protein. See Appendix-24 for more information. Do not sabotage your exercise efforts with insulin-spiking sports drinks full of glucose.

The 'Glycogen-Battery' Analogy

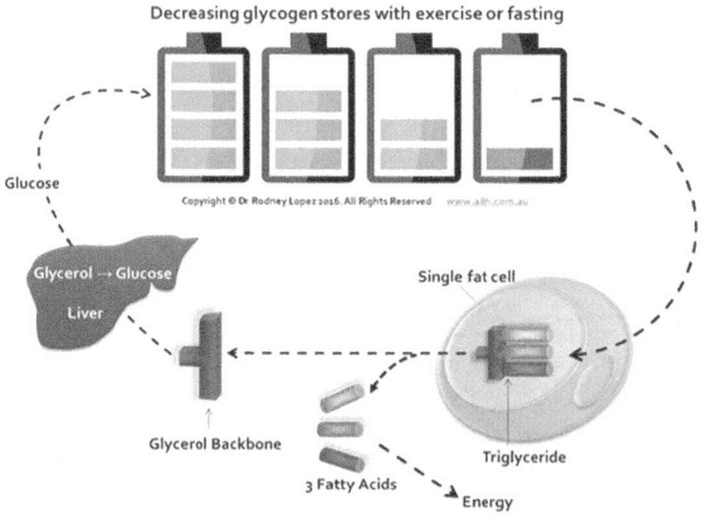

The benefit of glycogen depletion is enormous and is thought to be an important mechanism for improved glycemic (blood glucose) control, insulin receptor sensitivity and improved blood insulin levels. You absolutely pull the rug out from under you when you consume starchy (glucose-rich) carbohydrates before or after exercise and during the day. Keep on tapping into your fat stores by:

1. Using the intraday fasting system to be described soon
2. Stick to the Activ8Health Plan-A Diet that supports fat loss
3. Keep on depleting your glycogen stores by using Non-Exercise Activity Thermogenesis (NEAT or informal exercise) every day – 10,000 steps, stairs, fast/slow walking
4. Keep on depleting your glycogen by performing short 20-30 second HIIT exercises on a stationary bike in the morning or lunch break, do sprints 2 – 3 days a week in a park or street around your home. Just 2 – 3 of these 20-30 second bursts followed by 1 – 2 minutes of a very slow pace to recover in-between is all you need. This takes just minutes to complete.
5. You can do a HIIT session lasting less than 10 minutes in a gym while wearing your work clothes if you can quickly get into a gym during your lunch hour and you will still have time for lunch.
6. Use Super-Slow exercises described in Appendix-11 and 12 and in the exercise section to follow.
7. Perform a gym-based program one day a week to work the whole body or a split routine where you work one-half of the body on one day and then the other half on another day.

New findings on yo-yo dieting

An Israeli study has found a very interesting effect that may result in rebound weight gain which changes the body's setpoint. Changes in the gut microbiome with a poor diet, increased the loss of flavonoid polyphenols and these polyphenols that are found richly in veggies and fruit, can promote fat burning and weight loss. However, there seemed to be a 'gut microbiome memory' and so even though you can lose weight by switching to a healthy diet, the moment you consume an unhealthy, high fat Western diet, this bacterial memory kicks in and prevents fat loss by inhibiting flavonoid induced fat burning (Thaiss, Itav et al. 2016).

This study simply reinforces the fact that you cannot switch from an unhealthy diet, back to a healthy one and then back again to a less than desirable diet. Such yo-yo dieting plays havoc with your gut microbiome and we now know these organisms have a 'memory'.

Groups of microorganisms simply love the Western diet high in energy and fats and can't wait till the good times roll again with that feast signalling that they thrive on.

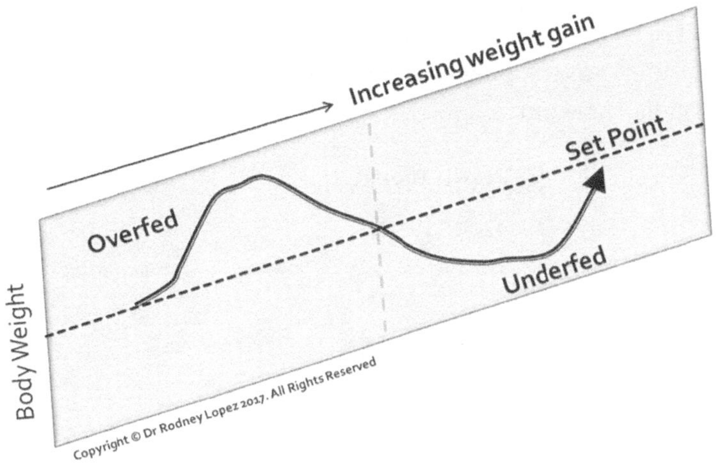

Is a weight setpoint is a fait accompli?

You may not be able to change your genetics or what your mother did regarding dietary intake while you were a foetus, but you have a powerful tool to change your weight setpoint, and that is to adjust your body composition through dietary and exercise strategies.

Ensuring calorie restriction and yet optimal nutrition plus exercising regularly will ensure your setpoint does not creep higher as shown in the diagram. Resistance training to increase muscle mass will help keep your weight set point low as well as your body fat percentage. Semi-starvation diets and then overfeeding will ensure a higher and higher setpoint. You need to be consistent and disciplined!

Insulin - fat gain enemy Number-1

Ask anyone about insulin, and they will know it has something to do with glucose and diabetes. However, insulin's actions go far beyond just the disposal of glucose into cells. Insulin has the following actions:

- Increases glucose entry into cells
- Increases glycogen synthesis
- Increases lipid (fat) synthesis
- Inhibits fat release from fat cells
- Increases amino acid entry into cells

- Increased protein synthesis through mTOR (mTORC1)
- Growth stimulating factor similar to IGF-1, IGF-2 and Relaxin
- Insulin blocks leptin signalling in the brain. Leptin is the 'satiety hormone' and curbs appetite in the hypothalamus. Ghrelin the 'hunger hormone' is opposed by Leptin.

When insulin levels are high, the Hormone-Sensitive Lipase (HSL) enzyme is strongly inhibited, as well as other enzymes like Adipose Triglyceride Lipase (ATGL). Fat release is a result of the hormonal interplay between Glucagon/Adrenaline versus insulin. These hormones are antagonistic. Glucagon and adrenaline can increase glucose release from glycogen stores and fat stores via the glycerol → glucose conversion in the liver (gluconeogenesis) that we have discussed.

Insulin powerfully 'locks' fat (triglycerides) in the fat cell

If you are trying to lose weight, then you need to target insulin and keep this as low as possible. If insulin levels are high, you will shut-off fat release. Two hormones critical to triglycerides (fats) mobilisation from your fat cells are Adipose Triglyceride Lipase (ATGL) and Hormone-Sensitive Lipase (HSL) --- the latter is **powerfully inhibited** by insulin thus trapping triglycerides in your fat cells ensuring that you gain a bigger belly or that those 'love handles' stay put!

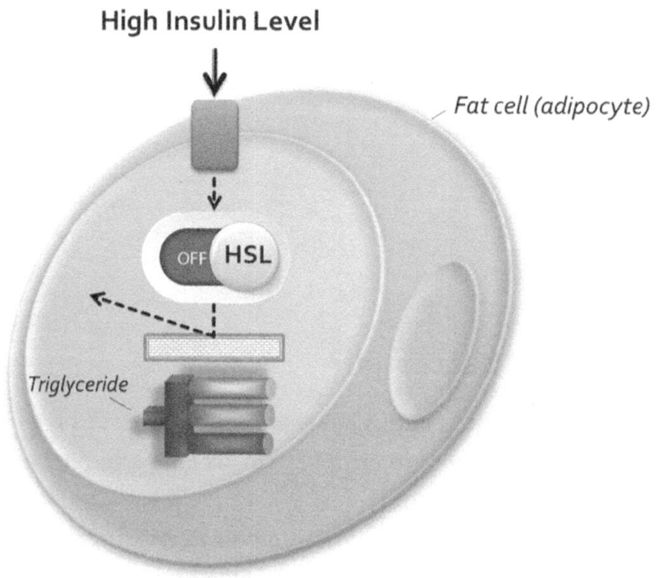

Insulin antagonises the effects of adrenaline and glucagon and works directly opposite to how these two hormones work.

Insulin is a **storage hormone,** and if this hormone is high, it will trap the triglycerides in the cell by powerfully blocking **hormone-sensitive lipase (HSL)** the 'magic' enzyme that helps break down the triglycerides in fat cells for release into the bloodstream.

You need to keep insulin levels low to enable fat to escape. This is biochemistry in action, plain and simple and an absolute scientific reality. Use science to guide you!

The Activ8Health Plan-A Diet is designed to ensure insulin levels stay low 24/7

So the key to fat loss is maintaining a very low level of insulin in your system and by doing so allow Hormone-Sensitive Lipase (HSL) to do its job and start to break up and release the triglyceride fats trapped in your fat cells.

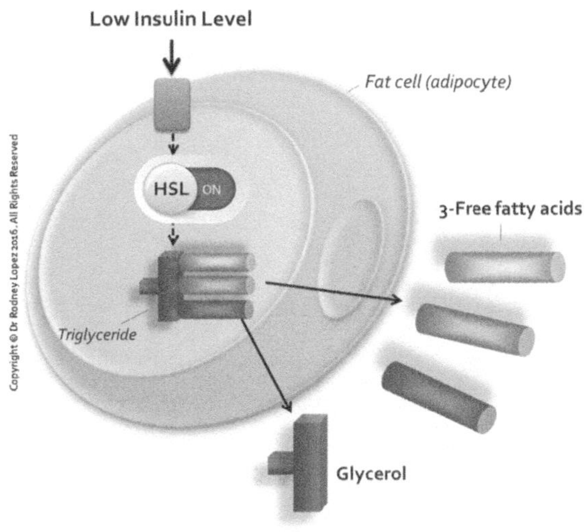

Food components that powerfully increase blood insulin levels are:

1. Starchy & Processed Carbohydrates
2. Protein
3. Dairy Products

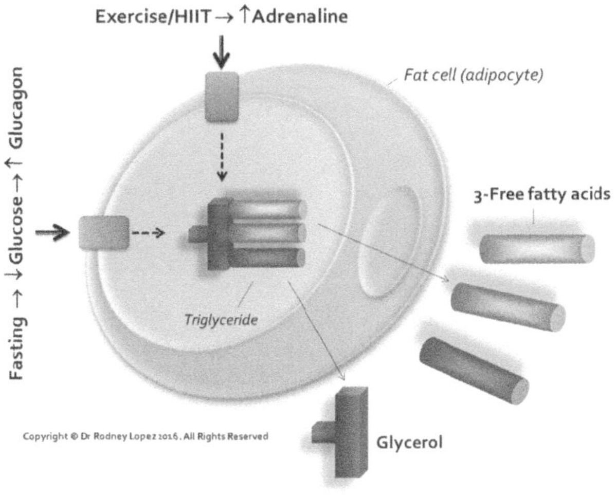

Keeping insulin levels low is the Holy Grail if you want to lose fat and become lean or stay lean. Insulin leads to energy storage and energy trapping for use when times are lean. The powerful anabolic effect of this hormone wants to keep stored energy in cells, and this could be glycogen or importantly fat stored as triglycerides in fat cells.

By intraday fasting, you produce prolonged dips in insulin and by easily increasing activity in your day through simple measures as discussed; you will blast away fat, become fit and stay lean and healthy throughout your life!

Although as mentioned, each fat cell has thousands of triglyceride molecules. For simplicity's sake, we are looking at just one (x1) triglyceride in one (x1) fat cell. Boost adrenaline by fast exercises like high intensity interval training (HIIT) and adrenaline levels rise rapidly and will powerfully mobilise fats (triglycerides) by stimulating **Beta Adrenoceptors** on fat cells. Glucagon responds to decreasing blood glucose levels in-between meals or intraday fasting to stimulate both the breakdown of glycogen in the liver and fat breakdown allowing the glycerol from triglycerides (fat) to be converted to glucose. We use the intraday fasting to lower insulin and glucose and increase adrenaline through exercise by performing NEAT/HIIT exercises.

Continually deplete glycogen, keep insulin levels low and lose fat

Key Points

- Diets fail because they focus on one component We want a diet that focuses on all the things that matter: micronutrients, phytochemicals, fibre, the right amount of protein, low-glycemic-index (not starchy) carbohydrates found in vegetables and fruit and the right fats
- Glycogen, a concentrated source of glucose in your muscles and liver mainly, can be decreased. This vital fight-flight response compound if depleted has to be replaced for emergency survival reasons.
- Starchy carbs, high protein intakes, dairy all increase insulin levels thus trapping fat in our fat cells (adipocytes)
- Intraday fasting ensures the hormone glucagon increases in the fasting state to draw upon glycogen in the liver and to increase fat mobilisation for energy.
- You found out that the non-exercise activity thermogenesis (NEAT) can increase significantly. NEAT and formal exercise increases adrenaline and this hormone powerfully mobilises the release of glucose from glycogen stores and triglycerides from fat stores.
- Insulin is a powerful storage (anabolic) hormone that wants to save energy in the body for times of famine. From an evolutionary perspective, energy conservation is hardwired in us. Keep insulin levels low and you can watch your fat stores start to disappear and change your body setpoint as a result.
- We provide a rich source of low-GI vegetable carbs in the Activ8Health diet. Remember, veggies are carbs but not the glucose and insulin spiking type.
- Constant depletion of glycogen through intraday fasting, NEAT, exercise associated with the Activ8Health Plan-A low insulin diet, will ensure a constant fat loss process in the body.

CHAPTER 9

Intraday Fasting (IF)

(IF2M or IF3M Fasting)

Intraday fasting = Nutrient shuffling in a day (it is not starvation or semi-starvation)

The concept of fasting is now well known, and many people practice the 5 & 2 diet where there are two days of fasting and 5 days of eating normally or at least normally for you. Intraday fasting is easier I feel, in that you are selecting just one meal to miss out on. It is all about ensuring you obtain all the nutrients and phytochemicals necessary for optimal health. It is not about semi-starvation or starvation! Fasting can be difficult for people, and many will indeed find it a difficult task long-term. What they may find easier to do is skip a meal 2 – 3 times a week but make up for the calculated protein intake at the next meal and to ensure you do not suffer from micronutrient deficiencies through the Activ8Health Plan-A and Plan-B type diets discussed in this book including prudent supplementation.

I have made the argument in this book that to benefit from a prolonged dip in blood Insulin/IGF-1 to dampen AMPK/mTOR signalling, may involve you having only two meals a day. The reason is that many people have insulin resistance in society and anyone with a large waist may indeed be suffering from insulin resistance meaning that blood parameters may never come back to normal before the next meal 6 to 8 hours away. Many people may look normal and thin on the outside and yet be fat on the inside. These are the so-called TOFI's (thin on the outside, fat on the inside).

Many devastating diseases can be avoided if people can conform to dietary restrictions and yet provide the body with all the nutrients it needs to prosper. Common and deadly diseases in society that include hypertension, prediabetes, diabetes, heart and vascular disease, stroke, dementia and many cancers are not an absolute mystery. They should not be accepted as a normal and inevitable part of life. Most if not all of these disease states can be avoided by disciplined dietary, and exercise practices and this includes intraday fasting.

As discussed, the Activ8Health Plan-A Diet supports fat loss through the glycogen depletion process aided by the use of NEAT, HIIT, Resistance Training and mixing it up with long walks or jogging as this 'mash-up' of a variety of exercises has been shown to be much better for telomere length than doing the same thing day-in and day-out. The Plan-A diet is also an optimal diet for everyday use by anyone wanting to practice calorie restriction yet optimal nutrition principles.

You can choose which of two paths you want to follow about food intake. You can either choose the path of constant feeding through three or more meals a day including snacks or choose a path where you give your body a chance to rest metabolically and thus support cellular repair and recovery. So the two choices are:

1. Constant feast signalling through incessant eating including unnecessary snacks stimulating cell multiplication at the expense of maintenance and repair processes

2. Intermittent famine signalling through intraday fasting to dampen down cell multiplication processes and stimulate the NAD^+/Sirtuin/FoxO pathways for cell repair and maintenance

Feast Signalling

The feast signalling pathway is the typical pathway that predominates in the Western world. The typical Western diet comprises large portion sizes of food with caloric (energy) values that are way beyond metabolic needs and protein intakes that are in all probability way too much for them. This type of food intake drives the feast signal pathway and this, in turn, drives cell multiplication.

This feast cell multiplication and energy storage process is simply Mother Nature preparing you for reproduction no matter how old you are. It is a hardwired response by the body when presented with a large caloric and protein intake. The evolutionary imperative is to keep you strong and for you to pass on your genes to the next generation. The feast signalling is a process that ensures both parents have all the energy reserves needed to look after their offspring (genes). Both the mother and father are made stronger through cellular multiplication that increases muscle mass and bone strength, ensures adequate energy stores of both glycogen and fat, and ensures they have enough vitamins, minerals and trace elements to look after the survival of their progeny as the child is carrying the precious cargo of genetic material from both parents.

This process though wears you out faster, shortens your telomeres and increases the number of senescent (old and dying) cells in the body. You age rapidly and program yourself for early demise as a result of this rampant food intake. Constantly stimulating cell multiplication increases the risk of genetic mutations that may accumulate to the point of malignancy. Path 1, the feast signal is summarised in the graphic.

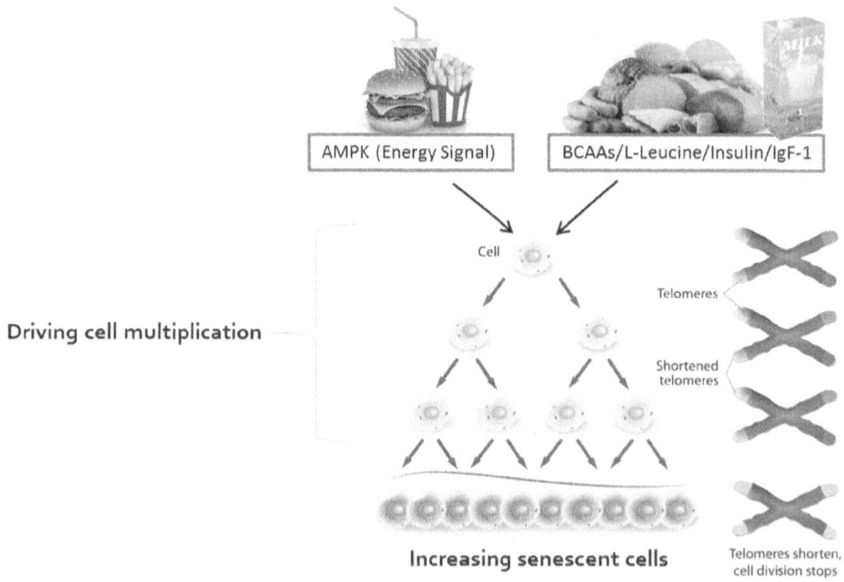

Famine Signal: Repair & Maintenance Mode

If you choose the famine signal pathway, then there are no cellular multiplication pressures and your body goes into a repair and maintenance phase. From an evolutionary perspective, what your cells are doing is keeping you in great shape for when the good times roll again so that you can pass on your genes.

Remember from an evolutionary perspective; we have had to deal with far more famine pressures than feast. You can achieve this signal by keeping caloric intake down, i.e. not having energy-dense foods and fast-foods, ensuring your body thrives on all the micronutrients it needs from vitamins, minerals, trace elements and a rich intake of phytochemicals for their hormetic effects on the body.

Aim to skip three meals a week eventually but rotate the days and meals skipped. For example, you could follow the suggestion in the table below, but the following week you could skip lunch on Monday, skip dinner on the Wednesday and breakfast on Friday.

The body loves to adapt to any changes made and so constantly varying the timing of the skipped meals can offset this.

Monday	Tuesday	Wednesday	Thursday	Friday
Skip Breakfast		Skip Lunch		Skip Dinner

Intraday fasting not only shifts you towards this cell repair and maintenance mode, but it also leads to significant glycogen depletion which you are now aware of, is vital for shifting fat. Enhance this glycogen depletion effect of intraday fasting by increasing exercise – NEAT, HIIT.

Intraday fasting is easy enough to achieve, but most Westerners will think they are dying because food has not gone into their mouths. Allow yourself to get over this hunger because once you start tapping into your fat stores during this fasting period a large amount of energy is released to drive your energy needs. It is the emotional response to not eating that many will need to overcome.

Remember, this process will only work if your body is not being deprived of nutrients it needs to survive. Intraday fasting is never going to be a starvation or semi-starvation system. It is about optimising macronutrient and micronutrient intake but not caloric intake and ensuring you give your system a respite to repair and maintain the cellular machinery and decreasing all those risks of rampant cell multiplication caused by overconsumption.

It is important to ensure you make up the protein that was missed in the meal not eaten. It is a myth to have to consume protein three times a day. A paper was written by experienced Australian nutrition experts. They stated:

> *"The body maintains a pool of indispensable amino acids which can be used to complement dietary proteins." (Marsh, Munn et al. 2012)*

Your body can store and distribute amino acids as it needs through proteins like albumin and other serum proteins. So do not concern yourself about having enough amino acids during the fasting interval as your body has the mechanisms in place to carry and distribute amino acids even when you haven't eaten.

Let's look at a three meal intraday fasting scenario (IDF3M)

This is a standard three meal pattern. It at least provides you with an overnight fast of 10-12 hours if lucky. What you eat at night in terms of the quality of carbs and quantity and whether you snack closer to your sleep time, will determine if you have a true prolonged drop in glucose, Insulin and IGF-1 during this overnight fast.

What undermines this possibility is that glucose and triglycerides may be elevated for 6 – 8 hours after eating and so, even if you ate at 7 pm, this glucose and fat will still be floating around at 1 AM or 2 AM in the morning. So you are not getting a prolonged, quality drop in all these factors overnight. It is the reason that having a meal late at night is so deadly especially if that meal is packed with simple carbs, lots of calories and fat.

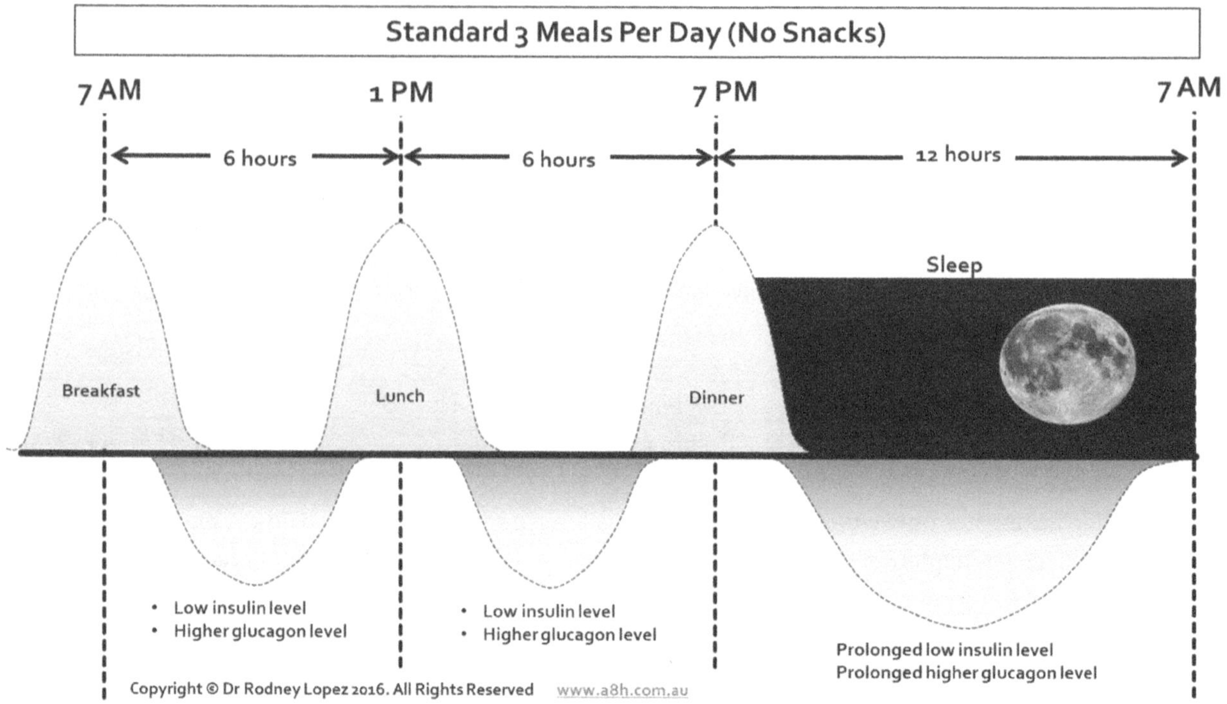

The type of graphic above has long been used in medicine as an aid to show patients what happens to blood glucose levels after eating and as a guide to instructing patients on insulin injections and their timing to keep these after eating glucose surges down in diabetic patients. The spikes above the line can simply represent all the changes that occur after eating such as a high blood glucose or blood fat levels and the Insulin/IGF-1 spikes that occur after food and essentially all the metabolic changes in the blood caused by food postprandially.

I have used this type of medical representation to show elevations in blood glucose with the standard three meals a day scenario showing the fasting intervals between these meals and a longer fast while you are asleep. These fasting moments between meals will see Insulin/IGF-1, blood glucose and triglyceride levels plummet in normal individuals but this may not necessarily be the case.

Can the standard 3 meal a day eating habit ever provide a famine signal?

It is unlikely that this will be the case. As indicated, the effects of any meal can last for 6 hours or more (Ceriello 2003). It means that your blood glucose and triglyceride levels may just be dipping before you eat the next meal.

Remember, if your waist circumference is not ideal (over 94 cm in men and over 80 cm in women of European descent) (WHO 2008), you may well have insulin resistance IR) and this may indicate that your blood glucose and triglyceride levels may never come down but stay elevated in your system 24/7 making this standard practice of 3 meals a day absolutely inadequate in light of how the longevity pathways work and the importance of a famine signal to trigger cell repair and maintenance.

There is a linear relationship between waist circumference and insulin resistance, and this means the bigger your belly, the greater the risk of insulin resistance and the greater the chance that your blood glucose and triglyceride levels may never come down by the time you have the next meal in a three meal a day scenario.

The three meals a day strategy may be appropriate for someone who trains intensely and needs the calories, but this still does not mean excessive calories as this will only harm the body. In my mind, a two meal a day strategy that includes all the protein you need and ensures micronutrient sufficiency will provide the dips in glucose and triglycerides and amino acid signalling to dampen down the AMPK/mTOR pathways.

A 2 meal intraday fasting scenario (IF2M) Skipping Lunch

Skipping lunch can be achieved easily by most people, and it doesn't have to be a complete fast if you are just beginning this journey. Around midday, I suggest boosting phytochemical intake by getting a low-glycemic-index vegetable juice with a small amount of fruit (See Appendix-4) which uses the Clean-15, Dirty Dozen concept to guide choice. Also allowable are healthy snacks during the fast that will not raise glucose or Insulin/IGF-1 levels significantly (carrots, celery, a few berries and a few nuts). You can view the 'Antioxidant Plates' for ideas on healthy snacking in this meal-free period. If you can go without any of these foods apart from the juice and phytochemical hit, then even better. You can always have these extras at times you eat.

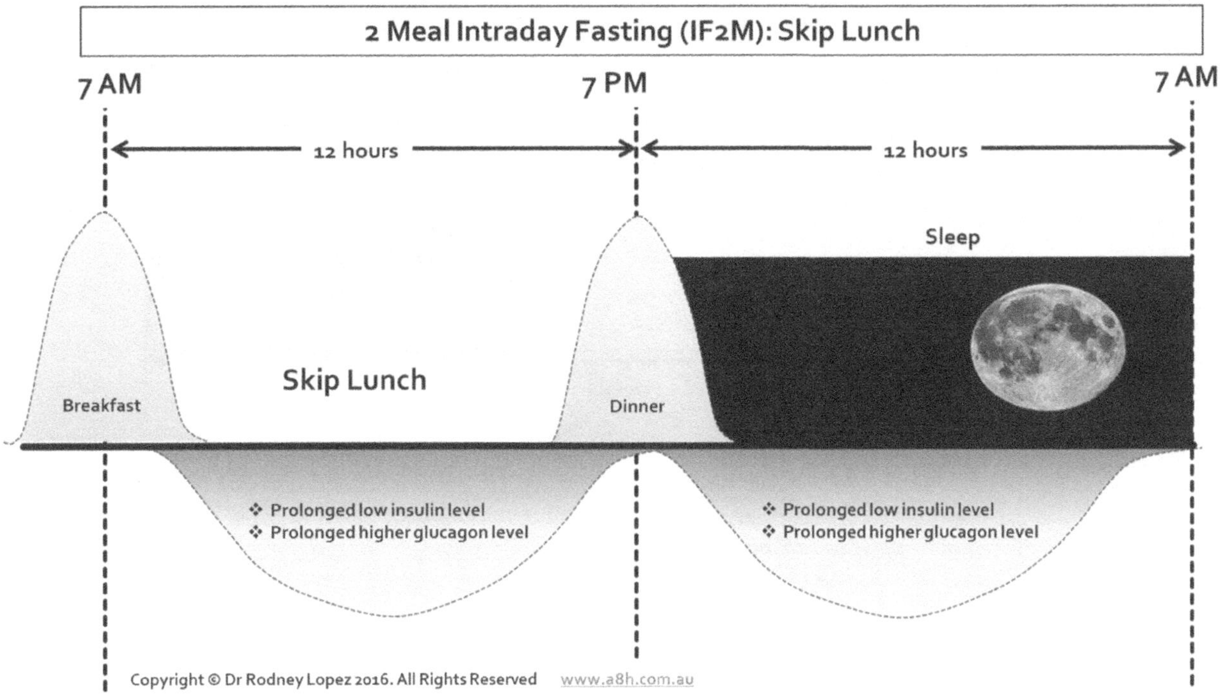

You could do this two meal, intraday fasting strategy two days a week or more if you feel you are capable of this. You will NOT die because you do not eat a meal. You have discovered now that high AMPK levels that signal low cellular energy can dampen down mTOR activity. Intraday fasting will provide this low energy (high-AMPK) signalling so important to health and longevity.

Caution: If you are feeling a little faint, have some nuts, seeds or low carb fruit and vegetables, and this can help greatly. If you are on diabetic medications or indeed any medication, then please check with your medical practitioner first before using intraday fasting strategies.

The prolonged dip in insulin levels between breakfast and dinner will activate hormone-sensitive lipase (HSL) to start the breakdown of fats (triglycerides) in adipose tissue cells. Glucagon will increase and begin to tap into your liver glycogen stores to supply your glucose-hungry brain which has an amazingly voracious appetite for glucose energy. In fact, 60-70% of total body glucose energy is used by the brain in any given day (Berg, Tymoczko et al. 2002) so you can see how vital it is that the body starts to mobilise your fat and existing glycogen stores to stabilise glucose levels. So this long intraday fast between breakfast and dinner is constantly creating that low glycogen 'battery' signal forcing your body to mobilise the triglycerides in fat allowing the glycerol backbone to be converted to glucose through gluconeogenesis in the liver and thus attempting to top up the glycogen 'battery'. This strategy will help chip away at that stubborn fat you have in all probability found so difficult to shift.

Try different variations on intraday fasting

Try other two meal fast variations. It may be far better to vary what you are doing to force your body to adapt and to take advantage of diurnal variations which could help greatly – for example, if you skipped the evening meal, you would have a time interval from 1 PM to 7 AM the next morning which is 18 hours of low to very low insulin levels because you are taking care of meal composition which keeps your average insulin levels way below others who eat insulin elevating meals. You can make up the protein deficit at lunchtime (or breakfast).

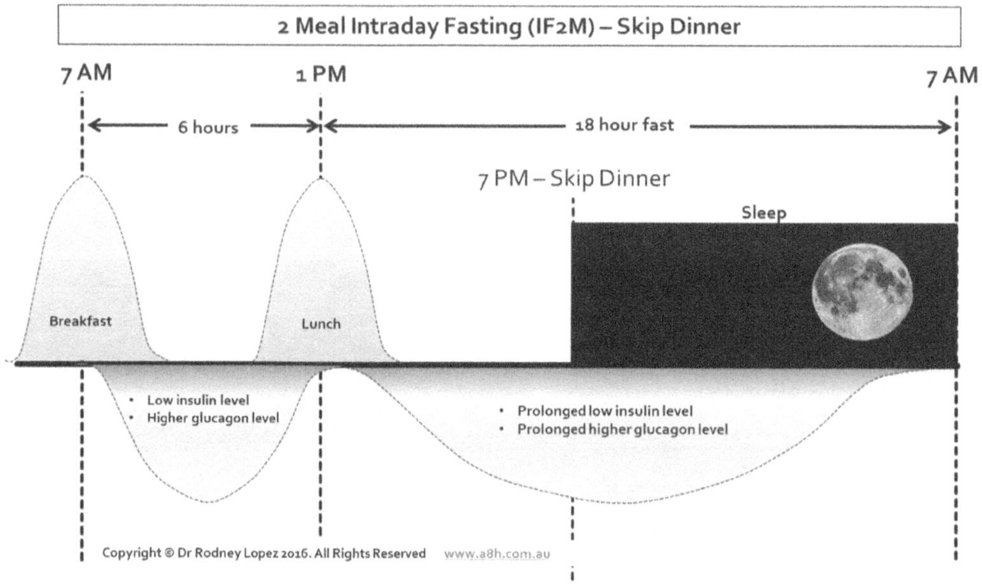

You could also skip breakfast to provide a long interval of very low insulin levels that dampen mTOR signalling for cell repair and maintenance. Make up the protein deficit at lunch or dinner. Vary the skipped meals where you skip breakfast on one day, lunch on another and then dinner on another day.

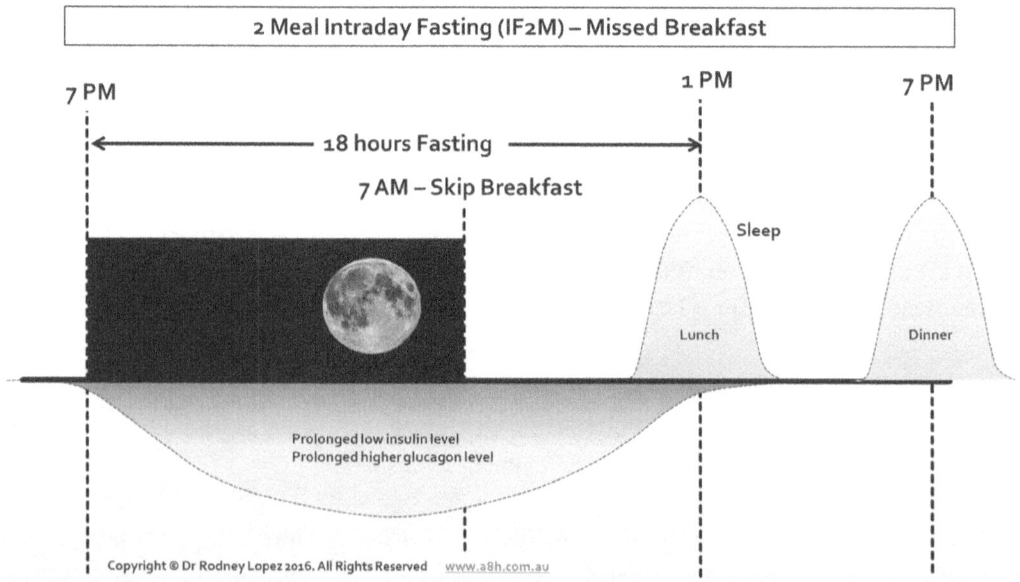

Non-stop eating and grazing: The Norm

The next graphic shows the way people usually eat. They constantly graze, and often this is mindless and could be out of stress or simply habit. People eat in the misguided belief that feeling hungry means, it is bad for your body when in fact this is a wonderful signal to your body to repair itself.

High carbohydrate and high-fat meals and snacks will mean that postprandial (after-eating) elevations in blood glucose, blood fats, blood Insulin/IGF levels will stay elevated for the vast majority of a 24 hour period. There will be little to no insulin dips and even that wonderful evening drop in insulin overnight is blunted because people will often snack close to bedtime or have their sugar-rich and perhaps fat-rich dessert after dinner and this will take away 6 hours or more of that wonderful overnight drop in Insulin/IGF-1 which is essentially your body's way of repairing itself during sleep time and this repair mechanism is destroyed by the constant supply of energy through eating inappropriate meals at inappropriate times.

This type of eating pattern will ensure that you will always keep your glycogen stores (the glycogen 'battery') filled to the brim. There is no incentive to tap into your fat stores as your glycogen levels are constantly high, and all you are doing is adding to your fat stores by eating and snacking constantly! Depleting glycogen is a great way to get rid of calories as energy is expended to fill-up these glycogen reserves. If the 'glycogen-battery' is full, then excess calories simply spill over into the fat stores.

The graphic on the next page shows how constantly eating pretty well destroys any chance of insulin levels dropping which prevents the famine signal of cell repair and maintenance kicking-in.

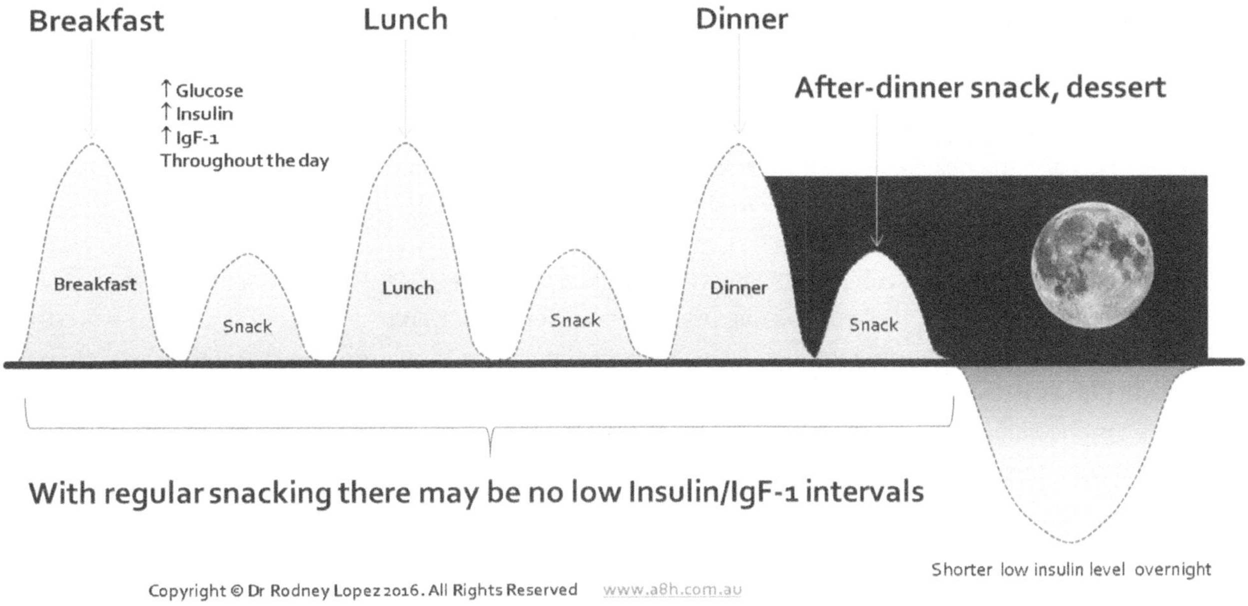

Should you just miss out on a meal every day at the same time?

As indicated, the body adapts rapidly to changes in diet or exercise and so doing the same thing every day may not produce the effect we are after. We do not want your body to think there is a famine every day as this may be counterproductive where metabolic rate is lowered and stays low as happens when individuals try to lose weight by lowering calories.

A scientific statement from the American Heart Association indicated from the research to date, that consistently missing out on breakfast was shown to have a detrimental cardiovascular effect and was associated with a higher body weight (St-Onge, Ard et al. 2017). This same paper showed that periodic fasting helped people to shed weight by 3 – 8% after 3 to 24 weeks of treatment (St-Onge, Ard et al. 2017)

Intraday fasting is NOT regularly skipping out on a particular meal but varying meals to skip up to 3 meals per week and to rotate the meals skipped from week to week to prevent any adaptations by the body that may counteract the benefits through regularly doing the same thing.

This program of intraday fasting which is essentially intermittent fasting is all about providing your body with **all the nutrients it needs** to function optimally, and by having the Activ8Health Plan-A or Plan-B diets, you are providing your body with a wealth of critical dietary factors. People who simply miss out on a meal like breakfast regularly, are not doing this out of knowledge or planning. The likelihood of them planning to make up deficiencies caused by the missed meal is extremely unlikely. No wonder these people do not do so well. The intraday fasting I am advocating in this book is vastly different to the scenario pointed out in the St-Onge paper on meal timing.

Starvation and Semi-Starvation Diets

Two influential studies, one on semi-starvation and the other a study on a starvation diet were carried out in the past. The first study of note was done at the Carnegie Institute, Washington in 1919 (Benedict, Miles et al. 1919). What the researchers were interested in the post-World War I (WWI) period was food conservation in a time of food shortages and whether this would impact metabolic rate to the point that it would impair intellectual capacity or muscle strength. What they found was when they reduced calories by around 30%, the metabolic rate dropped by a massive 30% as well because the body was trying to conserve energy due to a shortage of calories.

The Minnesota starvation rehabilitation experiment between 1944 – 1946 was a detailed study on starvation and was regarded as one of the most important research projects undertaken on this subject which was published under the title 'The biology of human starvation' in 1950 (Keys, Brožek et al. 1950).

Thirty-six healthy young men were chosen for the experiment, and caloric intake was lowered gradually. This study backed up the Carnegie Institute semi-starvation research and showed a huge 40% reduction in basal metabolic rate with rates of weight loss far lower than anticipated.

We are not restricting calories and nutrient intakes, we are just shuffling them around the missed meal! Intraday fasting is NOT missing out any of the nutrients your body needs in a day, and it is NOT starvation or semi-starvation. Intraday fasting is optimal nutrition with breaks in eating to relieve those constant pressures on cell multiplication and anabolic pathways through unnecessary nutrient intakes.

The missed meal's macronutrients, micronutrients and phytochemicals, are simply consumed at the next meal, so you are not missing out on nutrients.

Protein, as I have stated in the chapter on protein intake, does NOT have to be consumed at every meal as your body has mechanisms in place to provide amino acids at times you are not consuming any protein as I have indicated earlier.

You are walking a line between calorie restriction optimal nutrition (CRON) versus semi-starvation. We know the metabolic effects of semi-starvation where your basal metabolic rate can dramatically plunge so we want to avoid semi-starvation. Semi-starvation diets also have the great disadvantage in that they will result in you cannibalising your tissues to provide critical nutrients to vital organs like the brain, heart and kidneys. Keep in mind the triage mechanism of nutrient scarcity.

How can you prevent semi-starvation

Protein missed out on the fasting period during the day can be made up at the next meal or any meal you have in the day. What I suggest is to work out your visible protein meal portion which is outlined in the chapter on protein and then have the portion missed, at the next meal.

This strategy is fine as long as you keep the amount of protein in each meal to less than 20 - 25 grams. Researchers have noted that amino acid oxidation (burning off amino acids as fuel rather than being used for protein synthesis), occurs around 20 grams per meal of whole protein or 10 – 12 grams of essential amino acids (EAAs) (Atherton and Smith 2012). Another study stated the following;

> *"We report that increasing protein intake stimulates mixed-muscle and plasma albumin protein synthesis in a dose-dependent manner up to 20 g dietary protein, after which there is a marked stimulation of whole-body leucine oxidation and no further increase in protein synthesis (Moore et al., 2009)."*

This is easily achieved as even a 110 kg person only requires a total of 22 grams protein per meal when we take into consideration the hidden protein from fruit, vegetables, nuts and seeds and perhaps dairy or non-dairy sources of protein. This way your body never goes into starvation mode and will not cannibalise your tissues due to nutrient shortages. Keeping up with the high plant-based foods as suggested, will ensure you have an optimal intake of fibre, amino acids, phytochemicals, antioxidants, vitamins and minerals needed for optimal health.

Pitfalls in intraday fasting

In the section on protein intakes, you will find a guideline as to how much visible protein you should consume. Visible protein is what you can see on the plate. Hidden protein is something never considered and found in vegetables, fruit, cereals, legumes, fibre, seeds, dairy, nut milk and other foods, and you need to consider this hidden protein if you want to stay trim and avoid chronic disease.

The pitfall of intraday fasting as indeed all fasting regimens is that you will over-consume when you next eat. This could easily mean weight gain!

Autophagy, cell apoptosis and stem cell mobilisation: Renewing your body

By using intermittent fasting, what you are promoting is autophagy or cell death. Cells with ageing proteins and damaged cellular organelles (senescent cells), will have these damaged cellular components consumed and replaced in a process called autophagy to renew those impaired cells.

Other cells and organs can use the nutrients derived from the autophagy process.. However, cells that have been forced into a significantly weakened senescent state due to rapid cell multiplication and telomere shortening are programmed to die - a process called apoptosis.

When you go through the fasting stage and start to eat again, the nutrient stimulus mobilises stem cells to replace these dead and dying cells in effect renewing your body and organ systems to a far more healthy state of function.

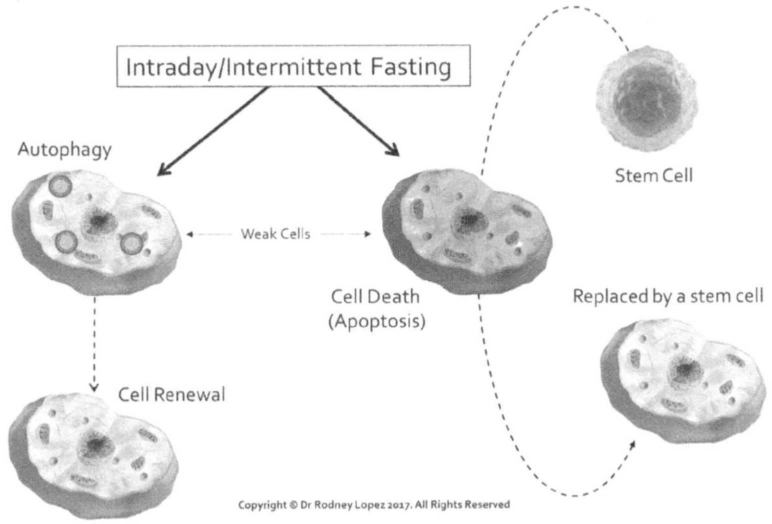

Ghrelin, Hippocampus, Neurogenesis

This whole area of fasting is shedding more and more light on the huge number of benefits conferred by diminished caloric intake. **Ghrelin is the hunger hormone**. Ghrelin is a 28 amino acid peptide hormone predominantly secreted by the stomach in response to lower dietary intakes and empty stomachs. Ghrelin secretion decreases as the stomach is stretched with food.

An exciting finding is that ghrelin stimulates hippocampal neurogenesis and synaptic plasticity (Kim, Kim et al. 2017). The hippocampus is associated with memory and spatial learning (Kim, Kim et al. 2017). So what is the evolutionary advantage of such a physiological effect of ghrelin on hippocampal neurone regeneration? One would think that with the search for food in our hunter-gatherer times that such effort would be mostly in a state of hunger where ghrelin levels would be higher. Ghrelin in having a positive effect on both memory and spatial learning would have obvious benefits for those wandering far and wide in search of food.

Meal timing & biochemical effects

It has been observed that overnight energy expenditure was greater in individuals having 2 meals a day compared to 6 meals a day (St-Onge, Ard et al. 2017). This same paper by St-Onge et al. commissioned by the American Heart Association (AHA) showed that HDL levels increased by a significant 17% from baseline if they consumed one meal a day rather than three meals a day where the HDL levels remained unchanged.

High-density lipoprotein (HDL) is the 'good' cholesterol. Now, this makes absolute sense with everything I have mentioned in this book about famine (repair and maintenance) signals. With one meal a day, most of the day will be in a fasting state triggering off the repair and maintenance signal.

An HDL elevation is a part of this repair process as HDL draws cholesterol from blood vessels and takes it back to the liver – a repair mechanism helping to remove the potentially damaging cholesterol buildup in the arteries, and this process can be seen as a repair and maintenance mechanism allowed to take place all because you are not bombarding your body constantly with calories and energy.

It takes 6 hours or more in a day for your body to truly decrease the postprandial (after-eating) shifts and longer if you have insulin resistance, where blood glucose and triglyceride levels never come. So if your fasting blood glucose or fasting blood triglyceride level is elevated or in the high normal range, then you will have trouble 24/7 and even more severe postprandial spikes in glucose and blood fats.

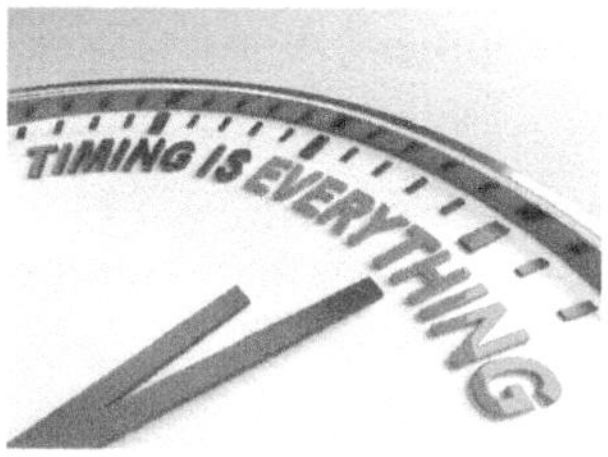

Ideally, you want to go beyond this 6 hour period to truly achieve a fasting state, and so you need to not eat for 8 – 10 hours or more. So how can this fit within a 24 hour period? Let's look at separating meals 10 hours apart in any given day:

First Meal	Second Meal	Third Meal
7 am	5 pm	3 am next morning

If you choose meals 10 hours apart, as you can see, you will be eating early next morning and if you do this (which is unlikely) what happens to the first meal interval? It becomes impractical. For this reason, I feel a strong case can be made for having two meals in a day provided you consume all the protein, phytochemicals and micronutrients your body needs (with supplementation), with a long enough interval between meals allowing the repair and maintenance mechanisms to occur.

Most adults can miss one meal. In its place you can have a vegetable-rich, phytochemical-rich juice, a small crudités platter or the antioxidant plates I have discussed at the back of the book can be consumed which will provide essentially low-calorie food choices that pack a micronutrient and phytochemical 'punch' and help you cope during a missed meal.

Deadly Dinners & the Dangers of Late Night Eating

If you choose a two meal strategy, then having more of your calories at breakfast seems to offer an advantage in comparison to individuals who consume most of their calories at night. The American Heart Association paper once again has shed some light on this. Having a higher calorie intake at breakfast resulted in a significant decrease in blood triglyceride (blood fat) level by a huge 33% whereas the blood triglyceride levels **increased by 14%** in those that had a higher caloric intake at dinner.

The authors of the paper by St-Onge et al. stated that the increased triglyceride levels in people who shifted their caloric intake towards the evening somehow **interfered with nocturnal lipid metabolism**.

Once again meal timing in research has not been assessed thoroughly enough and was not a factor even considered in so much past research and yet this makes great intuitive sense when you consider the body is winding down and that an overnight fast during sleep in all probability has been designed from an evolutionary perspective to enable a dampening down of the mTOR pathway, to allow the body to repair cells, proteins, DNA and to ensure damaging lipid profiles are dampened during this time.

This timing issue could have a profound effect on clinical outcomes for anyone who has cardiovascular disease by keeping triglyceride levels much lower.

Several cross-sectional studies have shown that eating late at night is associated with poor cardiovascular health, weight gain and increases in inflammatory markers keeping in mind that inflammation drives most of the chronic diseases in society (St-Onge, Ard et al. 2017). Late night eating was defined as having a meal within 2 hours of going to bed. In fact, the AHA study by St-Onge et al. pointed out that if you shifted your total energy intake (TEI) by just 10% to the evening meal, it was associated with a 3% increase in C-reactive protein (CRP) (St-Onge, Ard et al. 2017). CRP is a sensitive marker in the blood that indicates that there is inflammation in the body and is a strong indicator of future cardiovascular risk.

Just have a look at all the people that go out at night and have massive meals that may include huge sugary desserts quite late into the evening. Consider all the damage that is doing while they are asleep. Think about this with your children as well and shift caloric intake to ensure they do not eat large meals close to bedtime. A meal should be consumed 3 or more hours before bed, and meal composition is also critical using Plan-A or B guidelines to keep postprandial shifts as low as possible regarding glucose and blood fats and all those other damaging changes that occur in the blood after eating. Timing is King!

How do your cells handle glucose in the morning?

An interesting insight provided by one study and once again discussed in the St-Onge et al. paper. This showed that if you ate late at night for example at 11 pm rather than 6 pm, that your ability to handle glucose in the morning was poorer with elevated glucose being higher in your blood after your breakfast and all because you simply ate late at night.

Going back to first principles, if you can have a long enough fast between meals, what you are doing is making your tissues hungry for food (glucose). The GLUT4 glucose receptors are wide open after a fast and for that matter after exercise as both of these processes create a need for nutrients in the tissues. Having a carbohydrate-rich meal late into the night will mean that these GLUT4 glucose receptors are closed in the morning.

Glucose clearance in the morning is determined by how late you ate the night before

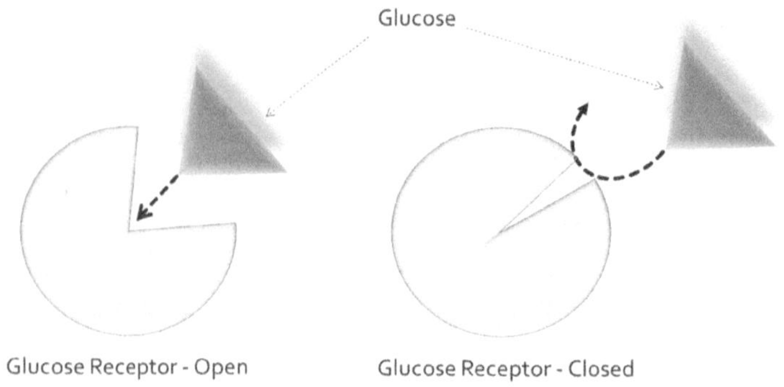

So the two-meal strategy to me is an excellent option provided you:

1. Ensure nutrient, phytochemical and protein adequacy for the day
2. Use simple supplements like a multivitamin and omega-3's even every second day
3. Ensure long gaps between meals without unnecessary snacking apart from a phytochemical juice or crudité plate or antioxidant plate
4. Ensure that you eat early in the evening by consuming an Activ8health Plan-A type meal at night 3 hours or more before bed. Avoid those glucose producing starchy carbs and desserts at night. Plan-A meals are designed to ensure low glucose and triglyceride levels anyway.

Just look at these amazing benefits of intermittent fasting

If you want to know that this strategy of intermittent fasting works including intraday fasting, then you just need to see the benefits as outlined in the excellent American Heart Association's commissioned St-Onge paper on meal timing (St-Onge, Ard et al. 2017). These incredible benefits include:

1. Body weight decreased in all studies on alternate day fasting or periodic fasting strategies by 3 – 8% even after three weeks.
2. Reduction in total cholesterol from 6% to an amazing 21%
3. Reduction in LDL cholesterol (the 'bad' cholesterol) from 7% to an incredible 32%
4. Reductions triglycerides from 16% to 42% especially if you had weight loss which is likely anyway on intermittent fasting regimens. This will have a significant impact on vascular disease.
5. Decrease in systolic blood pressure (the top figure in BP measurements) by 3% to 8%
6. Decrease in diastolic blood pressure (the bottom figure) by 6% to 10% in just six weeks, and these pressure changes were in conjunction with weight loss that is likely to accompany intermittent or intraday fasting
7. May prevent progression from prehypertension to hypertension a great fact for anyone with a family history of hypertension. Prehypertension is defined as a systolic blood pressure between 120 – 139 mm Hg or a diastolic blood pressure of 80 – 89 mmHg.
8. May decrease fasting glucose from 3% to 6% with the greatest decrease occurring in those individuals with prediabetes
9. May be effective in decreasing fasting insulin and fasting insulin resistance

Keep in mind that **<u>even small changes</u>** in weight, glucose levels, insulin, insulin resistance or blood pressure can have amazing effects on health outcomes and can prevent a range of diseases and keep you in the healthspan that all of us desire for as long as possible.

Sleeping and that overnight fast

You read so many articles on the importance of sleep and what is does to the brain and body. No doubt the reasons will be complex, but the fasting signal and cell repair and maintenance signal during sleep would have to be a prime reason for the need for sleep.

Sleep is counter-intuitive from an evolutionary perspective and would have put humans at great risk from predators in the early stages of our development. No doubt this vulnerability was an evolutionary pressure to keep together in groups for safety with sentinels to guard against being eaten in our sleep. A possible evolutionary answer to why people have varying sleep habits with owls that stay awake all night while others go to sleep early. This variation allowed for sentinels in the herd to protect others from being devoured in their sleep.

During sleep-time we are in a fasting state for 7 hours or more - well, at least most of us do not sleepwalk and raid the fridge, allowing damaged cells to repair themselves and this is a way that forces the body into that famine state triggering cell maintenance and repair as Insulin/IGF-1 levels are very low during this break from eating while we sleep. During this time, energy intake is nil, and the AMPK/mTOR pathway is dampened. We can rest and repair our bodies.

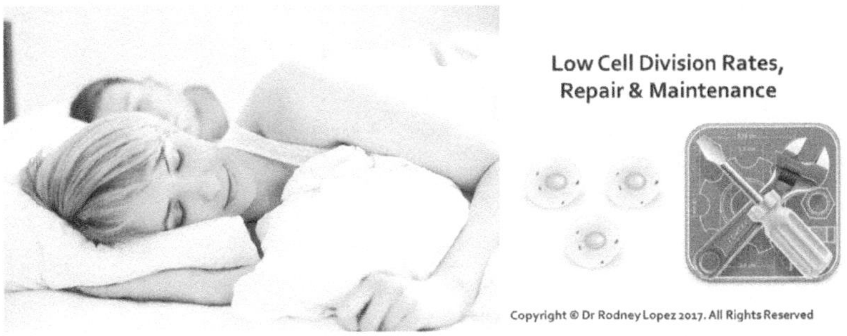

CHAPTER 10

Exercise

YOU CAN'T OUTRUN A BAD DIET!

That wonderful adage that 'You can't outrun a bad diet', has stood the test of time and scientific scrutiny. The tired argument of exercise versus diet as to which one offers the best solution to weight management is now dead and buried through extensive, thorough and technologically advanced scientific research across many species.

That energy regulation is tightly controlled in biological systems like a human body should be highly intuitive, self-evident and an inescapable conclusion of *a priori* reasoning when you consider that famine has always been nipping at the heels of humanity. Perhaps if we evolved on the savannas of Africa abundant with supermarkets, pizza parlours, sugar-soaked foods, unlimited soda streams and fast-food outlets, then energy considerations would have taken on a different meaning as food energy in this situation would be abundant, freely available and there would be no need to develop cellular systems that treated energy as a rare commodity. In this circumstance, we would have energy to burn!

However, this was not the reality in our evolution when our genetic code, cellular design, molecular capabilities and biochemical functionalities were forged.

Famine and starvation pressures were always a part of human existence posing existential threats around every corner of our development. Energy in this circumstance becomes a precious commodity that cannot be squandered but highly valued and preserved at all costs.

What seems to be the case from all of this energy expenditure research, is that no matter whether you are a hunter-gatherer traversing vast distances on the savannas of Africa in the hunt for food, or if you are a sedentary data-gatherer, sitting at a desk in a small corner of a concrete jungle gazing into a computer screen, both groups expend around the same amount of energy – believe it or not, adjusted for body size (Pontzer, Durazo-Arvizu et al.).

We burn the same number of calories no matter how physically active we are!

What the heading states, may be contrary to our beliefs about exercise being that master-blaster of fat and exercise being the enemy of muffin-tops. But this is not the case. Whether you are a hunter-gatherer on the plains of Africa or data-gatherer in the 'wild' unforgiving environment of investment banking, you will both burn the same number of calories in a day adjusted for body size.

For energy conservation and a metabolic rate setpoint to exist, some energy consuming systems need to be dampened down and others ramped-up to maintain that balance of fixed energy expenditure.

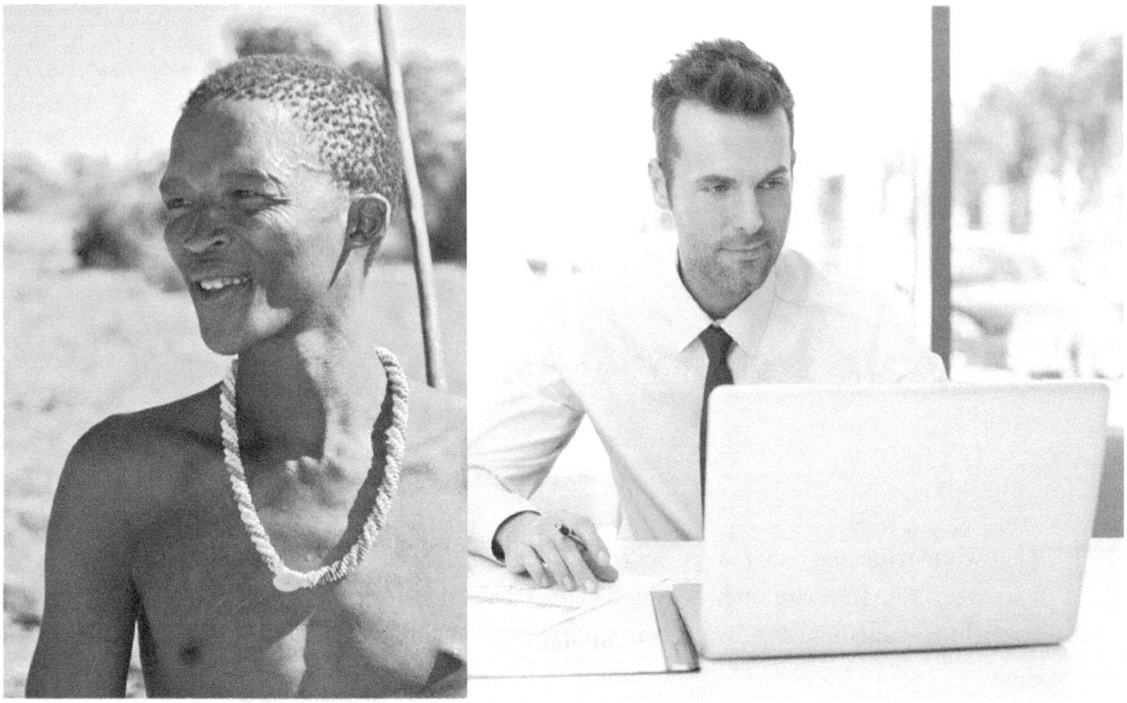

San Bushman By Ian Beatty from Amherst, MA, USA (IDBeatty_002219) [CC BY-SA 2.0 (http://creativecommons.org/licenses/by-sa/2.0)], via Wikimedia Commons

Deuterium (Hydrogen Isotope) and Oxygen-18 enriched water

Daily energy expenditures (kCal/Day) is measured through the use of these two radioisotopes mentioned above. This safe and accurate system measures the number of calories burned in a day. By analysing the concentration of these isotopes in the urine of participants, the daily rate of carbon dioxide production can be calculated providing reliable and reproducible energy expenditure rates in individuals across a range of highly active or sedentary lifestyles (Pontzer, Durazo-Arvizu et al.).

This technique has been used not just in human studies, but also in primates, and the same findings emerged regarding energy expenditures whether primates were in cages or the wild. An Australian study also showed similar energy expenditures in sheep or kangaroos kept in pens or allowed to roam free in the wild (Munn, Dawson et al. 2013). So how active we are doesn't seem to make a dent in our energy expenditures.

How can we make sense of these findings?

What these studies are showing is that exercise is not the way forward in losing weight no matter how much you exercise. These studies show that human obesity is not about energy expenditure as this is the same across cultures. It is all about dietary excess! Let's face it; we would be kidding ourselves if we think our efforts associated with daily living or in the gym, will come anywhere near that of a San or Hazda Bushman.

Imagine the effort and energy expended when chasing down prey on the plains of Africa. Our efforts will be dwarfed by the exertion required to not only hunt down their prey but to make the kill. Often it may take days to track down a dying animal after that animal's flesh is pierced by a poisoned dart, then finally finding that dead animal which could be a Giraffe, slaughtering it and then hauling those butchered heavy pieces of meat back across untold distances to their village. So it is not likely you will come anywhere near this gut-wrenching, prolonged intensity of exercise in Western life. And anyway, if your energy expenditure will be the same in the long-run, why bother?

Surely this can't be right! How can both groups expend the same energy?

So what is happening here? How are the two vastly different groups of hunter-gatherers and data-gatherers expending the same energy? As I have mentioned, we have energy balancing systems in place to get us back to a setpoint and the homeostatic state in our physiology.

When hunter-gatherers are on the hunt and expending large energy resources and consuming fewer calories in the process, they are essentially putting themselves in a semi-starvation state. This ***ratio of food and energy*** availability to activity level is an important factor for the total energy setpoint (Pontzer, Durazo-Arvizu et al. 2016). More research needs to be carried out to find out exact mechanisms, but this indicates that the metabolic rate drops and two studies on semi-starvation and starvation show without a doubt that energy expenditure drops 30% - 40% to conserve energy (and nutrient) resources.

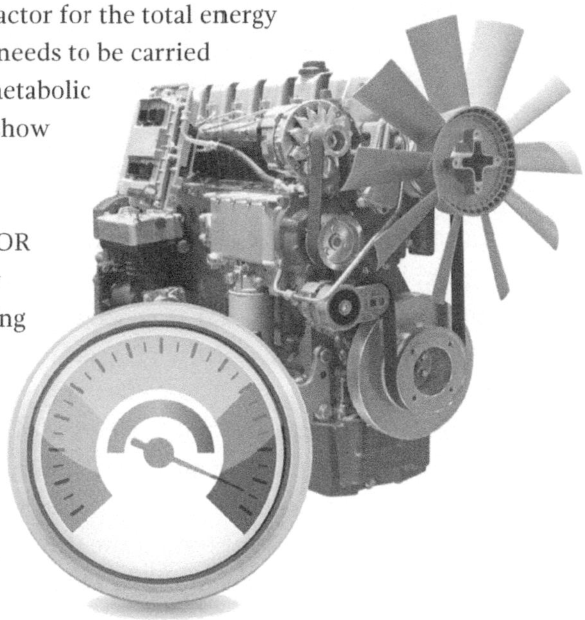

Also, cell multiplication processes through the AMPK/mTOR pathways are dampened down as ATP is consumed for energy purposes and AMP accumulates (our spent bullets), thus driving up AMPK. This high AMPK signal tells the mTOR pathway that there just isn't enough energy to create proteins or create new cells and in doing so, it allows your body to adapt to lower energy consumption and or increased energy utilisation through effort. The body moves into a far less energy-consuming cell maintenance phase avoiding the energy-consuming anabolic cell production process via the mTOR pathway.

Organ systems will also begin to wind down to conserve energy. Over time individuals involved in endurance aerobic activity will produce far more Type-1 (Slow-Twitch) fibres in their muscles that are highly energy efficient aerobically and these fibres will also adapt regarding mitochondrial density and increased energy efficiencies in the electron transport (respiratory) chain within the mitochondria regarding cell energy extraction systems.

So the seemingly large physical efforts of the hunter-gatherer in finding food are offset by energy consuming systems that are winding down in cells and organs pushing energy expenditure lower and more towards a particular individual setpoint.

The problem with revving-up the metabolic engine for too long

It all comes down to energy conservation and self-preservation. Burn off your energy resources, and you simply die! If you could just rev up your metabolic engine by exercise and have this elevated energy expenditure or raised metabolic rate continue unchecked, we would simply burn out. With unchecked high energy expenditures requiring enormous amounts of nutritional resources, **we would start to cannibalise or nutritional resources locked in muscle, bone and organ systems if we are not consuming the nutrients needed to prevent this happening during this high energy expenditure state.**

We can consider a car engine analogy where we plant our foot firmly on the accelerator and leave it there revving this engine to the maximum. This engine will overheat and then burn out.

Your body adapts to the level of activity and then shifts the metabolic rate back to your setpoint through complicated cellular and organ system responses that will conserve energy to offset energy-consuming processes in action.

This situation also happens post-exercise in the EPOC (Excess post-exercise oxygen consumption) period, where energy is expended to remove lactate, to fix the oxygen deficit caused by exercise, to create stem cells for increased lean muscle mass, expend energy in the anabolic processes after exercise to repair damaged muscle and adapt to exercise stress.

We consume energy to move back to a homeostatic state after exercise during EPOC. Energy balance is thus restored!

So then what is happening in the couch potato or the data-gatherer in an investment bank?

Why do these sedentary individuals have the same metabolic engine that is revving at the same rate of a hunter-gatherer? It is an interesting question and a puzzle that sedentary people have metabolic rates humming along to the same level as someone who puts in a tremendous amount of effort on the plains of Africa or in a gym. With exercise as a factor removed from the equation regarding overweight/obesity rates, we need to point at least one finger at our Western diet and an excess consumption of almost worthless, nutrient-poor calories.

I have explained about the highly researched AMPK/mTOR pathway in detail in this book. This pathway has far-reaching effects on your health as it profoundly affects metabolic processes and is a major factor in your healthspan and indeed your lifespan. Factors that drive this pathway towards cell multiplication at the expense of cell maintenance will require significant amounts of energy for all the cell building processes involved. You simply get fatter and fatter; develop multiple chins or folds of fat in your abdomen, increase cell numbers in your glandular tissues like the breast, pancreas or prostate and increase toxic intra-abdominal (visceral) fat all because this AMPK/mTOR cell multiplication pathway is being constantly stimulated by high-calorie, nutrient-poor Western diets.

High protein diets also stimulate this pathway greatly especially if animal meats are consumed to excess. I will expand upon protein dangers in this book.

So here you have an energy consuming process of cell building, and energy storage activities that will increase your energy expenditure and all you are doing is eating a very bad diet! No exercise needed for this energy-consuming convergence of cell multiplication pathways. Energy extraction in the electron transport chain in mitochondria will be less efficient, and energy will be wasted in sedentary individuals.

The gut microbiome and energy systems

The gut microbiome can change even with short-term alterations in diet. In the bowel, around 60% of the bacterial population belong to two phyla – Bacteroidetes or Firmicutes (Conlon 2014). There is a strong correlation between your gut microbiome and energy balance in the body (Riedl 2017). It is now a well-researched fact that with high energy intakes, your body's gut microbiome can shift to a higher proportion of the Firmicutes species of organisms that have the potential to harvest greater amounts of energy from food and transfer this energy surplus to your body for fat storage. Altering energy intake to a higher level has been shown to produce rapid decreases in the Bacteroidetes group of organisms (Riedl 2017).

So sedentary people on Western diets will move towards a population of more efficient energy extractors if there is enough energy available. The reverse is the case when there is energy scarcity.

In contrast to the sedentary data gatherer, a hunter-gatherer has a lower intake of solid foods and dietary energy including fibre. During a prolonged hunt and expending a great deal of energy, the combination of low energy input and high energy expenditure produces shifts in bowel microorganism composition and biomass. Changes in the bowel microflora of the hunter-gatherer, ensure less energy and nutrient needs in this gut organ and is thus one of the mechanisms for conserving energy and moving energy balance to a homeostatic state and one that helps ensure survival of the individual by decreasing energy and nutrient needs, provided that this process does not move beyond a critical threshold to sustain life.

After-eating changes in your blood seen as a threat to survival

Like the post-exercise EPOC effect that shifts all those changes that occurred in your body during exercise to a normal level again so too does your body have to shift the postprandial (after-eating) effects back to a normal homeostatic level.

The chapter on postprandial (after-eating) effects pointed out that the blood chemistry changes can last for 6 hours or more (Ceriello 2003). Blood glucose and triglycerides (fats) rise significantly after eating, producing many damaging effects including inflammatory processes in the body. To bring this food-related inflammation back to normal it takes energy to dampen down all the oxidative stress caused just by eating.

> *"Indeed, it now appears that our organism perceives each meal as an exogenous 'threat' stressful enough to mobilise homeostatic mechanisms to adjust to the stress of the postprandial state."* (Margioris 2009)

In the Western world, when are people not eating? When are they not in the postprandial (after-eating) state of raised blood glucose and blood fats? The answer is rarely. People feel they will die if they are a little hungry. They are constantly eating and grazing on snacks. People are consuming vast quantities of food in any given meal that will take 6 to 8 hours or more to digest and then distribute and metabolise the nutrient components.

It is likely that in large numbers of people in Western populations, the blood metabolic changes never goes back to normal with blood glucose and blood fats constantly elevated all because the interval between eating is never long enough for these to go back to normal.

All these food-related changes in the body after eating raises energy expenditure to get us back to a normal state. So just by eating constantly, raised energy expenditure in the data gatherer. Who needs to run after Giraffe's all day on a hot African plain?

Other energy consuming and conserving mechanisms in the data-gatherer will come to light in future scientific research.

So, is exercise futile and useless?

Definitely not! Exercise is critical to your survival, but by itself, it will not change your body composition without a solid dietary foundation.

For exercise to work to either lose fat or increase lean muscle mass, you need to have an optimal diet in place along with appropriate supplementation to support these body composition aims.

It is always diet first and exercise second! Increasing muscle mass can be a driver of metabolism. Lean muscle mass consumes energy resources just to keep this highly active tissue alive, and by increasing your lean muscle mass, you will stay strong throughout your life and drive your body fat setpoint lower to a much leaner you.

The take-home message from these studies on exercise and weight loss is that if done in isolation to dietary management, then the outcome is doomed as you can't outrun that bad diet! It is very hard indeed to burn off any excess calories that you consume. We all lead busy lives, and so need short, sharp exercise routines that are highly efficient and effective. In the section on 'Weekend Warriors' in this chapter, you will see that you can perform exercise routines that do not dominate your life and you can have almost the exact mortality outcomes as someone who seems to exercise incessantly and at an intensity that exhausts us just watching them. Working smarter but not harder is key!

So what is the answer?

First, ditch the idea that exercise can reverse excess dietary consumption habits. *You simply can't outrun a bad diet!* The evidence is in! Trying to lose weight through exercise alone is futile. **Combining an optimal diet with intraday fasting and exercise is the winning formula.** View this as a cycle of glycogen depletion, and then glycogen replacement. Review the glycogen 'battery' metaphor as this is vital if you want to stay lean throughout your life.

The essential components involved are shown below to not only keep you lean, but to increase muscle mass and prevent sarcopenia (muscle loss) that weakens you as you age and lowers your metabolic rate due to the loss of this highly active tissue as you age.

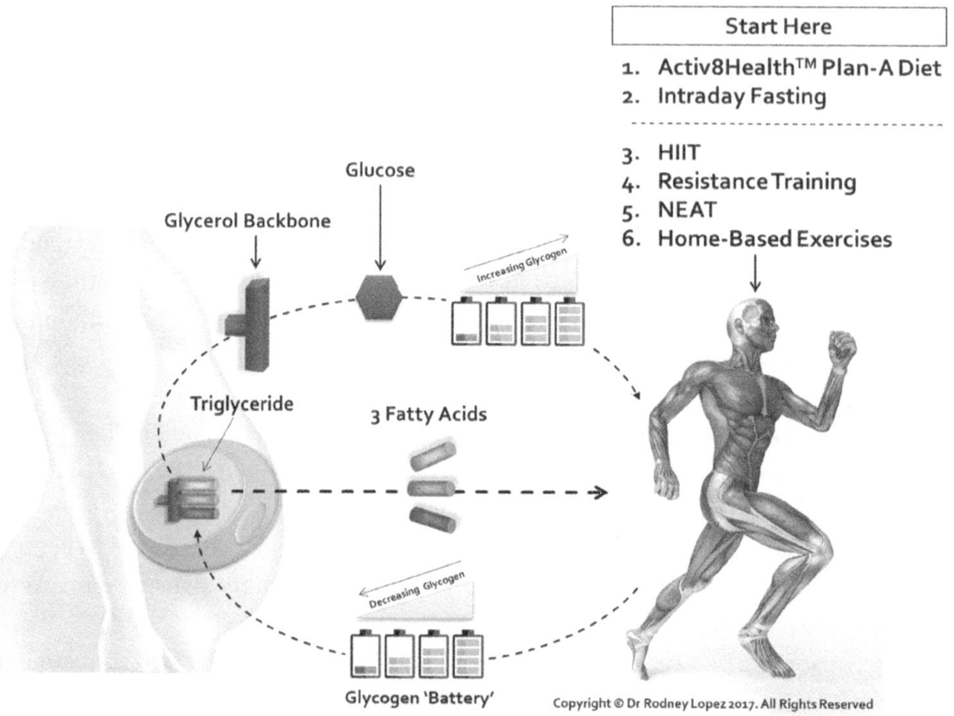

The Activ8Health Diet Plans

Designed to provide a wealth of micronutrients and to support fat loss. In Appendix 13, 14, 15, 16, I will give you an idea of what an Activ8Health Plan-A Blended, Activ8Health Plan-A Solid, and Activ8Health Plan-B Blended, Activ8Health Plan-B Solid diet is all about and how to use them.

Appendix 17 talks about personalising this diet to your needs and preferences which may include food sensitivities. Be guided by an accredited practising dietitian (APD), and this service is provided through the Activ8Health web portal (http://www.a8h.com.au).

It is important to know that any advice given by our Dietitians will need to be always placed in your clinical context and filtered by your medical practitioners who may or may not approve of the advice.

Most people only need an Activ8Health Plan-A diet for optimal health and fat loss. The Plan-B diet is for those engaged in frequent high-intensity exercise such as elite athletes who constantly deplete their glycogen stores and need these stores replaced efficiency and effectively without putting them at risk for long-term problems by consuming high glycemic index foods devoid of nutrients and phytochemicals.

The Orderly Recruitment of Muscle Fibres

Knowledge is King! – Thus spending a little bit of time understanding these concepts will pay dividends. Let's work our way through this. Essentially we should think of 3 types of fibres to make things easier. We have the Type-1 muscle fibres; the intermediates often labelled as Type-IIA's and then the Type-IIX fibres. These fibres differ in many characteristics including strength:

Type- I → Type-IIA → Type IIX

Weakest → Stronger → Strongest

All the fibres have potential to hypertrophy (grow bigger) but this potential increases from Type-I muscles fibres to Type-IIX's. The physiological characteristics of muscle fibres include but are not limited to; the number of mitochondria in the fibres, the blood supply, the type of energy extraction used (aerobic vs anaerobic), the myoglobin content of a fibre type and the type of Myosin Heavy Chains (MHCs). So there are many ways to distinguish a Type-I from a Type-IIA or Type-IIX muscle fibre and a large number of in-between muscle fibre types.

Type- I → Type-IIA → Upper Intermediates → Type IIX

Hypertrophy: ↑ → ↑↑ → ↑↑↑ → ↑↑↑↑

Dense muscle hypertrophy comes from engaging all of the muscle fibre types and encouraging their growth through increasing weight loads (slowly pyramiding-up, i.e. slowly increasing weight with each set). Super-Slow exercises help to force each muscle fibre to become involved. This form of exercise is described in more detail later.

The orderly recruitment of muscle fibres is where you tire out the weakest Type-I's, then move through the lower intermediates between the Type-I's and Type-IIA's and then to Type-IIAs and upper intermediates right up to the Type-IIXs. The weakest muscle fibres tire out first and then all the fibres up to and including the Type-IIX tire out in succession with the King of fibres the Type-IIX tiring out last.

Type- I → Lower Intermediates → Type-IIA → Upper Intermediates → Type IIX

You have to work very hard to get to the Type-IIXs. Home-based exercises with lower loads will arguably be unlikely to get to these fibres, but this is not the point of the home exercises. You will be helping deplete glycogen stores in the engaged fibres thus helping fat loss as I have amply described in this book. You are also encouraging muscle growth and maintenance of strength of all the muscle fibre types as you will hopefully perform at least, a one-day full-body gym routine using higher loads which will also involve Super-Slow movement to finish the routine for a particular muscle group.

The rest and recovery post-exercise section described soon show why just once a week routine for any muscle group is all you need if you take that muscle group to exhaustion.

Most glycogen is in the powerful Type-IIX muscle fibres

We have talked about glycogen stores in depth, and now hopefully you will see from the next graphic how the most powerful Type-IIX muscle fibres have the greatest amount of the fight-flight compound glycogen. The powerful upper intermediates and Type-IIX muscle fibres need instantaneous energy in the form of glucose to fight or run away.

You saw how the amplification process created by even one adrenaline molecule provides a multitude of glucose units rapidly for muscle contraction and you can stimulate the release of adrenaline through HIIT, box jumps and through loads you take to exhaustion.

The Type-I muscle fibres work best in an aerobic (oxygen rich) environment, and they extract more energy from muscle triglycerides (fat). Energy in the Type-I muscle fibres are extracted through aerobic glycolysis which is a very efficient system of energy extraction. The Type-I muscle fibres thus have a low glycogen level unlike the intermediates (especially the upper intermediates) and the Type-IIX muscle fibres that function best in an anaerobic (without oxygen) environment at high-intensity levels of exercise (Sprinting, HIIT, high loads taken to exhaustion or Super-Slow exercises to exhaustion)

	Type- I	→	Type-IIA	→	Upper Intermediates	→	Type IIX
Glycogen:	↑	→	↑↑	→	↑↑↑	→	↑↑↑↑

The upper intermediates and Type-IIX muscle fibres require some real effort to call them into action. Wimpy efforts will not be enough to engage these strong fibres. Super-Slow and the **Forced Orderly Recruitment of Muscle Fibres (FORM-f)** is an effective way to get to the powerful glycogen-rich fibres.

Prolonged aerobic exercise is not necessary!

High aerobic efforts such as running, swimming, treadmill, will only engage the glycogen-poor endurance Type-I fibres. By engaging the upper intermediates and powerful Type-IIX muscle fibres, you will increase strength and lean muscle mass. By increasing lean muscle mass, you change your body composition and hence change your weight setpoint.

Running for hours on a treadmill or hitting the pavements alongside a pollution-filled roadside makes no sense. Short, sharp HIIT bursts tap into the upper intermediates, and Type-IIX muscle fibres, simulating a fight-flight response and thus deplete glycogen in these glycogen-rich fibres. By taking them to exhaustion, you stimulate muscle growth (hypertrophy). Thus HIIT exercises followed by resistance training to exhaustion are a terrific synergistic combination for leanness and increased muscle mass.

Rapid vertical box jumps as an example, engage the upper intermediates, and Type-IIXs due to the explosive movement involved simulating the fight-flight response, and this is a great way to deplete glycogen in these muscle fibres as well in a gym setting.

The graphic below is a summary of the metabolic characteristics and energy substrates used by the various fibres.

Type- I	→	Upper Intermediates	→	Type IIX
Aerobic	→	Aerobic/Anaerobic	→	Anaerobic

Type- I	→	Upper Intermediates	→	Type IIX
Fat (Triglycerides)	→	Triglycerides/Glucose	→	Glucose/ATP/CP

The muscle fibres use different forms of energy from mainly fat (triglycerides) used for energy extraction in an oxygen-rich environment, to mainly muscle glycogen/glucose/Creatine phosphate (CP) use in an anaerobic muscle fibre environment.

Which form of energy each muscle fibre will use will depend on the intensity of exercise, and the blood and oxygen supply to those fibres.

High intensity exercise whether HIIT on a stationary bike, Super-Slow exercises taken to muscle exhaustion or intense muscle contraction, depletes oxygen levels in the muscle group being exercised, thus shifting this muscle group into an anaerobic state (low oxygen level) and this then shifts energy extraction into anaerobic glycolysis which occurs in an oxygen-poor environment that the upper intermediates and powerful Type-IIX's thrive on.

Anaerobic glycolysis is a less efficient use of energy (glucose) granted, but very fast! It is described in more detail below.

Energy Matters

Type-I muscle, endurance fibres have an abundant supply of blood and high oxygen-binding myoglobin which gives these cells a dark red colour in contrast to the fast-twitch Type-IIX muscle fibres that have low myoglobin content and are thus pale. Type-I's are rich in mitochondria which are the little energy factories in cells. So Type-I muscle fibres use a very efficient system of extracting energy called **Oxidative Phosphorylation** in an oxygen-rich environment. This is not to say that the Type-1 muscle fibres cannot hypertrophy because this is not the case.

Powerful Type-IIX muscle fibres will use a system called **Anaerobic Glycolysis** or the Glycolytic Pathway to extract energy rapidly which cannot be achieved through oxidative phosphorylation.

Type-IIX fibres do not have an abundance of mitochondria. The blood supply and oxygen supply becomes inadequate as a rapidly contracting muscle restricts blood and oxygen availability, and thus forces the most powerful muscle fibres to use glucose to extract energy in an anaerobic (without oxygen) environment and to use Adenosine Triphosphate (ATP) and Creatine Phosphate (CP) for quick sources of energy. Creatine Monohydrate is discussed in Appendix-25.

Efficiencies of energy extraction: Just look at the figures

The Type-IIX's can extract energy from glucose in an anaerobic environment 150% faster than the Type-I's can extract energy in an oxygen-rich environment (Hall, 2015). The Type-I's can extract around **36 MOLECULES of ATP** from just **ONE MOLECULE** of glucose (**1 to 36 ratio**) using oxygen in the process of oxidative phosphorylation whereas with the Type-IIX's, **64 MOLECULES OF ATP** can be produced in the same time interval but the catch here is that **32 MOLECULES OF GLUCOSE** are consumed in the process using anaerobic glycolysis which is a **1 to 2 ratio** (Salway and Granner 2004)

So this ratio for anaerobic glycolysis indicates that for every one molecule of glucose burned for energy, only 2 ATP molecules are produced in the very fast world of high-powered muscle contraction in an oxygen-free environment of the fight-flight response. Whereas in the cool and calm world of the Type-1's with time on their 'hands', one molecule of glucose produces 36 molecules of ATP. The powerful upper intermediates and Type-IIX muscle fibres are the energy 'gas guzzlers' in the muscle world.

Important: These figures may seem challenging but are the amazing clue for you regarding exercise efficiency. Tapping into the higher intermediates and Type-IIX's gives you the biggest-bang-for-the buck to cause glycogen depletion! You can take advantage of the high consumption rate of glucose by these fibres by targeting and engaging them. This means more fat will be raided to replace the lost glycogen but remember no carbs during or after exercise otherwise you will pull the rug from under this fat-loss process. Use the Activ8Health Plan-A diet only for fat loss and Essential Amino Acids (EAAs) during exercise.

The mega energy release from fat burning

Let's contrast the use of glucose as the substrate for energy production versus a fatty acid such as palmitate, the most common saturated fatty acid found in animals. Just one molecule of palmitate will be 'burned' aerobically by the Type-I and intermediate muscle fibres to provide **129 MOLECULES OF ATP** (Berdanier, Berdanier, & Zempleni, 2008).

No wonder muscle fats are used in the cool, calm endurance state of muscle action, but the energy production from fat is way too slow for the frenetic fight-flight muscle fibres.

Energy from fat is what you will be burning when you perform intraday fasting. Get over those hunger pangs to tap into your super-rich energy fat stores.

Destroying this amazing advantage of glycogen depletion by the 'gas guzzlers'

What's the use if you take all that effort to engage these high-end muscle fibres, deplete them of glycogen and have all this lost glycogen replaced in an instant by drinking glucose-rich sports drinks or worse still, by having a croissant or cream bun or any other starchy carb you can think of soon after exercising.

All these carb-rich foods will likewise destroy this advantage and all because you are consuming a vast amount of glucose that rapidly and efficiently replaces the lost glycogen in the muscles you have just exercised. How many people do you see in gym gear in cafes often found around gyms for a good reason, with sweaty hair and sweaty exercise gear consuming their sugar-rich reward for all that exercise?

For mere mortals who are not elite athletes constantly and dramatically depleting our glycogen stores, this is the last thing you want to do as an everyday Joe or Joanne trying to keep lean. Force your body to replace that lost glycogen through your body fat stores by only consuming EAAs in water before, during and immediately after exercise. Read about how to use EAAS in Appendix-24.

Sports drinks full of glucose is the last thing you need to consume around exercise. The glucose is avidly and rapidly absorbed and shunted towards glycogen synthesis to fill the exercise-induced glycogen void in muscles and liver.

It is well known that as far as sports drinks go to support muscle protein synthesis, that you only need essential amino acids (EAAs) in water. It has been shown that glucose does not increase muscle protein synthesis (MPS) or decrease muscle protein breakdown (MPB) and that all you need are EAAs for this purpose (Atherton and Smith 2012; Borsheim, Tipton et al. 2002). By providing your body with the EAAs before, during and just after exercise, you are assisting muscle repair mechanisms and protein synthesis for muscle growth. Let your fat refuel that low glycogen battery!

The Activ8Health EAAs have the added benefit of L-Citrulline to help keep blood vessels in the muscle dilated through nitric oxide (NO) production thus allowing more oxygen and nutrient delivery because of this nitric oxide (NO) induced blood flow. See Appendix-23 & 24.

The Activ8Health EAAs have been formulated to have not only added L-Citrulline but L-Glutamine + L-Arginine but at low enough doses so as not to trigger rapid oxidation (burning) of these amino acids as energy enabling them to perform their intended functions such as increasing Nitric Oxide (NO) and to support muscle protein synthesis. Pushing large doses of amino acids upregulates enzymes and biochemistry pathways that facilitate oxidation or burning of amino acids as fuel.

The bonus of EAAs is that they do not require any digestive power but are rapidly absorbed into the bloodstream, and this prevents blood being shunted away from freshly exercised muscle to the gastrointestinal tract (GIT).

As a guide using 0.1 g of EAAs per kg body weight has been shown to increase muscle protein balance (Williams 2005). So a 70 kg person will need 7 grams of EAAs in total. Simply add this to water and fill with around 700 ml of plain water. Have 1/3 immediately before exercise, 1/3 during exercise and the remainder immediately after exercise. Just add the EAA powder to a sports drink bottle with a metallic mixing ball and add the water when you get to the gym to keep this fresh.

Only have a glucose-rich drink if you are an elite athlete that has to replace glycogen rapidly. This is not the case for the vast majority of people out there struggling with weight issues and poor dietary choices. You have a small window of opportunity around exercise and 1 – 3 hours after exercise to boost protein synthesis in muscle (Williams 2005).

Shutting down the energy ('gas') guzzlers

It is for this reason that these powerful muscle fibres are also shut down after engagement for days after as I will discuss in the rest and recovery part of this chapter. It is the reason why engaging these Type-IIX fibres in a gym setting pretty well mandates that you do not engage them again for days to a week after taking them to exhaustion as you risk injury and overtraining. These muscle fibres have to recover their energy stores and repair the damage that has occurred through exercise training.

This lasting muscle injury is beyond doubt and not subject to interpretation or conjecture – it is what it is! Rest is thus an absolute requirement based on physiological processes and markers of muscle damage post-exercise. Avoiding Sarcopenia

You should fight against sarcopenia, which is the loss of muscle as you age and do this throughout your life by resistance exercises. By engaging the powerful upper intermediates and Type-IIX muscle fibres, you will ensure you stay strong throughout your life and particularly in your senior years. Importantly, you should have this exercise monitored by an Exercise Physiologist to avoid injury with exercise.

With ageing, you predominantly lose the powerful Type-IIX muscle fibres. This unfortunate process of muscle attrition and in particular Type-IIX muscle fibre loss due to the ageing process may begin as early as your mid to late 20's depending on your diet and lifestyle. The Type-IIX's can fall from an average of 60% in sedentary young men to as low as 30% in the elderly over 80 years of age (Evans and Campbell 1993)

Rep ranges - using weights

What I suggest is to start off with a light weight that is very easy for you and perform 12 or more reps as a warm-up. Pyramid-up, i.e. increase the weight slightly and then do 12 more reps at this weight and then pyramid-up again and repeat. Then end that exercise on 12 reps reaching exhaustion at the 12th rep, and this will maximise hypertrophy.

The hypertrophy rep range is often touted as being between 6 – 12 reps but many exercise physiologists favour the 12 rep range as this will be a lighter load and less likely to cause injury. In saying this, at the end of this chapter I have indicated that low loads to exhaustion can have the very same effect so this thinking may indeed be flawed. High rep ranges can take up a lot of time, and lower reps like 12 reps keep the routine flowing. Starting off with lower loads and pyramiding up has its advantages. These include:

1. Warming the muscle up and preparing the muscles, tendons and ligaments for higher weight loads by increasing blood supply, warming up the soft tissues and helping you adjust your grip, symmetry, stance, i.e. making proprioception adjustments before increasing your weight thus preventing injury.

2. The lower loads and higher reps are helping deplete glycogen in muscle fibres lower down the line from the Type-I's to the Type-IIA's.
3. Engaging all the lower order muscle fibres thus increasing hypertrophy in those fibres.
4. Reaching a load where you can reach exhaustion on the 12th rep is great for hypertrophy but not an absolute necessity for hypertrophy as lower loads to exhaustion have been found to be as effective. This concept is explained further at the end of this chapter.
5. Finish each set of an exercise on a Super-Slow where you start in a position where the eccentric phase is called into action first so that you double-up on the eccentric and reach exhaustion. This Super-Slow set squeezes out that glycogen depleting effort even more and forces the movement through the muscle fibres that escaped exhaustion with the normal rep ranges described in points 1 to 4.

What is an eccentric contraction?

Dr Ellington Darden's 'Body Fat Breakthrough' book provided an astonishing insight into a method that was counterintuitive and yet highly effective (Darden 2014). The technique involves slow and purposeful movements that concentrate greatly on form that **accentuates the eccentric contraction** component of any exercise.

This super-slow technique can be incorporated into virtually any resistance exercise whether you use free-weights, machines, and cable or body-weight exercises.

So what is the eccentric phase of a contraction? If we look at say a biceps curl with a weighted bar if you curl that bar towards the body, this is the concentric phase of the contraction where the muscle shortens. However, when you allow the bar to drop away from the body, you are now in the eccentric phase where the muscle is being lengthened (stretched). Another example would be the leg press where you push the weighted plate away from your body and in doing so, you are contracting the muscle i.e. the concentric phase. However, when you allow the legs to come back towards the body, you will feel that lengthening or stretching in your quadriceps and this is the eccentric phase of the leg press exercise.

This eccentric phase is really where the action is. This phase results in more microscopic tears within the muscle and requires more effort as long as you do not allow momentum to help you. These microscopic tears are really what matters in terms of repair and mobilisation of muscle stem cells to form new muscle fibres and increase muscle mass through adaptation. Body sculptors and bodybuilders concentrate on this phase and often use spotters that help to resist these eccentric movements to increase loading and increase muscle stress, metabolism and microscopic tears and post-exercise muscle inflammation that helps stimulate muscle growth (Tidball 2005).

Super-Slow exercises and the orderly recruitment of muscle fibres

By doing any exercise whether this is a biceps curl, chin up, leg press or shoulder press, if you can do these extremely slowly, then what you are forcing the muscle to do is move through the orderly recruitment of muscle fibres. Super-Slow exercises are essentially the **Forced Orderly Recruitment of Muscle Fibres (FORM-f)**. Even if you just get to the upper intermediates that are also rich in glycogen (glucose) stores, you are winning. You are more likely to get to the Type-IIX's if you try to push beyond the point of exhaustion to get those last few reps in before you just can't do anymore. This takes discipline but is worth the effort!

The 'Dirty-30' Accentuated Eccentric Super-Slow Exercises

You can double the time you spend in the eccentric phase by starting your Super-Slow exercise in the eccentric position start-point, then performing the concentric movement and finishing your set for any muscle group in the eccentric phase of the movement. So this allows for twice (2x) the valuable eccentric movements in a particular muscle group being targeted. As Dr Ellington Darden states, you can start off with a 10:10:10 second time interval i.e. 10 seconds for each movement --- so 10 seconds eccentric, 10 seconds concentric and finish on a 10-second eccentric movement. So if we use the biceps curl again to shed light on this, raise the bar to the top towards the body. This is the starting point. Lower for 10 seconds (eccentric) then move towards the body for 10 seconds (concentric) and then away from the body again for 10 seconds (eccentric).

So you can see that you are doubling the time in the eccentric phase. It doesn't matter whether you begin with a 5:5:5-second routine as you need to gradually build up to the 'Dirty-30' as this takes time, effort and dedication to exercise form to get to this point.

Exercise is not a race! You need to condition your muscles, tendons and ligaments gradually before performing any strenuous activity.

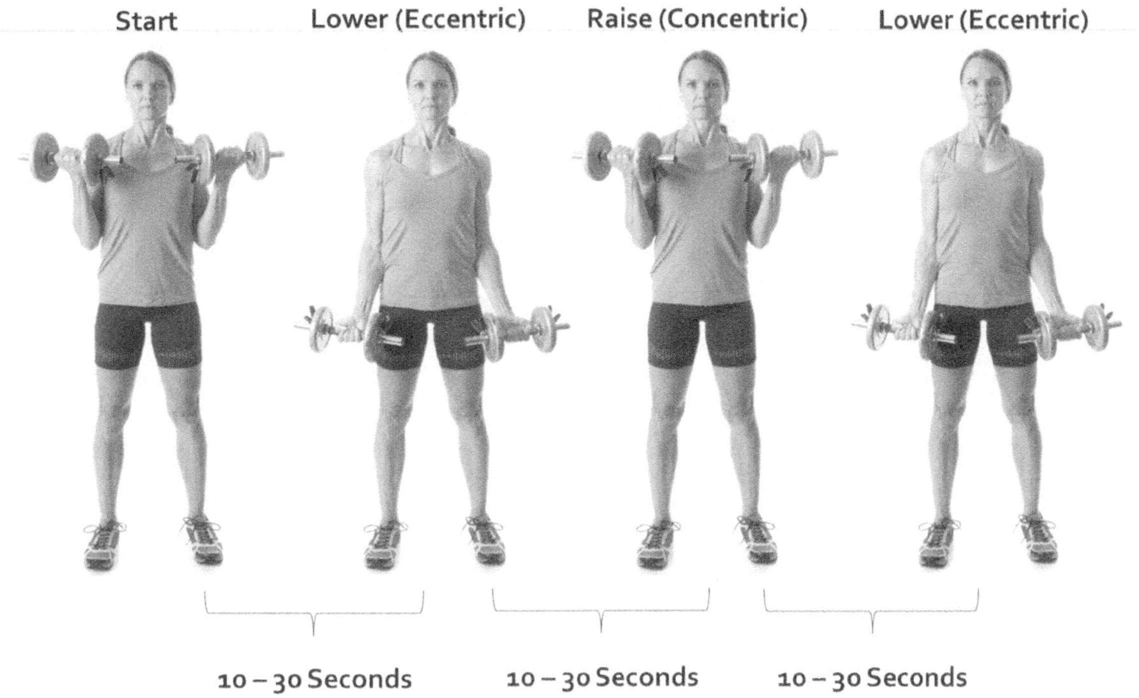

Remember you can do all of these Super-Slow exercises with a squat, a shoulder press, leg press, chest press etc. Just learn what the concentric and eccentric components are of each exercise and remember begin with the eccentric position so that you can double the eccentric moves with every exercise. This is how you will tap into those powerful upper intermediates and Type-IIX muscle fibres and engage them meaningfully. This is how you will keep on tapping into those glycogen stores, and if you do the right thing with your diet by consuming the Activ8Health Plan-A Diet as described, you will keep fat levels in your body very low indeed in the healthy range and blast away abdominal fat throughout your life.

These Super-Slow exercises are not easy as you will find out. Just do any resistance exercise at your usual pace for 2 or more sets and then finish with a Super-Slow set to exhaustion to finish that particular muscle group and then move on to the next exercise and do the same thing. An exercise physiologist or personal trainer will be able to let you know the phases of any exercise movement. You can use this strategy for any resistance exercise whether you are using your body weight, resistance bands, cables or free weights.

Kettlebell Squat to Upright Row

If we look at a Kettlebell Squat to Upright Row, the concentric contraction will be getting up from the lower position, and the eccentric contraction will be going down which stretches the muscle quadriceps muscle. This exercise can be divided into two parts:

1. The squat movement
2. The shoulder movement

With the shoulder movement, the concentric movement is lifting the Kettlebell up, and the eccentric phase is the weight being brought down. So, as you bring the weight down from the shoulders and then squat, this whole movement will be in the eccentric phase of the movements. So this is an excellent exercise that involves a multitude of major muscle groups. You can see how Super-Slow can be incorporated in many home-based exercise routines that should all be completed from starting with the HIIT session on the bike as a warm-up to a resistance exercise like this Kettlebell Squat to Upright Row and all completed in 10 minutes before you shower and you getting ready for work.

Using multi-joint exercises that engage as many joints in one move is always good value in the home or gym setting. Thus as you can see with this Kettlebell Squat to Upright Row, that you are engaging the ankles, knees, hips, wrists, elbows and shoulders in just one move along with axial loading of weight vertically down the spine. This axial loading is great for bone health.

You can also make this exercise a **Kettlebell Squat Press** using one hand. Follow the moves below but finish by raising the one hand holding the Kettlebell above the head. Adding this movement produces a greater challenge and is a truly multi-joint exercise.

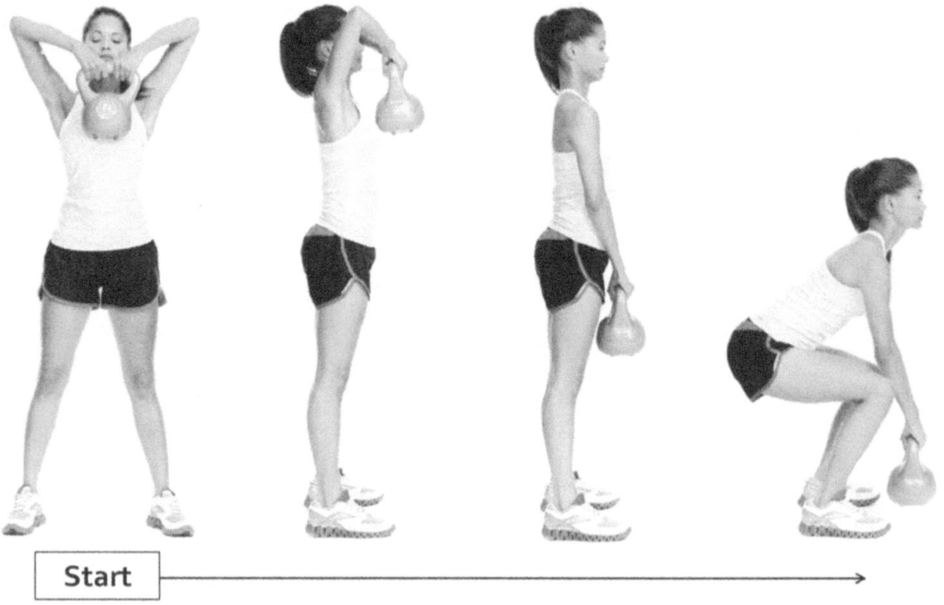

With a home-based exercise program what I would do is warm up first with a HIIT session on a stationary bike of 2 to 3, 20 – 30-second bursts of the fast phase followed by 1 – 2 minutes of a very slow phase to catch your breath before the next fast phase. Then follow this up with resistance exercises using resistance bands which are a great choice for beginners or even advanced exercisers or you can use free weights, kettlebells or even body weight exercises. As with the gym-based exercises, just perform any resistance exercise at a usual pace and then end on a Super-Slow movement.

With resistance bands, as long as you can take the exercise to exhaustion you will have moved through the classes of muscle fibres getting to the upper intermediates and possibly the Type-IIX's by pushing that exercise a little further as I have mentioned by squeezing in an extra rep or two beyond the point you feel you can't. Bands are easy to pack in a suitcase if you travel as they are extremely light and take up next to no space.

The Big-5 gym-based exercise program

A great place for beginners or intermediate gym goers is to ensure the Big-5 exercises are used either on their own or incorporated into a gym routine. These 5 exercises engage a large number of major muscle groups across multiple joints thus helping to deplete glycogen stores effectively using a small grouping of targeted exercises. So in essence, the Big-5 works the whole body with just 5 exercises. Apart from an effective home-based exercise program I suggest going to the gym 1 day a week (whole body routine) or 2 times a week (doing a split routine - upper body one day, rest then lower another day). This would be a wonderful way to add variety to your exercise regimen and to increase loading on your muscles.

Like variety in your diet to increase bowel microbiome diversity, diversity of exercises is also vital to prevent muscle adaptations that make a particular exercise less demanding and to call into action the various parts of a muscle group through various exercises. It is very hard to match the variety or loading possibilities provided by a gym and so even a full body exercise routine just once a week in a gym can work wonders on your body composition and physique and change your body composition setpoint.

Value your muscle mass and think about your skeletal muscle as a precious resource because like it or lump it, it starts to diminish over your lifespan and once it reaches a critical point, you will barely be able to get yourself out of a chair or walk upstairs in your older age. You now become dependent on others to do the basic of tasks in your old age. You need to stay strong as you get older.

Thus doing a home-based exercise program even 2 days a week along with a full-body gym routine like the Big-5 once a week or a split routine twice a week will be perfect. These recommendations take into consideration energy conservation and muscle repair needs. Resting for one week after a gym session should be minimum before exercising a particular muscle group again. You can test this by performing an exercise at a particular load one day and then go in again the next day and try to do the same routine with the same load. I'm sure you will find you will not be up to the task because the upper intermediates and Type-IIX's have been subdued because the body cannot allow energy guzzling muscle fibres to keep on working and thus deplete the body of precious storage energy.

Muscle glycogen cannot be in a constant state of depletion as it is an evolutionary imperative that these glycogen stores are available for the next threat. So resting is mandatory to repair and recover. Resting and recovering of a worked muscle group, is the basis of the split routine. The rest and recover part of this chapter will hammer home the point of how important it is to rest, repair and allow your muscle to grow.

For those not used to gym-based routines, starting off with the Big-5 once a week is a good option. These five exercises pretty well cover all the major muscle groups. Ideally, you will want a fresh routine every 2 – 3 months, but this will be a good start. Once again getting a full functional assessment by an Exercise Physiologist will be important before you begin any exercise routine. If you are medically fit then you are good to go. Remember, Exercise Physiologists can provide safe yet progressive programs to challenge you and your muscles.

The gym protocol

1. A warm-up on a stationary bike or rowing machine
2. Perform a HIIT session of 2 - 3 x 20 or 30 seconds of the fast phase pedalling on a stationary bike with 2 minute slow intervals in-between the fast phases. Why bike? Because time after time, engaging the quadriceps femoris group of muscles, a large glycogen-rich group of powerful muscles, has shown significant health benefits.

3. Do some dynamic stretches before resistance training
4. Commence the Big-5 exercises (or other Exercise Physiologist guided exercise resistance program)
5. Pyramid up (increase weight incrementally) --- choosing very light weights initially and perform 10 – 12 reps. Increase the weight slightly and do another 10 – 12 reps and then increase the weight again and do another 10 – 12 reps. Aim for exhaustion on this last set at around 10 – 12 reps. You will need to choose appropriate weights, and this will be trial and error initially. Your Exercise Physiologist will be able to help out here.
6. Finish on a super-slow set at a weight that allows a slow 10 seconds on the concentric and eccentric phases. You can even do a 5-second Super-Slow routine for each of the moves, to begin with. Remember to begin with the eccentric phase so that you can complete twice the amount of time in the eccentric phase of the movement. Then move onto the next muscle group and repeat steps 5 and 6 for this particular muscle group. The Super-Slow exercises help to diminish glycogen even more in all the muscle fibres which may or may not include the Type-IIX's.
7. Do not go back to aerobic exercise after resistance training – see below.

The Big-5	Exercise	Muscles worked
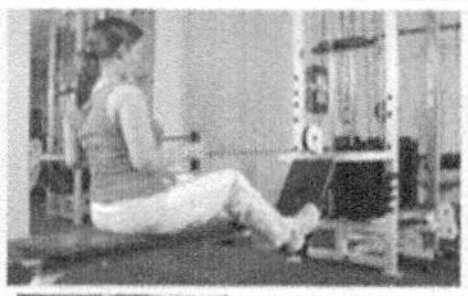	Seated row	Forearms, biceps, triceps, lattisimus dorsi, the rhomboids, paravertebral muscles, core muscles
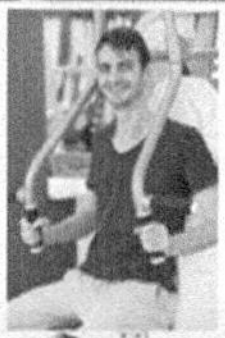	Chest press	Pectoral muscles, deltoids (shoulder), forearms, biceps, triceps
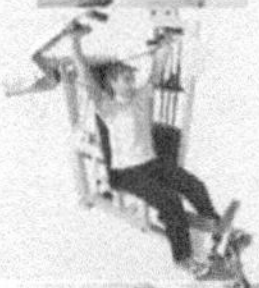	Overhead press	Shoulders, with strong involvement by the triceps and pectoral (chest) muscles, core muscles (stabilization)
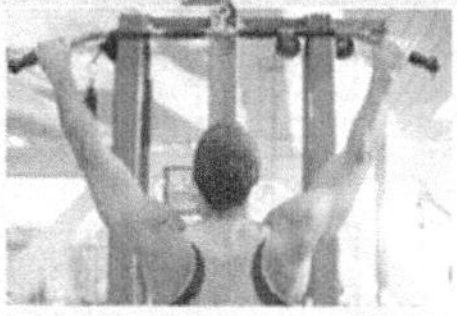	Pulldown	Upper back, pectoral, forearms, biceps, triceps, shoulders , core muscles (stabilization)
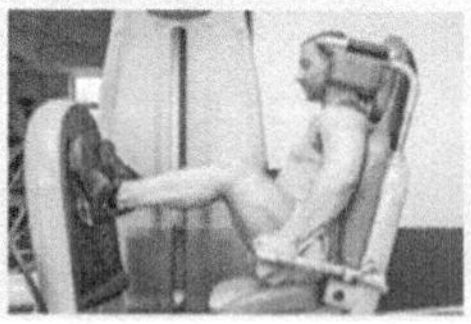	Leg Press	The lower body from waist and lower back to ankles, strong activation of buttocks, quadriceps, hamstrings, calves, core

Do not go back to aerobic exercise after resistance training. AMPK shuts down mTOR muscle synthesis

You can end on some dynamic stretches but never go back to an aerobic exercise after the resistance training. The reason is that you will have ramped up mTOR signalling for protein synthesis. If you finish on an exhaustive aerobic exercise, what will happen is that you will increase AMPK by chewing up your ATP and increasing AMP levels. Remember. High AMPK indicates to the body that energy levels are very low. If energy levels are low (high AMPK signalling), it shuts down the protein synthesis pathway through mTOR as the body is saying; 'I do not have enough energy for energy-expending processes like building muscle protein'.

So not clever to finish a resistance training routine and then run like mad on a treadmill!!! – It is all about molecular signalling and to engage in exercise intelligently; you need to be aware of these molecular signals to get the most out of any exercise routine.

The Big-5 using cables, free-weights or machines

The Big-5 can be executed using machine-based resistance training, cables or free-weights. It is best to get a professional to design an exercise routine to incorporate multi-joint, compound moves using a variety of equipment so that you do not spend hours in a gym and can finish a routine in 45 – 60 minutes to cover the points I have mentioned. This is the smart way of exercising. The concentric and eccentric movements of each exercise in the Big-5 are shown in the next graphic to help you with the Super-Slow finishes for each exercise.

The Big-5	Exercise	Muscles worked
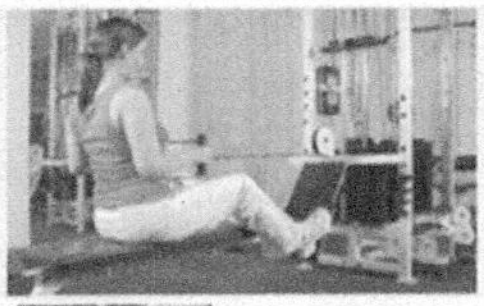	**Seated row**	**Concentric:** Pulling towards you **Eccentric (slow):** Movement away from you
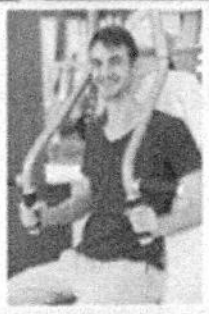	**Chest press**	**Concentric:** Pushing away from you **Eccentric:** Movement back towards the chest
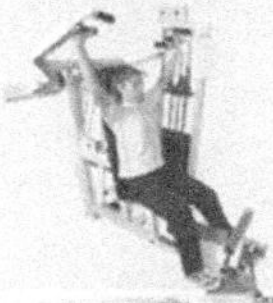	**Overhead press**	**Concentric:** Pushing up away from you **Eccentric:** Movement back down
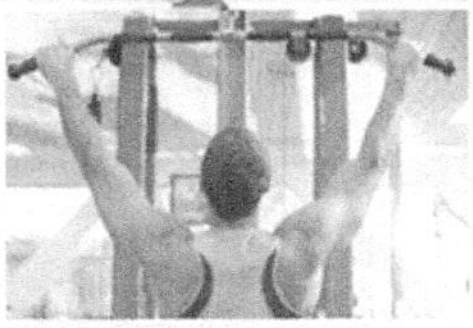	**Pulldown**	**Concentric:** Pulling downwards **Eccentric:** Movement back up
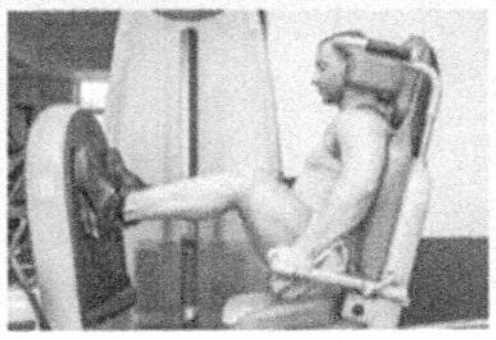	**Leg Press**	**Concentric:** Pushing away from you **Eccentric:** Movement back towards you

Results without exhaustive exercise - The smart Activ8Health protocol

People seem to think that it is not exercising unless you put in an exhausting effort in a gym or you pound the pavements dripping with sweat jogging ceaselessly. A study in the Journal of the American Medical Association (JAMA) stated that:

> *"1 or 2 sessions per week may be sufficient to reduce all-cause, CVD, and cancer mortality risks regardless of adherence to prevailing physical activity guidelines." (O'Donovan, Lee et al.).* CVD = Cardiovascular Disease

Elizabeth Blackburn, who won the Nobel Prize for telomere research in her excellent book 'The Telomere Effect', also stated that in terms of telomere length, a powerful marker for cell aging, that there is no difference in telomere length between those engaging in low to moderate exercises in comparison to those who engage in ultramarathons (Blackburn 2017). What this shows is that short, sharp and effective exercise is all you need to benefit your body and increase your healthspan!

I am afraid that I am time poor and what I want is a smart, quick and practical way to keep trim and strong. I will reinforce here that depleting glycogen stores are your key to fat-loss success supported by the Activ8Health Plan-A Diet.

The Quadriceps Femoris Muscle Group

One powerful grouping of muscles is the quadriceps femoris group (the 'quads'). It is this group of muscles you want to target through HIIT and increasing NEAT activity by brisk walking, walking up flights of stairs carrying your heavy briefcase, or using a stationary bike that truly targets this grouping of powerful, glycogen-rich upper leg muscles.

So why the quads? Because this grouping of muscles is vital for the flight-fight responses helping you leap out of harm's way. Which other group of muscles can you think of that can spring you out of trouble or enable you to sprint away rapidly? For this reason, these groupings of very long and powerful upper leg muscles have high glycogen content, and this makes sense. This fight-flight response activates the Type-IIX fibres in the quadriceps femoris muscles (the 'Quads').

HIIT with sprinting or on a stationary bike simulates the fight-flight response as do box jumps. Targeting such a large grouping of muscles and in particular, the absolutely glycogen-rich upper intermediates and Type-IIX fibres in this muscle group help you effectively deplete a significant amount of glycogen with relatively minimal effort.

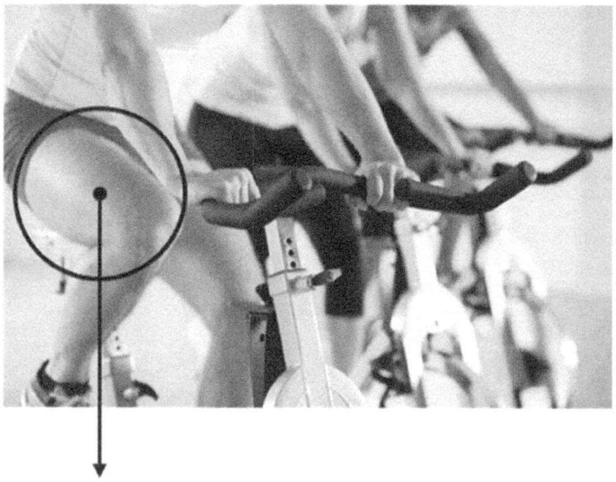

Quadriceps femoris muscle group

In biopsy studies, the quadriceps femoris muscle had significantly higher levels of glycogen than the deltoid muscle (Hultman 1967). It makes sense for such a powerful muscle group that keeps us upright and can spring us out of trouble when necessary. Squats as an exercise are often hailed as a king of exercises for the impact it has on the whole body. Make sure you exercise the Quadriceps Femoris group effectively, and you can also use the Super-Slow exercises to truly challenge this powerful muscle group, remembering that it is the downward move that is the eccentric move in a squat or the legs moving back towards the body on a leg press machine.

One study showed a huge **48% increase in glucose clearance** in nonobese diabetic patients with just a **16% increase in Quadriceps strength** (Ishii, Yamakita et al. 1998). Quadriceps training means effective glucose clearance for the whole body. Even though around 50% of this large quadriceps femoris muscle group is made up of Type-1 muscle fibres, i.e. the endurance fibres that keep us upright and walking all day (MacIntosh, Gardiner et al. 2006), the remaining 50% of the muscle is made up of the most powerful intermediates and Type-IIX muscle fibres which are the Holy Grail of body sculptors and bodybuilders.

So training the quadriceps has a tremendous effect on the whole body through improved glucose clearance and this is a major benefit for anyone with prediabetes or diabetes. Individuals who suffer these glucose disorders will do well to concentrate on quadriceps exercises through HIIT, box jumps and strength training with an emphasis on the eccentric contractions.

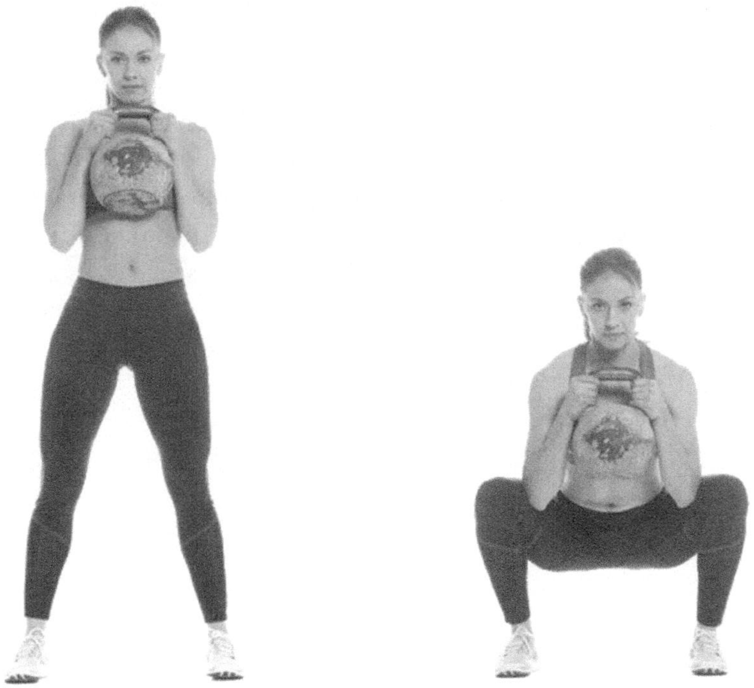

The graphic above shows the squat targeting the huge quadriceps femoris muscle group. Using Super-Slow exercises, the downward movement as mentioned is the eccentric phase and thus you need to start upright and slowly descend as this will stretch the muscle as you slowly go down, slowly get up and then slowly go down again to get twice the eccentric effort and you will finish in a safe position to put the weight down as no doubt this will be a challenging exercise.

Remember you can start with 5 seconds of each movement 5:5:5 and building up to 30 seconds of each slow movement 30:30:30 - a great challenge indeed.

How effective do you think short bursts of activity are?

It is easy to dismiss short bursts of high-intensity exercise as being of minimal value because we are all conditioned to think that we need to work very hard for anything worthwhile in life and that there is no reward unless there is a lot of pain. But this is definitely not the case. Efficiency counts!

As far back as 1986, pioneers in the study of high intensity training (HIIT) on human physiology, discovered that even **a short sprint lasting 30 seconds** will **deplete glycogen in the vastus lateralis**

muscle of the quadriceps femoris (thigh) muscle by a massive 25% and will also **deplete the ATP levels in this muscle by an amazing 37%** (Cheetham, Boobis, Brooks, & Williams, 1986).

It just shows the tremendous energy-consuming process involved in short, intense exercise typical of the fight-flight response. I am hoping you can see how powerful those lunchtime sprints or short 10 minute HIIT sessions in a gym nearby during your lunch break can be regarding glycogen depletion allowing you to shift that fat that seems so stubborn.

Without this knowledge, shifting fat is very difficult as people destroy their efforts with what they put in their mouths after exercise. Carb-rich foods with exercise just sabotage any effort by providing all the glucose you need to fill in the glycogen stores lost --- such a pity. Ditch those glucose-rich sports drinks. The Activ8Health Plan-A diet is a vital part of this strategy enabling you to lose fat to provide the glycerol that fills in that glycogen 'hole'.

The weekend-warriors: Moderate exercise just as good as vigorous

Professor JoAnn Manson is a professor of medicine at Harvard Medical School, Brigham and Women's Hospital has described two reports coming out of England and Scotland in the peer-reviewed Medscape online resource for physicians. These studies were assessing the amount of exercise needed to decrease all-cause mortality. Current guidelines recommend a gruelling 30 minutes of exercise most days with a total of around 150 minutes a week which is 2.5 hours a week. In this busy world, many people would find this extremely difficult, and we also have to keep in mind that many people just hate exercise but may well engage in exercise if it is brief yet physiologically effective and time efficient.

The study involved quite a large cohort of people who were assessed and comprised of 63,000 men and women who were asked about their exercise habits and whether this was either moderate or vigorous activity. These individuals were placed into one of four (4) groups (O'Donovan, Lee et al.):

1. Those who did not engage in moderate or vigorous physical activity
2. Those who met the standard guidelines and exercised for 75 – 150 minutes a week at least three (3) times a week
3. Weekend warriors who compressed the standard guidelines into one (1) to two (2) sessions a week.
4. Those who did some moderate to vigorous physical activity but less than the guidelines

It was very interesting that those in groups 2, 3 and 4, were ALL found to have significant reductions in cardiovascular disease (CVD) and all-cause mortality in comparison to the sedentary individuals in group 1 who did no exercise.

Those in groups 3 and 4 who performed exercise below the standard guidelines had around a 30% reduction in all-cause mortality in comparison to those in group 2 who complied with the recommended guidelines – group (2) individuals had a 35% reduction in all-cause mortality. So as you can see, the difference is negligible, and this well and truly reinforces that you do not have to exercise your heart out to enjoy the benefits of exercise. The researchers stated the following:

> *"Weekend Warrior and other leisure-time physical activity patterns characterized by 1 or 2 sessions per week may be sufficient to reduce all-cause, CVD, and cancer mortality risks regardless of adherence to prevailing physical activity guidelines." (O'Donovan, Lee et al.)*

Isn't this a wonderful opportunity for you! With such a short 20 to 30 second effort, you are creating such a huge impact on your metabolism not only locally within the muscle group exercised but throughout the body. This short 30-second fast movement (Sprint/HIIT) will result in the following wonderful effects on your body. A stationary bike and squats target your quadriceps very efficiently.

However, going back to the benefits of high intensity short burst exercise. The following applies:

1. Decreasing glycogen stores improve insulin sensitivity in your body as your muscle cells become more efficient in taking up glucose through either increasing insulin receptors or increasing insulin receptor sensitivity or both to ensure glycogen stores are replaced efficiently and rapidly due to that evolutionary imperative to keep glycogen stores at an optimal level for the fight-flight response. Diabetics or those who suffer from insulin resistance, i.e. the pre-diabetics or women with PCOS can add years to their life by doing these types of exercises.
2. It will diminish your ATP stores. Remember, we described the ATP as the active bullets that are 'fired' in the body to supply energy leaving the spent shells (AMP) to build up. As AMP levels increase, so does the AMPK energy sensor to replenish the energy balance in the cell. But also remember, a high AMPK is a low energy signal, and this means that your mTOR system will be inhibited so that you move into repair mode rather than protein synthesis, growth or cell multiplication. All exercise – aerobic or resistance training will decrease energy stores post-exercise with higher AMPK levels unless you have destroyed this effect by guzzling glucose-rich drinks during exercise and eat carb-rich foods after exercise.
3. It improves aerobic fitness over time (VO2max). Aerobic fitness is associated with longer telomeres (Blackburn 2017). This effect was not shown with resistance training which has other valuable benefits though.
4. Increased telomere length. The exercises that created amazing increase in telomerase were (Blackburn 2017):
    - ✓ Moderate aerobic endurance activity
    - ✓ High-Intensity Interval Training (HIIT)

   Resistance training did not increase telomere length, but the effects of resistance training are amazing in terms of balance, strength, metabolic rate and insulin sensitivity. It improves systemic glucose uptake and let's not forget resistance training increases muscle mass that requires a lot of energy to survive even in the resting state thus changing your weight setpoint to a much lower one and you have achieved this through a change in your body composition by the use of resistance training.

Exercise also increases autophagy

Autophagy was described under intraday fasting as an important process in cell renewal. The term autophagy derives from the Greeks meaning 'self-eating'. It is a process of self-cleaning where large internal cellular structures such as damaged organelles (mitochondria, lysosomes, Golgi apparatus etc.) are cannibalised and reused. For example, protein structures are broken down into amino acids, and these can then be supplied to other parts of the body that require essential and non-essential amino acids for synthesis. This mechanism is thought to have been developed to survive starvation pressures but this system has evolved to help replace damaged and struggling cells, and this could also help prevent cancer by repairing or eliminating cellular damage that could result in malignancy.

It is interesting that exercise can increase both telomerase and autophagy. Remember, telomerase is the enzyme that elongates telomeres, and longer telomeres are associated with health and a longer lifespan (Blackburn 2017). We now have another two great scientifically measurable reasons to exercise, and the great news is that an effective exercise program does not have to be an exhausting one that takes up a lot of your time. Exercise has powerful effects on cancer outcomes and enhanced autophagy no doubt has a role in this.

Rest and Recovery Post-Exercise

I have mentioned the importance of rest and recovery to not only enable your muscles, tendons, ligaments and bone to adapt to the stress of exercise but also to acknowledge that exercise causes damage to tissues. It is this damage and inflammation post-exercise that stimulates cell growth and mobilisation of stem cells to form new and stronger tissue. By not recognising that you need to rest and repair, you expose yourself to injury and ill health as a constant stress on the body has an impact on your immune system as well.

Creatine Kinase (CK) is a muscle enzyme that is involved in the creation of phosphoCreatine (PCr) a molecule used for rapid ATP creation. This enzyme is released after muscle damage and is a marker for a heart attack as levels rise in the blood after the heart muscle has been damaged. However, this also occurs after exercise and CK can rise dramatically after a bout of exercise and especially so in untrained individuals. A marked elevation in CK levels are often seen in general practice in someone who has exercised intensely a few days before a blood test, and this then creates concern about rhabdomyolysis which is a severe form of muscle injury. More often than not it is not rhabdomyolysis but just a marker of skeletal muscle injury caused by the exercise and the vast majority recover without any problems This CK rise occurs especially so **after intense eccentric contractions**.

Of significant interest with muscle injury and CK release into the bloodstream, is that the increase may not begin until 48 hours after the bout of exercise and may not peak until 4 – 6 days after exercise (Clarkson and Hubal 2002).

Magnetic Resonance Imaging (MRI) has turned out to be a powerful tool in determining muscle injury after exercise. A T2-weighted MRI image reveals oedema (fluid) in tissues and oedema (US edema) is a marker for leaky, damaged tissues and inflammation. MRI has revealed prolonged T2-weighted oedematous changes post-exercise (Clarkson and Hubal 2002).

These two scientifically validated indices of muscle damage should be more than enough to show you that rest and recovery is vital for your muscles to grow and for you to avoid injury.

A word of warning: Just two weeks of inactivity can increase your risk of chronic illness

The research was conducted at the University of Liverpool by Dr Dan Cuthbertson et al and the results were presented at the European Congress on Obesity (ECO) in Porto, Portugal (17-20th May 2017). The findings were published on the university's website, and the authors stated that;

> *"just two weeks of inactivity in young healthy people can reduce muscle mass and produce metabolic changes that could lead to an increased risk of developing chronic diseases such as type 2 diabetes, heart disease, and potentially premature death." (Cuthbertson 2017)*

Exercise is thus non-negotiable. Do not engage in exercise on a weekly basis and you face an early death. Having a short healthspan where you are struggling just to survive due to early onset disease is to me early death because life becomes meaningless when all your thoughts and efforts are simply dealing with the symptoms and limitations of a disease process. Smart, efficient exercise in the least amount of time is highly achievable as outlined in this book.

Core Strength - Often Ignored

A great way to view your whole body is to consider the upper, middle and lower body as 3 links in a chain with the middle link (the core muscles) as the crucial link around which all other movements depend. A weak core weakens the whole body. If you think about it and imagine any sport or any home task you perform like picking up an object to raking a lawn or sprinting, it will all revolve around the strength and stability of these core muscles. Many muscles are involved in this core region from your upper abdomen to your pelvis but simply viewing that middle part of your body as the core is important enough as a visual cue to know which area you are training and to ensure you do not ignore this area in any workout.

The core muscles if they become weak cause a herniation-like effect where the content of the internal abdomen i.e. your bowels and body fat will bulge out causing that large belly effect and even those 'muffin-tops'. Keeping all of these muscles toned will provide you with the strength to perform all the other exercises or sports effectively and help your posture and physique. Focus on the core in all your training. Make this a primary training target.

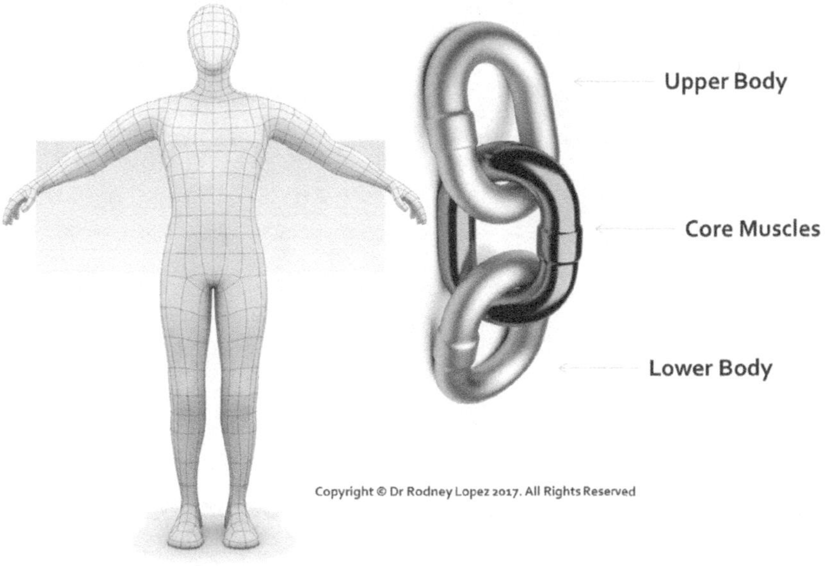

Using cable machines are a great way to work the core from beginner to advanced. You can work the upper, middle and lower abdomen through cable twists from standing or kneeling cable crunches. Your oblique's are tremendously engaged in these twisting motions as well as a large portion of your back muscles that are also a part of the core. Performing wood-chopper rotational type body twists starting with the bar set at a high level then mid-level and finishing at a low level, pretty well engages all the core muscles front and back. Use these twisting motions with various loads and also incorporate Super-Slow finishes.

Performing all exercises with optimal form is vital to ensure you do these exercises efficiently and so getting some professional advice from an Exercise Physiologist will be helpful. Neglecting the core and just training your arms and legs and simply performing crunches, will never give you that toned and balanced physique you are after. You may be working hard and getting nowhere. Core training seems to be less sexy than training the 'guns' in men or the 'butt' in women – however, an overall sexy physique is all about the core.

Sexy or not, the core is critical for anybody as back pain is extremely common and the vast majority of back problems stem from a very weak core. Remember, the core involves not only the abdominal muscles and obliques but also the back. Ensure a significant part of your training includes working all the core group muscles in every gym session.

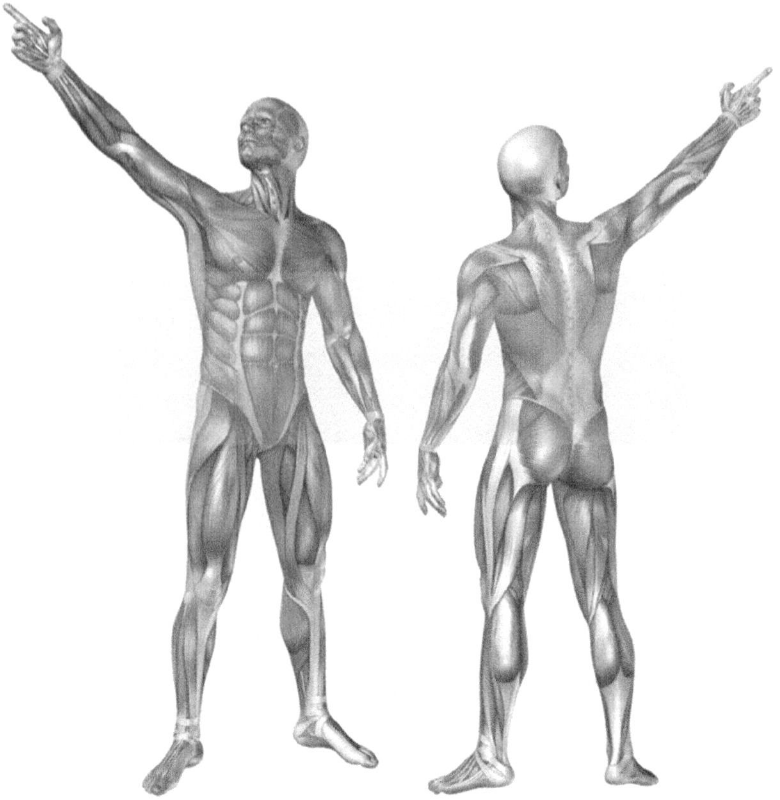

Heavy loads (weights) versus Lighter Loads to Exhaustion

Sometimes what seems intuitive just isn't so! One enlightening paper stated:

> *"increases in MPS are negligible with RE at 20–40% (1RM) but maximal at 70–90% of one-repetition maximum when workload is matched (according to load × repetition number). However, low-intensity exercise performed to failure equalises this response." (Atherton and Smith 2012)*

RE is simply resistance exercise and MPS is 'muscle protein synthesis'. So what this is stating is that if you used low loads then there is limited muscle protein synthesis but higher loads would stimulate this effect. The important point with the statement above is that low-intensity exercise, e.g. using lower loads or Super-Slow exercises to **exhaustion** where you just can't do another rep produces this same muscle protein synthesis (MPS) responses as per the high load weight training. It is fantastic news and must certainly make you happy that this is the case where you can work smarter and not harder. Lower loads to exhaustion will also be a lot safer and result in fewer injuries.

Home-based exercises can also be effective provided you work your way through them as suggested and perhaps finish off on an exercise with a Super-Slow set to exhaustion. Gyms offer a great deal of variety and loading options.

Key Points

- Exercise without the right dietary strategy in place is futile.
- Get an all-clear from your doctor before commencing exercise
- Get a functional assessment by a qualified Exercise Physiologist (EP) before commencing any exercise to avoid injury
- A graded program is always wise.
- Get new programs every 3 months
- Do home based exercises say twice a week
- Gym-based exercises once a week (whole body training) or split routine twice weekly
- Super-Slow exercise should be incorporated for **Forced Orderly Recruitment of Muscle Fibres (FORM-f)**.
- The Activ8Health™ Plan-A diet is designed for fat loss and to stay lean.
- The Activ8Health Plan-B diet is for those elite athletes who deplete glycogen stores regularly in a week.
- Remember, you can power your day with the use of fat. Just 1 molecule of palmitate, a fatty acid can produce 129 ATP molecules (Berdanier, Berdanier et al. 2008). ATP drives all energy consuming processes in the body. Contrast this to just 36 molecules of ATP produced from 1 molecule of glucose.
- Exercise can increase telomerase and telomere length.
- Aerobic fitness and not strength training is associated with an increase in telomerase but strength training is vital for a long life
- Weekend-Warriors and those who perform moderate to strenuous exercise less than the standard recommendations do almost as well as those who perform exercise three times a week for 150 minutes or more!
- Exercise also enhances autophagy (controlled digestion of cell organelles and membranes.
- Low load exercise to exhaustion can produce the same benefits as high load exercises in terms of muscle protein synthesis (MPS)
- Rest and recovery is critical as markers of muscle injury have been shown to be prolonged and a full week's rest is vital before exercising the same muscle group.

CHAPTER 11

Dangerous Protein

Protein is a very misunderstood and misused macronutrient. A high protein intake is never a good idea for a multitude of reasons. One of the greatest dietary 'sins' is to consume a lot of protein in the belief that this provides a metabolic advantage. The other huge error of judgement is to think a high protein intake is a healthy thing to do. A protein intake beyond your metabolic needs can be a deadly risk. The reasons for this increased risk will be outlined in this chapter.

Many people have a lot of protein because of the scientifically recognised increase in thermogenesis (heat production in the body) caused by this macronutrient after eating, in contrast to carbs or fats. In other words, your body needs to use more energy to metabolise protein than it does for fats and carbohydrates but what people do not know is that this effect is relatively minor in the scheme of things.

If you look at how we use energy in the body, i.e. our total energy expenditure (TEE), then you will see that the thermic effect of **ALL** food is around 10%. Thus, protein is simply a part of this thermic effect percentage. Protein's thermic effect is a relatively small and relatively fixed in comparison to say the NEAT (non-exercise activity thermogenesis) component of exercise that can be significantly increased and can produce a far greater thermic effect than just consuming excess protein.

High protein intakes put the brakes on autophagy

Protein is a significant driver of cellular multiplication through the AMPK/mTOR pathways. Such rampant cell division pressures prevent your body from repairing cellular components and DNA damage, decreasing telomere size, increasing the population of senescent cells in your body and increasing SASP (inflammatory) signalling. Protein has an abundant amount of energy powerful lowering AMPK and powerfully driving up mTORC1 activity through potent anabolic amino acids like L-Leucine. So protein essentially is a powerhouse anabolic (cell-building) macronutrient.

Autophagy ('auto' = self & 'phagy' = eating, so autophagy is self-eating), is a vital function in cells where damaged cellular proteins and organelles like ageing mitochondria are broken down and the nutrients reused by the body. As mentioned previously, autophagy may have been a mechanism that provided an evolutionary advantage in starvation where cell components could be cannibalised for reuse by other cells and organ systems and where damaged cells or cellular components are removed from the system and the components reused for the health of the body as a whole.

mTORC1 signalling is recognised as the most important factor in autophagy (Laplante and Sabatini 2012). mTORC1 is the major switch between anabolic (building) and catabolic (breaking down) processes. If you can suppress mTORC1 signalling, you ramp up autophagy mechanisms. So by eating copious amounts of protein, you are preventing autophagy and allowing crippled cells to accumulate in your body simply and you thus prevent these cells with numerous protein and DNA defects to simply hang in there and perhaps become cancerous. Each cell division may produce a DNA defect, and so these cells are often just one DNA defect away from malignancy. Consuming vast amounts of calories and protein just drives these cells closer and closer towards cancer.

This mTOR inhibition of autophagy adds to the ageing process where muscle, tendon, ligaments, organ systems and other tissues become weaker and less efficient because defective cells and defective cell components just accumulate. How many senior people injure muscles or snap their tendons so easily? They are not being replaced by younger cells through stem cell mobilisation and differentiation or regeneration of those impaired cells. So if you want to look good all your life, this process is happening in your skin as well.

A high protein intake in this light is not a good idea as you can see. Think about large steaks on your plate or those massive hits of protein you have around exercise often 30 grams or more.

Autophagy plays an important part in the cell maintenance phase during famine or fasting signalling when Insulin/IGF-1 signals are low and this almost invariably correlates with low energy and low protein signalling. Intraday fasting as suggested in this book helps your body stay young by promoting autophagy during the fasting period. Intraday fasting lowers mTORC1 signalling and ramps up autophagy.

However, pure protein is not only a source of energy in itself as amino acids can be used for energy production, the amino acids in protein, and in particular the branched-chain amino acids (BCAA's), are potent protein nutrient sensors and stimulatory signals for the mTOR pathway.

Animal protein provides the 'perfect storm' as the energy in this protein source is high due to the combination of a wealth of amino acids, a high-fat content and a rich source of BCAAs that powerfully drive mTOR keeping in mind one of the BCAAs is L-Leucine.

So in animal protein, we have an abundant supply of energy (lots of fat energy to produce ATP and hence low AMPK energy signalling). We also have an abundant supply of amino acids (protein adequacy, mTOR signalling) to drive the AMPK/mTOR pathway into a frenzy of rapidly multiplying cells which is ongoing, unless intakes are reduced through portion control and through intraday fasting a few times a week.

Protein can increase your fat stores! Not an arguable point! It is a reality!

That protein can cause fat gain in an obesogenic society is an important piece of information. It amazes me that protein is rarely discussed as a cause of weight gain as if only carbs or fat increase body fat levels. This myth should be busted!

As I have mentioned, if you think that protein cannot increase fat levels in your body then think again. Maybe, this quote should be printed and placed on the fridge door:

> *"In spite of the exhortation by some popular weight-reducing diets to eat large quantities of protein, it should be remembered that surplus dietary protein can be converted to fat. For protein to be converted to fatty acids and triacylglycerols, the essential precursors for fatty acid synthesis, namely a carbon source, acetyl CoA, and biosynthetic reducing power as NADPH, must be formed." (Salway 2006)* Triacylglycerols is another term for triglycerides.

This particular biochemistry text is used in universities around the world, and one which I have relied upon to understand complex Biochemistry pathways in my post-medical studies in nutritional science. This important quote from an important text is stating: **excessive protein intake can and will increase body fat and worse it can increase your cancer risk if you are under 65 years of age four-fold (4x).**

The fact that young people in the pursuit of body perfection consume vast quantities of protein because their trainers tell them to do so can undermine their goals and put them at great risk of long-term health problems. Pointless shining brightly in your youth and then suffering chronic illness and premature death at a time your career is thriving in your 40's and 50's and when you have a young family depending on you. Why not shine brightly throughout your life by knowing the dietary factors that conspire to put you in an early grave.

Remember, I am a bona fide medical practitioner who has practised medicine at the coalface of primary health care where all the dreadful diseases of society present. Choose the wrong foods, and you pay the price in many ways. Food is not benign! Having a high protein intake while trying to build muscle mass and muscle definition is a contradiction in terms. That any trainer or nutritionist can state have a high protein intake to build muscle mass and look 'cut-up' is oxymoronic advice! Such advice may condemn someone to long-term ill health.

You do not need much protein to achieve your aims; you need an optimal amount of protein for your level of activity and body composition goals. See Appendix 17 & 19 for help at hand. Look closely at Appendix-24 and essential amino acids (EAAs) for exercise.

Protein intakes, insulin levels and leptin

It is becoming more and more apparent that the problem of overweight and obesity is essentially a biochemical problem induced by changes in hormonal signalling inherently triggered by nutrient components.

Insulin/IGF-1 is a major culprit because of the effect it has on the mTOR pathway and how insulin stores and locks fat in your adipose (fat) tissue. Insulin as I have stated also blocks the action of leptin on the hypothalamus in the brain and this stops you from being satisfied as leptin is the satiety hormone saying enough-is-enough – stop eating! What is appreciated is that factors that raise insulin level become problematic when it comes to weight gain. What seems to be very misunderstood is the effect of protein on insulin levels after eating.

There is a marked insulin response to eating protein with amino acids like L-Leucine which is a powerful **insulin secretagogue** (stimulator of insulin secretion) (Newgard 2012). *One of insulin's many actions is to allow amino acids into cells for protein synthesis.*

Of great interest in the Western world is the huge prevalence of prediabetes which is a insulin resistant state. Protein intake is concern because of the insulin increasing effect making matters worse and demanding more insulin from a struggling pancreas. An equal concern is how rich animal and complete proteins are in Branched Chain Amino Acids (BCAAs) which includes Leucine, isoleucine and valine, and these BCAAs may synergise with fatty acids to increase insulin resistance producing higher insulin levels (Newgard 2012). More on BCAAs later.

A high protein intake in an obesogenic society, riddled with prediabetes/insulin resistance, is putting many lives at great risk from a raft of serious disease states.

Choosing an optimal protein intake level

An optimal protein intake, however, is vital for good health. So what type of protein is best for your health and at what level should we be consuming protein? Because of important research, we now know that our age is also a part of the equation in determining protein intake. As I have discussed, animal protein is associated with a higher risk of chronic illness through the various mechanisms outlined, and so you need to consider this in planning your diet and protein intake.

We know that red meat is a carcinogen. 'Feed the man meat' is the type of indoctrination that needs to be erased from the mind. Plant-based sources of protein can provide a wealth of protein and BCAAs. You need to strongly consider your visible protein sources both in type and quantity. There are many plant-based visible sources of protein that could easily be used instead of animal-based protein. Fatty fish is always a good choice regarding visible protein as long as you stick to the portion size mentioned.

About protein needs, you need to slot yourself into one of three groups: Based on the University of Southern California study (Levine, Suarez et al. 2014):

1. Those in the 50 – 65 year age group who had high protein intakes increased their risk of cancer **4-fold** during the following 18 years with a 75% increased mortality risk.

2. Those 65 years of age and over had lower mortality levels when they increased their protein intake due to naturally diminishing body IGF-1 levels and loss of muscle (sarcopenia) at this age and beyond. So from 65 years of age and beyond, you need more protein!

3. All ages had much higher diabetes mortality when protein intakes were high, and in fact, a 5-fold increased risk of mortality. So, not a good idea if you are a pre-diabetic or diabetic and consuming a high protein diet. I discussed the mechanisms of risk above. A high intake of protein is defined as a protein intake beyond that necessary for an individual's weight, age, health and lifestyle factors. An Accredited Practicing Dietitian (APD) is in the best position to guide you. Go to www.a8h.com.au and search for a practitioner who can be of help to you.

Why use 65 years of age as a cut-off point?

A landmark study by Levine et al. was different to existing protein-based research and was very clever in that it looked at age as a factor. This age factor made all the difference in teasing out important factors that determined long-term risk with excessive protein intake. So why choose 65 years of age as the cut-off point? Because at this age, IGF-1 levels and BMI decline significantly. At this age, you begin to lose muscle mass and become weaker and weaker.

As I have mentioned Insulin/IGF-1 are powerful anabolic buddies. So at 65 years of age in most people, this loss of anabolic drive affects organ size, liver and renal function and impairs the function of all cellular and organ systems due to this age-related decline in the anabolic drive. So in this age group, increasing Insulin/IGF-1 is a good thing as we increase mTOR signalling to drive protein synthesis, increase muscle mass, stabilise organ size and increase bone density. We have gone back to being babies in this regard requiring this cellular reproduction and protein synthesis drive.

The dangers of high protein intakes in the pre-diabetic or diabetic

One of the greatest health threats in the Western world, and increasingly in developing countries, is the emergence of prediabetes and diabetes in epidemic proportions. I have mentioned in this book that in Australia, it is estimated that around 16.4% have prediabetes over 25 years of age (Twigg, Kamp, Davis, Neylon, & Flack, 2007). With a population of 24 million people, around 4 million are in a pre-diabetic state.

Prediabetes by definition means that you are somewhere between normal and a full-blown diabetic state. This definition is, however, an artificial and misleading definition as this pre-diabetic state can cause horrendous cumulative damage over time to your vascular system and organ systems like your kidneys and brain. A huge opportunity in preventative medicine is being ignored in this insulin resistant state.

So this figure for prediabetes does not include those with an established diagnosis of diabetes, and this is around 1.5 million people added to this tally of insulin resistance and abnormal glucose metabolism. In fact, there are many undiagnosed people with diabetes, and so this figure could well swell to 3 million people with diabetes or over.

According to the highly respected Garvan Institute of Medical Research in Australia, around 275 people develop diabetes every day! So in total, around 7 million people in Australia have an abnormality with insulin sensitivity and raised glucose levels in the fasting state and postprandially (after-eating). This figure represents a tremendous number of people primed for early disease including many cancers, a high risk for cardiovascular disease and Alzheimer's Disease.

Very little is done about this pre-diabetic state. There is a high probability of reversing this medical problem with diet and lifestyle interventions, and yet the 'experts' argue over whether prediabetes should be considered a disease state and why? Governments are loathed to classify such a huge group as having a medical problem! Once you classify them as having a problem, you now have to pay for all the interventions, tests and medical visits. You can see why this important disease state is neglected, and it all comes down to $$$. How many of these experts would ignore their pre-diabetic states, and if they do, they are not experts are they? They have bought into their propaganda and their early demise.

According to the American Diabetes Association, 29.1 million Americans in 2012 suffered diabetes around 10% of the population and a staggering 25.9% of seniors had diabetes. As I have mentioned previously, more frightening is that 86 million people in the United States of America had prediabetes. There is a high cumulative risk for converting from a pre-diabetic state to overt diabetes over time, and this is a 70% conversion risk according to an American Diabetic Association expert panel (Tabá, Herder, Rathmann, Brunner, & Kivimäk, 2012).

The distinction between prediabetes and diabetes may be a moot point in any case as many studies are showing how devastating prediabetes is regarding cardiovascular risk. This risk is a high 2x increased risk, and this is similar to the risk diabetics face of 2x – 3x the risk of normal individuals acquiring cardiovascular disease (Ford, Zhao et al. 2010). Risk starts at much lower levels of blood glucose than stated by mainstream medicine.

So, the study by Levine et al. showed that there was a tremendous 5-fold risk of increased mortality in people with diabetes with high protein intakes and all probability, this mortality risk extended to pre-diabetics as well. So why does protein cause such a deadly effect in people with diabetes? It is most likely because a pre-diabetic state is one where there is insulin resistance, and the body tries to compensate by forcing the pancreas to secrete greater amounts of insulin to overcome this impaired insulin sensitivity due either to insulin receptor malfunction or post-receptor signalling defects. We are fully aware that protein causes a robust increase in insulin secretion by the pancreas because one of the functions of insulin is to allow amino acids to enter cells for protein synthesis and this ties in with insulin's anabolic effect on the body. Thus, high protein intakes in this group of individuals with diabetes and no doubt prediabetes only tips a struggling pancreas into failure and beta-cell burnout thus hastening the progression from a pre-diabetic state to full-blown diabetes.

You may recall that by the time a pre-diabetic's glucose level rises and has been measured and diagnosed, 30% of their pancreatic beta-cell mass has vanished, and by the time they are diagnosed as a full-blown diabetic, 80% of this beta-cell mass has gone (Rea and Tien 2017)!

Overstimulation of the Insulin/IGF-1 pathway driving mTOR signalling can lead to many diseases of Western civilisations (Melnik, John, & Schmitz, 2011). Not only protein but grains and dairy can increase Insulin/IGF-1 signalling putting you at long-term risk.

So, are you at risk for prediabetes?

You are at high risk for prediabetes or diabetes if you have a family history of the disease. Having just one brother or sister with diabetes increases your risk 4-fold. If you are overweight with abdominal fat and lead a sedentary lifestyle, then you are at increased risk. Anyone in their mid-40's onwards has an increased risk of being pre-diabetic or diabetic. Just taking a look at your waist can tell you if you are at risk of insulin resistance as a large waist circumference is an indicator of insulin resistance as I have discussed. You can now see how significant the risk is with most people in Western worlds and high protein intakes only magnify this risk. Moving away from high animal protein intakes to more plant-based sources can greatly reduce mortality risk (Levine et al., 2014).

Check your blood through standard tests for glucose and fasting insulin levels and better still ask for a **glucose tolerance test (GTT) with insulin checked at all stages of blood collection - an insulin response test.** This test is a great way to see if you are insulin resistant, or if you are pre-diabetic or indeed a full-blown diabetic. Blood glucose levels are a late-stage marker for diabetes. Insulin levels rise much earlier. By doctors only checking glucose and then congratulating you on how good your level is, they are signing your early death warrant. Your doctor can organise this test, but unfortunately, many general practitioners are unaware of the insulin response GTT and may look at you cross-eyed if you request this particular test.

Yet, this insulin response test may just save you from prematurely dying from cardiovascular complications.

Quality protein and well timed

Now you may be anti-soy, anti-dairy, anti-meat and these are your personal choices. I am not a fan of dairy but see tremendous benefit in whey protein esp. whey protein isolate (WPI) because the hormonal danger is removed in the fat that is discarded making WPI a very low-fat protein source. Some people push Whey Protein Concentrates, but this is higher in fat and carbs and lower in protein concentration than WPI and is seen as the poor cousin to WPI.

The higher fat content in WPC may harbour bovine oestrogen. However, like all protein sources, whether this is plant-based or animal-based, it can provide that protein adequacy signal for cell proliferation, and so this is no excuse to overdo it on protein whether plant-based or whey-based.

What is not negotiable is someone not getting an optimal amount of protein in a day with all the required essential amino acids (EAAs) and all the micronutrients they need.

An optimal intake of protein can be difficult indeed if you are a vegan or vegetarian unless you supplement, as plant-based sources are often deficient in many micronutrients needed including Vitamin-

B12, Zinc, Carnosine, Omega-3's, Iron, Taurine and Vitamin-D. These micronutrients are critical for health. So you choose your protein sources but do so with knowledge and a true understanding of the nutritional deficiency dangers you face from your choices.

My feeling is stick to the RDA (RDI) as a baseline from lean, organic white meat such as chicken or turkey, cold water oily fish and whey and you top this off from protein acquired from vegetables, fruit, nuts, seeds, small amounts of legumes and tubers.

The preference now is to avoid red meat due to the cancer potential. I always try to talk people into getting their protein from seafood as much as possible, as seafood is rich not only in quality protein but in essential omega-3 fats and a vast range of micronutrients that include choline, iodine, zinc, Vitamin-B12 Vitamin-D and Vitamin-A. It may be prudent to go lower than the RDA because of the added protein from various sources we do not even consider.

We need to consider our protein intake in the following light:

1. **Visible protein** --- what you know has protein on your plate ---fish, seafood, chicken, meat, meat substitutes, soy protein sources or whey protein you put into a blend or a shaker.

2. **Hidden protein** --- in nuts, seeds, fruits, vegetables, tubers (yams, sweet potato, turnips), grains (rice, wheat, rye, barley, pseudocereals (amaranth, buckwheat, Chia, Quinoa). Dairy can be included here as many people do not consider dairy as a rich source of protein.

It is the hidden protein that can truly blow-out our protein 'budget' and tip you over into protein excess that can, over time lead to ill health and cancer. The amount of protein we consume needs to be dramatically overhauled, because of that hidden and overlooked protein sources.

Just three servings of cooked vegetables (1 ½ cups) provide a little over 3 grams of protein (USDA). It is recommended that around 8-10 servings of vegetables (predominantly) and three servings of fruit is consumed not just the 5 & 2 servings. If we have this intake through the recommended servings of cooked vegetables, salads, nuts and seeds, we will be consuming around 23 grams of extra hidden protein from these food sources. This figure of 23 grams is variable and will depend on your intake of various foods. Only a full dietary analysis will enable you to make a more accurate determination – See Appendix 19.

Determining protein intake based on lean body mass or whole body mass?

How one determines protein intake is a fundamental question and comes down to whether you should determine this based on lean body mass or absolute body weight (Rand, Pellett, & Young, 2003). However, using the lean body mass method may be more appropriate for the younger individual than the older person and why? Because the seniors have a recognised lower level of lean muscle mass and protein utilisation and thus require higher intakes of protein (Rand, Pellett, & Young, 2003).

However, working out lean mass through mathematics (unless you use a DEXA scan), can be confusing for many and too costly to have the scan done for some. Thus sticking to the recognised RDA for the younger adults and a higher intake for the older people makes life that much easier and practical and more likely to be adopted by people and medical practitioners advising their patients.

1. Less than 65 years of age – use 0.80 grams of protein per kg whole body weight minus 23 grams for hidden protein from fruit, vegetables, nuts and seeds.

2. Over 65 years of age – use 1.0 gram of protein per whole body weight and do not subtract the 23 grams of hidden protein from fruit, vegetables, nuts and seeds.

If you add dairy or non-dairy foods, this increases the hidden protein consumed.

Hidden protein sources

The following table outlines an ideal intake of various components, but this can only be a guideline. One of my Dietitian's estimates that the figure of 23 grams could be anywhere between 15 – 20 grams but these figures vary based on the food databases used and the type of foods studied. Protein content may vary from region to region as well due to a range of agricultural practices and climate. Thus getting too fixated is not logical as the composition of food is quite variable with no perfect figure that can be derived. The principle of hidden protein is an important concept in light of the ever-increasing data gathering on the dangers of a high protein intake and especially if this protein is coming from an animal source. Increasing plant-based protein is vital to your health.

Source	Serving	Protein/Serve	Recommended servings
Vegetables –cooked	½ cup	1.27 grams	3 servings = 3.81 grams protein
Vegetables –salad	1 cup	1.72 grams	5 servings (cups) = 8.6 grams protein
Fruit	Medium size	0.47 gram	3 servings = 1.41 grams protein
Nuts (Mixed) Dry roasted	30 grams	5 grams	30 grams nuts per day = 5 grams of protein
Raw pumpkin seeds	15 grams	4 grams	1 serving 15 grams of seeds per day = 4 grams protein. Protein varies between different seeds
Total Protein		**23 grams**	

If you aim to have these foods in the quantities suggested, then you need to take into consideration all this hidden protein and adjust your visible protein intake accordingly. To not do so simply adds to the excesses of food intake and we know protein is fat producing. We are just programmed to have large portion sizes that are unnecessary and dangerous to our long-term health. Dairy should be kept to a minimum regardless, and I prefer people avoid dairy for the reasons outlined in this book.

In the elderly, protein intake needs to be guided by kidney function and what is termed the glomerular filtration rate (GFR) which can be approximated using a simple blood test. The test should also look at blood levels of urea and creatinine to assess kidney function. Excess protein in someone with a diminished kidney function could lead to renal failure.

An interesting thought is that excessive protein and carbohydrate intakes lead to excessive acid loads on the kidneys (see Appendix 9). Over time this excessive renal acid load leads to a loss of muscle mass, organ size and osteoporosis due to the fact your body has to neutralise these acid loads at the kidney by 'robbing' components from bone and muscle to offset this damaging acidity over time. Kidney shrinkage and diminishing renal efficiency is the result. So, at a time you need an increased protein intake, your lifetime dietary mismanagement prevents you from doing so!

Let's see how this pans out for a 70 kg adult

We know that the higher the intake of plant-based foods, the lower your risk for chronic disease and lower mortality rates from all causes. We want to thus consume more plant-based foods beyond the recommended 5 & 2 recommended by government sources -5 servings of vegetables and 2 servings of fruit. The biggest positive impact on your health comes from consuming more vegetables rather than fruit, but fruit also has a raft of phytochemicals and nutrients that are beneficial provided you choose fruit with low fructose levels.

So if we look at say a 70 kg individual, then the recommended serving if we go by the RDI of protein at 0.8 g/Kg of weight, this means that this individual consumes 56 grams of protein daily (70 kg x 0.80 = 56 grams protein). That only 10% of energy should come from protein is suggested (Costill, Wilmore, & Kenney, 2012), and so this seems right.

We still need to that that hidden protein into consideration and so 56g + 23g = 79 grams of protein consumed a day if this hidden protein is not considered making 1.13 grams of protein per kg of wholebody weight. We have overblown our protein budget with the added negative of a powerful protein sufficiency signal on mTOR. All we need then is a powerful energy signal to drive cell multiplication and trigger fat storage. Do Westerners ever have a shortage of food energy? Remember, more protein equals more fat storage in our bodies.

In essence, this individual should be consuming 56 grams minus the protein from the hidden extras of 23 grams, and this leaves 33 grams of **visible** protein from meat, meat substitutes, whey or fish per day which is visible protein on your plate or in a scoop. **This means 11 grams of visible protein per meal x 3 meals in a day or 16.5 grams of visible protein twice daily if you practice two meals in a day with intraday fasting.**

The table that follows gives a guide to the amount of visible protein for various whole body weights. These visible protein portions should be consumed per meal, keeping the number of meals to 2 - 3 meals per day and if one meal is missed in the process of intraday fasting, the next 2 meals should make up the missed protein portion as it does not matter when you consume protein as your body can store and distribute the necessary amino acids to the body as required. Missing a meal does not mean missing out on your protein needs in any given day!

These suggested intakes are for sedentary to moderately active people and not labourers or bodybuilders. If this seems like it is too small an amount of protein, it just shows how modern Western diets have skewed our minds about portion sizes. A multitude of diseases can be traced back to an overconsumption of food and overstimulation of cell reproduction through the AMPK/mTOR pathways in a large majority of people who suffer from these disease states (Cordain, Eades et al. 2003, Melnik, John et al. 2011).

Visible protein portions (under 65's):

Weight	0.8 g protein/kg/day	Minus Hidden grams of protein	Grams visible protein per meal 3 times a day
50 kg	40 g	23 g	6 grams protein per meal
60 kg	48 g	23 g	8.5 grams protein per meal
70 kg	56	23 g	11 grams protein per meal
80 kg	64	23 g	14 grams protein per meal
90 kg	72	23 g	16 grams of protein per meal
100 kg	80	23 g	19 grams of protein per meal
110 kg	88	23 g	22 grams protein per meal

The RDI for females is 0.75 grams of protein/kg/day, and for males, it is 0.84 grams of protein/kg/day. The 0.8 is an average amount. Remember, this suggested visible portion is contingent upon you consuming the valuable foods suggested that have hidden protein. For those over 65, it is easy enough to calculate what you need. Have at least 1 gram per kg of weight so if you weigh 50 kg then you have 50 grams of protein per day. Because those over 65 years of age need extra protein, do not subtract the hidden protein as you need the extra for reasons discussed above.

Using the table on the next page provides a guide. It is an estimate of what 10 grams of visible protein looks like on a plate. Trying to measure food to the gram is always counterproductive as this takes a lot of time and effort and is not sustainable. Being accurate is not necessary and in fact counterproductive. Small protein excesses are never going to be a problem. It is the consistent consumption of high protein intakes day-in and day-out that is problematic and so slightly overdoing protein in any given meal should not be considered such a danger that you need to become fixated or obsessive enough to count every gram. It is far better to have a little bit more than less protein. Many variables determine individual protein needs from genetics to lifestyle, exercise considerations, the microbiome, stress and medications to name some of these. No known infallible algorithm takes into consideration all the factors needed to derive an accurate protein intake --- so why obsess? Who in real life bothers to work out how much protein either visible or hidden is on a plate. This chapter will at least guide you towards a safer level of protein intake without an obsessive approach.

At a practical level, you can keep tabs on your body composition through electronic body composition scales, DEXA assessments at 12-month intervals or more and check waist measurements to see how you are tracking with your food portions. Adjustments may be necessary but what is needed is an easily implemented guide that is practical for everyday food consumption. You can see instantly from the table that 10 grams of visible protein is a very small amount indeed!

I am not a fan of eggs or soy or for that matter mercury-riddled tuna but have just provided a glimpse of the portion size of various foods needed for 10 grams of protein. For those that do not do dairy, do not do meat, do not do legumes and so on, you need to choose foods according to these guidelines. The Activ8Health dietitians can help you in this regard (www.a8h.com.au)

10g Visible Protein Portions

Food	Amount
Baked Beans	200 g (small tin)
Beef, Lamb, Pork (Lean) - cooked	35 grams
Chickpeas	¾ Cup
Chicken, breast tenders, oven roasted	65 grams
Eggs	2 small eggs
Nuts and Seeds	60 grams
Pasta – cooked	300 grams
Perch, dry cooked	55 grams
Quorn (Vegan & Vegetarian Options)	~ 100 grams
Salmon, wild, dry cooked	50 grams
Salmon, canned, 110 grams	½ Can (50 grams)
Sausages (beef, chicken) Chopped	½ Cup
Soy milk	400 ml
Turkey, breast, roasted	35 grams
Trout, Rainbow, dry cooked	50 grams
Tofu, silken, firm & Soy 'meat'	120 grams
Tuna, canned, 100 grams	½ Can (50 grams)
Wholegrain cereal	3 cups (90 grams)
Supplements	
Free Form Amino Acids (EAAs)	10,000 mg (10 grams)
Protein Power (high-protein whey or hydrolysate)	15 – 20 grams (1 Tablespoon)

The myth of food combining

Plant-based protein can suffer from lower levels of some amino acids such as leucine, lysine, methionine and tryptophan (Marsh, Munn, & Baines, 2012).Your body holds onto a pool of essential (indispensable) amino acids to use at times you are not eating (Marsh, Munn et al. 2012), and thus it is a myth for you to have to consume protein at every meal or even to combine proteins to ensure protein adequacy.

Amino acids can be carried to tissues by proteins like serum albumin (Kragh-Hansen 1981), but also in the form of other serum carrier proteins. What is necessary with a plant-based diet is variety. So choose from a wide array of fruits and vegetables and never have the same thing daily and ensure you have a variety of nuts and seeds in a day. It is also interesting that the gut microbiota contains a higher proportion of the branched-chain amino acids (BCAAs) which are essential amino acids. What this suggests is that the microbiome may manufacture these essential amino acids or perhaps prevent their breakdown (Neis, Dejong et al. 2015).

Branched Chain Amino Acids (BCAA's) and Chronic Disease

Of great interest is the consumption of branched-chain amino acids (BCAAs) and the development of insulin resistance and diabetes. In fact, there is a staggering 5-fold increase in diabetes risk with high levels of BCAAs consumed (Neis, Dejong, & Rensen, 2015). This finding ties in with the same level of risk at

5-fold which was also discovered with high protein intakes in diabetics, by Levine et al. in the University of Southern California study (Levine et al., 2014).

Remember, that animal-based protein is rich in essential BCAAs. The BCAAs - **Leucine, Isoleucine and Valine**, are both direct and indirect nutrient signals. They are powerful signalling molecules at mTORC1 (the mTOR pathway), especially L-Leucine but as I have described in this book on feast signalling, this pathway also needs an energy signal like AMPK to drive protein synthesis and cell multiplication. BCAA metabolism may be impaired in obesity, and this can lead to even more accumulation of BCAAs in the body and toxic metabolic intermediates (Yoon, 2016). There is 'crosstalk' between the BCAAs and lipids to produce insulin resistance.

> *"..these findings suggest that chronic elevations in BCAA and related metabolites may synergize with a similar slow rise in circulating fatty acids to drive a state of chronic hyperinsulinemia. This constant secretory pressure on the β cell may ultimately contribute to β cell dysfunction.." (Newgard 2012)*

L-Leucine is a **direct nutrient signal**, and it works to prevent muscle breakdown (catabolism) and to inhibit autophagy (Yoon, 2016). Autophagy to refresh your memory is the process by which damaged components of a cell such as the organelles, damaged cell proteins or cell membranes are broken down for nutrient and protein **recycling** or to ensure removal of damaged cells. By L-Leucine preventing autophagy, it may contribute to damaged cells surviving and hence increasing the risk of cancer states with high protein intakes (Levine et al., 2014). Remember a high L-Leucine amino acid intake is a direct surrogate signal for a high protein intake and along with a high-calorie intake equals a feast signal for cell multiplication at the expense of cell repair mechanisms.

It is tempting to think that animal proteins and plant proteins differ greatly regarding their essential amino acid (EAA) and BCAA levels. An excellent article puts this to rest showing that various sources of animal protein including meat, chicken, herring, eggs and milk versus soy, kidney beans, peas, peanuts, oat and wheat, had very similar levels of EAAs and BCAAs (Gilbert, Bendsen, Tremblay, & Astrup, 2011).

Young gym-goers may be placing themselves at risk by consuming large amounts of BCAAs.

Protein-to-Energy Ratios Count!

Of significant difference is the amino acid content of animal-based proteins versus plant-based proteins and the **protein-to-energy ratios** provided by each protein source. Proteins acquired from animal-based sources have a much higher protein-to-energy ratio than that from plant-based protein sources (Gilbert, Bendsen, Tremblay, & Astrup, 2011). Remember, for feast signalling and rapid cellular multiplication where abnormal cells may form, you need an energy signal and a protein nutrient signal. Animal protein with all that fat and high protein content provides the perfect storm regarding a powerful combined energy and protein adequacy signal for cell multiplication at the expense of cellular maintenance and repair with animal protein having an abundance of BCAAs.

Plants provide the protein signal but not the high energy signal (low AMPK signalling), and this puts the brakes on cell multiplication and feast signalling.

Plant protein - putting the 'brakes' on protein synthesis & feast signalling

According to the Australian government's Nutrient Reference Values for Australia and New Zealand (www.nrv.gov.au): *"all of the necessary amino acids can be provided in the amounts needed from plant sources."*

Plant-based sources of protein, however, are limited in many amino acids such as grains which lack lysine or legumes and soy that lack the sulphur-containing amino acids methionine and cysteine (Gilbert, Bendsen,

Tremblay, & Astrup, 2011). Threonine is lower in cereals in comparison to animal-based products (Young & Pellett, 1994). Even though soy protein is regularly touted as being a complete protein with all the essential amino acids (EAAs) the body needs, the overall EAA content is around 85% lower than milk (Gilbert, Bendsen, Tremblay, & Astrup, 2011).

Having a wide variety of plants, nuts and seeds, enables you to meet your amino acid needs. The very important point with plant-based proteins and the limiting amino acids in plant proteins is that it puts the **'brakes'** on protein synthesis and cell multiplication as the body has to adjust its cellular anabolic and cell reproduction responses to these plant-based amino acid limitations. This slowing down effect of plant-based proteins on the mTOR pathway is vital to optimal health and helps decrease the risk of the vast majority of the chronic disease states that plague the Western world as shown in study after study on vegetable intakes and health. It is in all probability why plant-based protein sources are far superior to animal-based proteins regarding long-term health.

So is one animal protein type better than another?

Each protein has its strengths and weaknesses. It is naïve to think of one animal-based protein source as being better than another because we know from the Levine et al. study that there is increased mortality risk from the consumption of animal protein whether this is from meat, fish, dairy or poultry. The authors stated this was not the risk with plant-based sources of protein.

Factors involved in health risk regarding red meat consumption includes the high protein-to-energy level inherent in animal proteins or the high saturated fat levels that increase lipopolysaccharide (LPS) inflammatory responses even after a single fatty meal. **Heme (also Haem) iron is thought to be a risk for bowel cancer in red meat.**

With dairy as a protein source, the risk is in the GI-Insulin Dissociation where disproportionally high Insulin/IGF-1 levels occur in relation to the relatively small carbohydrate content of the dairy food. The oestrogen content of milk may also be hazardous to hormone-sensitive organs like the breast and prostate.

Fish intake cannot be seen as safe in comparison to red meat but may be relatively safer due to the higher omega-3 level and lower protein-to-energy ratio plus lower L-Carnitine levels in comparison to red meat (see below). Omega-3 levels in fish is a great positive to use fish as a protein source. However, omega-3 content will depend upon the type of fish consumed as it is the small, oily fish that have a high omega-3 level, not the white fish like Perch, Dory or Barramundi that people usually consume.

We must not forget that we have polluted oceans where large fish like tuna or shark are riddled with highly toxic compounds like mercury or dioxins and other biohazards. A large portion of fish cannot be considered a good thing as you increase both protein-energy and branched-chain amino acid (BCAA) intakes. Keep protein portion sizes down at all times regarding animal protein irrespective of the type of animal protein being consumed.

Grains and legumes as a protein source? Not a good idea!

Trying to get your protein intake from grains whether these are whole grains or not or legumes, means you will be consuming a high carbohydrate load. This high carb intake increases the effects of glycation on the body and produce Advanced Glycation Endproducts (AGEs) postprandially (after-eating). The high carb load also stimulates a high Insulin/IGF-1 response driving the mTOR pathway if you try to get your protein needs just from grains or legumes.

Another inconvenient truth

For those who love their red meat, the news is getting more and more grimmer by the minute. Red meat includes **beef, veal, pork, lamb and mutton**. A study published in the British Medical Journal in 2017 was one of the largest of its kind including data from over half a million people in America, aged 50 to 71 years involving more than 7.5 million American person-years of observation (Godlee 2017). This study revealed that there was a 26% increased risk of premature death in those who consumed the most red meat. In fact, mortality from nine different diseases was increased as a result of red meat consumption.

Heme (or haem) iron it seems is a major culprit in cancer risk, but other risks described below also matter. One paper noted the incredibly important association between red meat consumption and the major killers currently so common in society, and this includes an 11% increased risk for stroke, 11% increased risk for breast cancer, 15% increased risk for cardiovascular mortality, 17% increased risk for colorectal cancer. Colorectal or bowel cancer seems to be increasing in incidence in younger adults and 19% for advanced prostate cancer (Wolk 2016). These figures were for the consumption of 100 grams per day of **unprocessed red meat** with risk starting at 50 grams per day.

The risk of disease with red meat consumption is staggering. Just looking at just one disease state and then using that percentage to approximate how many lives can be saved in any given year by avoiding red meat consumption is a sobering thought.

How many of you reading this book know of someone who died from breast cancer or bowel or prostate cancer or died from a heart attack or stroke? Red meat could be seen as a weapon of mass destruction (WMD) killing vast numbers in the population, but with every paper that comes out that highlights the risk, the industry muddy's the waters by getting in their 'big guns' to produce research that sheds a positive spin on red meat consumption.

Gullible and ill-informed government members will have the hood pulled over their eyes or perhaps they ignore these frightening statistics because of bias or that warm and fuzzy feeling of eating a dead animal as they have done through their lives. Even more cynical, is the thought of allowing these disease states to flourish and increase in incidence all because of keeping an industry alive because it provides jobs and props up export dollars at the expense of human lives.

It is up to you to view these concerns being put forward by highly credible researchers and published in some of the best medical journals on the planet. Avoiding red meat in childhood may just slash rates of cardiovascular disease in adulthood. Remember the casualties of the Korean and Vietnam wars discussed in the chapter on postprandial effects. These young men fought in the pre fast-food era where 77% of these casualties had advanced vascular disease at the age of 22 years? The staples of their diet included – red meat, dairy and grain-based foods. Smoking would have hastened the effects.

Our ancestors ate meat at most once a week (Godlee 2017), because hunting and killing animals was a dangerous task that also involved huge energy expenditure. Red meat consumption in our society is vastly different to our ancestors because red meat is so readily available and overconsumption is the norm.

Of importance, the 2017 study showed that replacing the consumption volume of red meat with white meat such as chicken, turkey or fish decreased all-cause mortality risk. So there are choices, but many studies are pointing in the direction of consuming more plant-based protein choices. The Activ8Health system indicates to do just this and if you have animal meat, to keep the visible portion to that calculated in the book and to consume a high plant-based diet that provides a wealth of non-animal protein in your diet. My advice is to avoid red meat and stick to the white meat alternatives at the Activ8Health recommended intakes.

'Red meat consumption is linked to higher risk of death from most major causes'

Medscape published a review of an article with the title above which was also in the BMJ authored by Zosia Kmietowicz - BMJ 2017; 357 doi: https://doi.org/10.1136/bmj.j2241 (Published 10 May 2017). Medscape is a web-based resource for medical practitioners and professionals and publishes peer-reviewed articles for the medical profession online. The Medscape review is at (http://www.medscape.com/viewarticle/880662). Registration is necessary.

Data from 537,000 individuals aged 50 – 71 was examined and what was found was that people, who ate the most red meat, had a: *'26 percent higher odds than those who ate the least of dying from a variety of causes.'*

Of interest in this same study was the fact that those who ate mostly white meat that included poultry and fish *'were 25% less likely to die of all causes during the study period.'*

The numbers involved in this study were massive, and many other large studies have shown similar findings. It is pointless waiting for more and more research to come out condemning red meat for you to make your mind up that this form of food should be avoided. No food is essential. However, micronutrients are essential for optimal health and if you can't get zinc or Vitamin-B12 because you are avoiding red meat, you can get an abundant amount of these micronutrients from fish like sardines where 3.74 times the RDA for Vitamin-B12 can be obtained by consuming just 100 grams of sardines including 11% of the RDA of highly bioavailable zinc ((USDA).

Supplementation is not a dirty word as I have often mentioned in this book. Supplements can be used to 'fill-in-the-gaps' irrespective of the highly right-wing views of so-called 'experts' who dramatically highlight the "risks" of supplementation but are absolutely silent on the dramatic real and tangible risks of consuming whole foods like red meat.

High protein intakes and bodybuilding

The concern in bodybuilders and gym goers is that they not only consume a large amount of protein but also take supplements like essential amino acids and BCAAs. It is also interesting that there may not be a problem with higher intakes of protein or EAAs/BCAAs in healthy but **actively exercising** individuals (Campbell et al., 2007). It may be because dedicated protein synthesis is occurring in muscles, tendons, ligaments and bone due to the intensity of the exercise consuming these amino acids. Amino acids are thus being diverted to this purpose and not to generalised mTOR pathway stimulation affecting cellular reproduction in other organ systems. It is interesting that the phosphate content of protein food may negate the bone losing effects of the higher protein intake (Campbell et al., 2007).

The key words above are "actively exercising", and this means **regular intense exercises**. For those who visit gyms or exercise less intensely and less frequently, the intake of food, protein and BCAAs may be a long-term hazard. What about someone who decreases the intensity of exercise but continues using the same quantity of protein or amino acids? Young men may wax and wane about exercise but still maintains their protein or BCAA intakes in their downtimes in the belief that these nutritional components will stimulate protein synthesis when not exercising. This strategy is not wise!

Bone is significantly affected by weight-bearing exercises resulting in bone building. Around 50% of bone is made up of protein (Type-1 Collagen), and thus bone becomes a 'sink' for amino acids being consumed by the actively exercising individual – once again the operative words are **actively exercising individuals**. High protein intakes or high EAA/BCAA consumption may not be too good for a sick bodybuilder that may be suffering from prediabetes or diabetes, remember the 5-fold increased mortality risk with high protein consumption in this subgroup of people (Levine et al., 2014). The subtle long-term effects of these extreme diets on those who intensely exercise are not well studied. Most research focuses on the adverse outcomes of anabolic steroid use rather than the side-effects of nutrient overconsumption. Once food, in general, is seen to have toxic, cumulative and long-term effects, only then will these subtleties be investigated fully.

L-Carnitine, TMAO and cardiovascular risk

Here is another nail in the coffin for animal-based protein. A beautifully designed and well-executed study on L-Carnitine was carried out on meat eaters and a vegan who was happy to eat meat for the cause of research. L-Carnitine is an amino acid involved in the metabolism of long-chain fatty acids in the mitochondria to extract energy from these lipids. About 75% of L-Carnitine can be obtained from food or biosynthesis can occur from the amino acids lysine and methionine (Steiber, Kerner, & Hoppel, 2004). L-Carnitine is found predominantly in animal protein products, but smaller amounts are found in fruit and vegetables as well. Cooked steak, for example, has 525 umol of carnitine per 100g of meat whereas avocado has 4 umol/100g and asparagus and cauliflower have around 8 umol/100 grams of food (Steiber, Kerner, & Hoppel, 2004). The amounts in milligrams are below.

L-Carnitine is a trimethylamine compound that in meat eaters is altered to trimethylamine-N-oxide (TMAO) which is a pro-atherogenic compound - an arterial plaque promoter, leading to vascular disease as shown in mice studies. This conversion to TMAO occurs due to specific gut microbes that colonise the bowel in omnivores. Providing L-Carnitine to a vegan produced negligible blood TMAO levels initially, but animal studies have shown chronic L-Carnitine ingestion alters gut flora with increasing levels of TMAO produced as a result of **continued** meat consumption.

Vegans and Vegetarians have been consistently shown to have low L-Carnitine blood levels, and this is undoubtedly one mechanism that protects them from cardiovascular disease. High TMAO levels prevent reverse cholesterol transport (Koeth et al., 2013) leading to atherosclerosis which in turn leads to heart attacks or strokes or peripheral vascular disease.

This research was important because it was long thought that the saturated fat component of meat was the culprit in atherosclerosis but meta-analyses did not seem to back this up. We now have an entirely different mechanism that can produce vascular disease from animal protein through L-Carnitine, not saturated fat. What this study also reinforces is the tremendous capacity of the bowel organisms to adapt to changes in diet for the better or worse regarding long-term health. Fine-tune your meal composition, based on knowledge to minimise long-term health risk.

The concern is the use of L-Carnitine supplements by gym goers or by individuals wanting to augment 'fat-burning'. It is important to note that choline found in lecithin is a trimethylamine containing compound is an essential nutrient, and it is vital you have this daily. However, you should limit lecithin consumption to 1 teaspoon (5 grams) per day only. I have discussed choline metabolism in this book, and it may be wise to revise this section in the light of this knowledge on TMAO production.

Protein Source	TMAO Level^ (mg)
Beef	80
Pork	24
Milk (whole)	8
Fish (Cod)	5
Chicken Breast	3
Avocado	2
Asparagus (6 spears)	0.2
^ http://lpi.oregonstate.edu/mic/dietary-factors/L-carnitine	

This level of L-Carnitine in meat versus plant-based sources may be an important reason for the difference in cardiovascular disease between the two groups and perhaps provides a guide as to which protein sources need to be avoided for cardiovascular health.

Animal protein intake and weight gain, weight re-gain, amino acid oxidation

High protein intakes are probably the reason why many people fail regarding dietary attempts to lose weight. Not limiting protein intake during acute weight loss dietary programs and during maintenance phases, adds to the increased risk of chronic disease and fat gain or regain, if appropriate intakes of protein are not factored in. Consuming too much protein from animal sources only results in significant amino acid oxidation which means the amino acids are burnt off as energy or used to create other compounds like fat. Studies found that a 95% increase in amino acid oxidation occurred when the protein source was an animal in origin (Westerterp-Plantenga et al., 2006).

It makes no sense to use an expensive protein source such as meat, poultry or fish for energy (oxidation). There are far less expensive dietary sources of energy in cheap carbs or fats/oils. You want just enough protein for protein synthesis in your body and amino acids in protein diverted for the creation of neurotransmitters, hormones, signalling molecules or antioxidants as needed by the body. You do not want to use protein for energy – it is a waste!

Protein Leverage

There are many other considerations regarding protein intake levels. The 'Protein Leverage' hypothesis is an important one to consider. That protein is critical to life and thus prioritised in energy intakes has been studied as a cause of overweight and obesity in society. If protein intakes or amino acids are deficient in any diet, then there is a drive to over consume to meet the protein or amino acid requirements of the organism. The authors of one study on protein leverage, stated that if the level of protein in the diet was 10% or less of total calories, then the intake of food needed to offset this i.e. the amount of food you would need to eat to get all the amino acids necessary to maintain life

"may not be physically feasible." (Gosby, Conigrave, Raubenheimer, & Simpson, 2014)

What is the maximum amount of protein the body can use?

From sophisticated studies on amino acid utilisation in the body, it is stated that the maximum amount of protein that can be utilised in the body is 1.7 g/kg body weight (Wilmore, Costill, & Kenney, 2008). This figure is an important ceiling for bodybuilders, and it is pointless going beyond this ceiling as study after study has shown greater amino acid oxidation beyond this intake. Protein, as stated above, is a very expensive macronutrient to be used as just fuel for energy.

Above this ceiling of 1.7g/kg body weight, amino acids are burnt off as energy and not utilised for protein synthesis. Excessive protein may cause a strain on the kidney as many people in society may be pre-diabetic or diabetic or have hypertension, and these disease states can damage the kidneys, greatly making them susceptible to high protein intakes. This ceiling of 1.7g/kg body weight has been shown time and again in many studies as the upper limit for anyone including bodybuilders, and yet you see time and again, recommendations that go way beyond this upper limit for muscle building.

Most people just need the RDA for protein intake as recommended in this book and to use EAAs before, during and after exercise.

Professor Louise Burke is a highly respected Australian sports nutritionist stated that:

> *"10-20 of a good-quality protein seems the ideal size of a protein recovery snack. There is substantial increase in protein synthesis with a 10g protein serve, but the response seems to level out at 20-25 grams. In fact, more than 25 g of protein will lead to increased use of protein as a fuel source which negates the purpose of consuming protein" (Burke, Cox, & Deakes, 2010) .*

In a 2009 study by a few of the most published authors in exercise physiology such as Mark A Tarnopolsky, and Stuart M Phillips tried to find the optimal dose of protein needed for protein synthesis post-exercise. They stated:

> *"We report that increasing protein intake stimulates mixed-muscle and plasma albumin protein synthesis in a dose-dependent manner up to 20 g dietary protein, after which there is a marked stimulation of whole-body leucine oxidation and no further increase in protein synthesis" (Moore et al., 2009)*

Eggs - are these a good choice of protein?

The eggs in Western supermarkets are a far cry from free-range hens wandering around in the wild consuming a variety of wild nuts, seeds, insects, worms and other organic matter they come across. Chickens like humans are thus omnivores and not vegans! Cage fed hens or even commercial free-range chickens are fed grains – so chickens are forced to be vegans.

These grains are the source of omega-6's which are pro-inflammatory essential fatty acids. The adage is 'you are what you eat' and thus if the food intake is skewed towards an overconsumption of grain foods with poor micronutrient bioavailability and a high omega-6 content, then guess what? The yolks in eggs are going to be rich in omega-6, and arachidonic acid, the precursor to all the inflammatory eicosanoids (see Appendix 2). The micronutrient content of that egg will suffer as well.

Dr J. David Spence wrote an important letter to the editor of the journal Circulation (Spence 2002).. Dr Spence is the director of the Stroke Prevention & Atherosclerosis Research Centre (SPARC) located in the Robarts Research Institute, Canada. Dr Spence stated that egg yolk increases LDL by about 10% but what is not recognized or stated in all the media presses and advertising about eggs, is that **egg yolks increase oxidised-LDL (OxLDL) by 34%.**

Oxidised-LDL is very damaging to the lining of your arteries as it seeps under the blood vessel lining to increase inflammation in this location and can activate enzymes that can cause rupture of vascular plaque and even cause death (apoptosis) of the cells lining the blood vessels increasing risk of more and more damage to the blood vessel lining called the endothelium (endothelial dysfunction).

Dr Artemis Simopoulos is a founding member of the International Society for the Study of Fatty Acids and Lipids (ISSFAL) and president of the Centre for Genetics, Nutrition and Health, in Washington DC. She carried out a study on the difference between eggs from chickens from the island of Crete that ate an omnivorous diet that included worms and insects and also included plants like purslane versus eggs from supermarkets from hens fed grains. It is interesting that Purslane is a plant that is rich in alpha-linolenic acid (ALA) a short chain omega-3 essential fatty acid that can be converted into long-chain omega-3 essential fatty acids like EPA and DHA compounds found in high concentrations in cold water fish and krill oils. So these island hens had a varied diet of highly nutritious food. It is not surprising that this food intake was reflected in the nutritional composition of the yolk.

Simopoulos found a staggering difference between the eggs from Crete and supermarket eggs and one major difference was the omega-6 to omega-3 ratio. This study showed a whopping omega-6 to Omega-3 ratio of 19.54 which means 19.54 more omega-6's than omega-3's in supermarket eggs compared to the Greek egg which had an almost equal level of omega-6's to omega-3's (Simopoulos & Sidossis, 2000).

Omega-3 eggs are now increasingly available in supermarkets, and the yolks are higher in omega-3 essential fatty acids and the reason for this is that the hens are fed flaxseed (linseed) instead of cereal grains. Flaxseed is rich in alpha-linolenic acid (ALA), and this changes the character of the essential fatty acid composition in egg yolks.

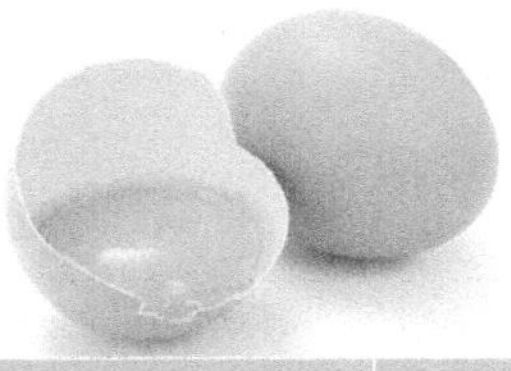

Fatty Acid Composition	Greek Egg (mg)	Supermarket Egg (mg)
Total Omega-6	23.02	33.81
Total Omega-3	17.66	1.73
Omega-6/Omega-3	1.3	19.54

Simopoulos, A. P., & Sidossis, L. (2000). What is so special about the traditional diet of Greece. *Mediterranean Diets. World Rev Nutr Diet, 87*, 24-42.

Eggs and cancer risk

Many large-scale studies have shown distinct associations between egg intake levels and cancer risk. In a prospective study, 27,607 individuals were followed up to assess the link between egg consumption and prostate cancer incidence between 1994-2008. They studied men without prostate cancer who then went on to having distant cancer spread or died of prostate cancer. What was stated was something unbelievable and the conclusion was:

> *"Men who consumed 2.5 or more eggs per week had an 81% increased risk of lethal prostate cancer compared with men who consumed less than 0.5 eggs per week (Richman, Kenfield, Stampfer, Giovannucci, & Chan, 2011)"*

The authors went on to state:

> *"In conclusion, consumption of eggs may increase risk of developing a lethal form of prostate cancer among healthy men."*

Please note the term 'healthy' men and this would have to be of concern to every man reading this. No matter where you go in restaurants, cafes or clubs - eggs seem to be in many of the choices on the menu or in the sauces. Eggs are a Sunday staple with people loving their scrambled eggs on toast or eggs Benedict. These traditions are so entrenched in the West so the feeling is how can the consumption of eggs be problematic? Eggs are promoted as being healthy, and many men consume eggs every day. Look at the statement above. We are talking about 2.5 eggs a week not 7 or 10 or more eggs a week the egg board would love you to have.

The risk from eggs may be coming from the very high omega-6 intake from the yolks or perhaps from hormones or other growth factors yet to be discovered in eggs.

It is doubtful that much research will go into finding what the killer factor is in eggs because of powerful lobby groups and yet if we could find this factor or factors, it could be the saviour of the industry as this factor (or factors) involved could potentially be removed through genetic modification which in this case would save countless millions of lives. Anything bad for the prostate will in all probability be bad for female breasts as these two glandular tissues respond to very similar hormonal signals and other influences.

Likewise, a study from Uruguay showed a significant risk of a multitude of cancers including breast, prostate, colorectal, pharynx, oropharyngeal cancers and aerodigestive tracts (lips, mouth, upper oesophagus, nose, tongue, throat, vocal cords and trachea) through the higher intake of eggs (Aune et al., 2009).

It is an absolute credit to independent researchers like these who look for risk irrespective of commercial concerns to help save lives. Are eggs essential to your life? Absolutely not! You can get all the nutrients from other sources including supplementation. Our taste, preference and traditional practices all drive our consumption so how silly is it to think a food like eggs could be dangerous to our health? People's eyes need to be opened, and I have written this book for this very purpose.

Harvard University's School of Public Health states:

> *"While a 2008 report from the Physicians' Health Study supports the idea that eating an egg a day is generally safe for the heart, it also suggests that going much beyond that could increase the risk for heart failure later in life."(https://www.hsph.harvard.edu/nutritionsource/eggs/)*

The Nurses' Health Study and Health Professionals Follow-up Study also showed a higher cardiovascular risk in those with diabetes, and if this is the case, then this would almost certainly apply to the millions of additional people with prediabetes.

This Harvard statement is at odds with the statement by Richman et al.

Whey protein

Whey has many advantages in that it is rapidly absorbed. It is a complete protein containing all the essential amino acids (EAAs) and is high the branched-chain amino acids (BCAAs) that include L-Leucine a powerful driver of protein synthesis through mTOR signalling. There is a high concentration of cysteine in whey, and this is a sulphur containing amino acid that is associated with higher cellular glutathione levels. Glutathione is a powerful antioxidant generated by the body.

Indeed, whey is a dairy product, and the concern is whether whey has the disadvantage of the high oestrogen concentration found in milk especially in the last trimester of the cow's pregnancy. For one thing, steroid hormones like oestrogen are highly lipophilic (Zambito 2007). Both free oestrone and oestrone sulphate (US sulfate), are highly bound to fat with free oestrone markedly lower in low-fat milk. Estimate of free oestrone bound to fat range from 55% - 80%. (Macrina, Ott et al. 2012) Lipophilic means that a molecule is 'fat-loving' and transported in fat molecules.

It is important to be aware that the sex hormones like oestrogen and testosterone are formed from the fatty substance cholesterol, which is water insoluble. So hormones are fat-based compounds but also carried by proteins and lipoproteins. Whey protein isolate (WPI) is very low in fat and thus low in hormones as the fat these hormones love to cling to (hydrophilic compounds), have been discarded leaving the WPI powder with a very high protein content of 90% or higher (Hoffman and Falvo 2004).

It is not the dose but the effect

As an aside, there are so many articles out there that vehemently state that bovine oestrogen or IGF-1 levels are so low in dairy that they could not possibly cause problems. Dairy is unlikely by itself to trigger cancer, but it may help pull the trigger along with other factors in place. Most things in life are multifactorial, and a single cause is highly unlikely. Dairy is 100% not essential for you to live as every component thought to be valuable like calcium can be found abundantly in other foods. It is up to you whether you want to take the risk and continue a food that is not essential to your life. The concentration of a hormone regarding end-effects on cells or organs is irrelevant as hormones are amazingly powerful compounds that affect cell systems far greater than their weight or volume. Infinitesimally small amounts in our systems pack an enormous punch (Cone, 2012).

It is thus extremely naïve to defend dairy based on absolute levels of these hormones. We need to as well, consider exposures to the hormones in dairy at vulnerable times of human development in a foetus or the very young with rapidly multiplying cells during the process of growth or in people who have existing pre-cancerous cells. Deleterious effects based on timing in a developing human and epigenetic imprinting is rarely even considered in research, and only history will shed light on this ignorance. No doubt denizens of this future planet will look back historically in disbelief at how we took food for granted and accepted dietary norms without question. Epigenetic priming can occur early in life and may only take effect later in life. The research as it stands is a very blunt instrument that is not able to tease out these complex long-term possibilities. Oestrogen in whey is extremely low and well below the body's intrinsic production of this hormone even in men.

Whey and the Incretin Effect

Back to whey. Most of the fat is removed along with the steroid hormones, in a high-grade whey protein isolate (WPI). Not to say that you can consume vast amounts of whey protein as whey can also produce a robust Insulin/IGF-1 response in your body after consuming it.

In fact, whey has a powerful incretin effect as well. The two known incretins thus far are glucagon-like peptide 1 (GLP-1) and glucose-dependent insulinotropic polypeptide (GIP) that can powerfully increase insulin release from the pancreas. Both of these incretins can be broken down by the enzyme dipeptidyl peptidase-4 (DPP4), and pharmaceutical companies have created DPP4 inhibitors to allow the action of the incretins on the pancreas to produce insulin, and this is beneficial to people with diabetes who suffer from diminishing insulin production.

In fact, whey protein can increase GLP-1 production by a staggering 298% (Jakubowicz et al., 2014).

Whey also has the potential if consumed before a meal, to lower after eating glucose levels. A highly significant 28% reduction in after-eating blood glucose level has been observed with a uniform reduction early and late in the postprandial (after-eating) period (Jakubowicz et al., 2014). By keeping glucose levels down, you decrease postprandial (after-eating) glycation of body proteins as has been discussed in this book and by doing so, you prevent the ageing effect of glucose.

Whey has also been shown to suppress appetite powerfully. The incretins slow down nutrient absorption by decreasing stomach emptying thus slowing down the effects of food after eating. Incretins promote satiety i.e. a sense of fullness. Through such a large surge in GLP-1, you can see how protective whey protein is in so many ways, provided that you do not consume more than is necessary.

However, whey has an advantage in the post-exercise period where your body is craving amino acids for cell growth, and if you want to maximise protein synthesis and increase lean muscle mass, then this high Insulin/IGF-1 response is a great advantage after exercise. However, do not overdo it!

After periods of fasting, your body also craves glucose and amino acids, and this is the case in the mornings where you have fasted in your sleep overnight. The amount of whey you would use has been calculated in this chapter based on your weight and the protein acquired from hidden protein in fruits, vegetables, nuts and seeds.

Whey is a double-edged sword. It is rich in the branched-chain amino acids (BCAAs), and as you have just discovered BCAAs may have disadvantages in those with prediabetes or diabetes. BCAAs are, however, important signalling molecules for protein synthesis. Remember, protein is not evil as we need this for a multitude number of reasons. Where protein becomes evil is when we consume vast quantities beyond our optimal intakes, and this is the downfall of Western diets and overconsumption attitudes – if a little is good, then a lot must be so much better. Not!

Whey protein has a high sulphur-containing amino acid component as I have touched upon and in fact an almost 4-fold increased level of the sulphur-containing amino acid cysteine. Cysteine is an important precursor molecule for glutathione one of the major antioxidants produced in the body to fight off free-radicals generated from food intake and the various metabolic processes. So whey can abundantly provide the necessary building block for glutathione synthesis that protects your cells from oxidative stress.

Whey has been shown to provide a calorie restriction type effect on the body through various mechanisms.

The rich BCAA component has been shown in animal studies to increase mitochondrial biogenesis (new mitochondria being formed) keeping in mind your energy levels and muscle function depend upon the mitochondria being able to supply your body with ATP the driving force for cell metabolism (D'Antona et al., 2010). Please see Appendix-10. Not all whey proteins are equal with many formulations having artificial sweeteners, flavourings or high sugar levels and not all are from grass-fed cows or of high grade. It is important that the whey you use is organic and pesticide, herbicide and hormone free. It is the Wild West out there in terms of supplementation, but honourable manufacturers do exist, and practitioner-only products also exist that are of high quality.

For those wanting to watch their calories, there is a distinct alternative, and this is the Essential Amino Acid (EAA) power that can be used before, during and after exercise to stimulate protein synthesis throughout the gym session without adding calories to the mix. In fact, if you have enough EAAs that contain 3 – 4 grams of L-Leucine in the amount used (10-12 grams of whole EAAs), then this provides a complete postprandial (after-eating) protein stimulus comparable to eating a protein containing meal (Norton and Wilson 2009).

Remember though, EAAs do not contain all the other micronutrients provided by fruits, vegetables and other plant and animal proteins. Thus you should think about using EAAs in the Peri-Exercise period. See Appendix-20

KEY POINTS

- Protein is eaten to excess and is problematic
- Protein can be converted to fat and this is an incontrovertible biochemical fact – hidden protein needs to be taken into consideration
- Protein also produces a high insulin response after eating
- High protein intakes are associated with a 4-fold increased risk of cancer in those under 65 years of age.
- There is an upper limit of around 25 grams of protein per meal
- An upper limit of 1.7 grams per kg of body weight is a ceiling
- Some proteins are associated with cancer as shown with eggs or dairy
- Whey is over 90% protein, rich in BCAAs and Cysteine
- Whey, does not have the high energy to protein to fat ratio
- 3 – 4 grams of L-Leucine provides the anabolic stimulus of a full meal
- All proteins can cause harm if consumed beyond that which is necessary
- Plant protein sources have a lower energy to protein ratio thus decreasing the risk of driving AMPK/mTOR pathways
- L-Carnitine can lead to TMAO increasing the risk of heart disease. Red meat is rich in L-Carnitine and plant sources are very low in this compound
- Plant protein sources decrease the risk of cancer
- Choose lean proteins and grass-fed forms
- Choose cold water, oily fish for their omega-3 content as a protein source as often as you can

CHAPTER 12

Antioxidants

A recent estimate of the number of human cells in the body is 37.2 trillion cells (Bianconi et al., 2013). Now, each cell could have between $10^3 - 10^4$ (1000 to 10,000) mitochondria (Milo and Phillips 2015). Thus, the mitochondrial numbers in the human body is a colossal $37.2^{12} \times 10^3 = 37.2^{15}$ in all our cells. Just taking the lower figure of 10^3 mitochondria per cell, we have an astronomical figure of one quadrillion mitochondria (1,000,000,000,000,000 mitochondria), in the human body give or take a few hundred million.

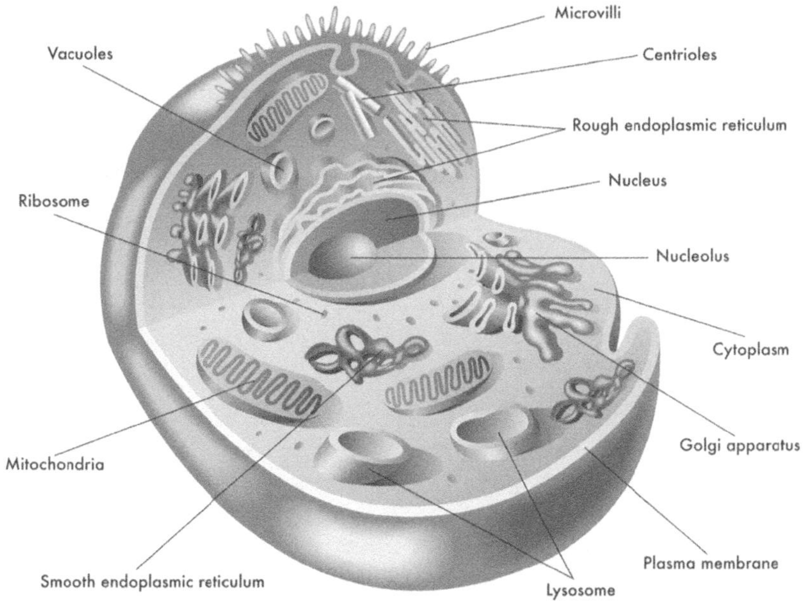

The mitochondria are the amazing powerhouses of cells that are essentially factories for converting food to energy. Mitochondria extract the energy in food and drive this extracted energy towards the production of adenosine triphosphate (ATP), the currency of energy in cells that enables muscle contraction, allowing you to move parts of your body or to blink an eye. Cells requiring a lot of energy (ATP) function have more mitochondria like skeletal muscle, liver and heart cells.

ATP energy drives protein synthesis and a myriad number of other cellular reactions. This was discussed in the chapter on the AMPK/mTOR pathway topic. Along the inner membrane, the mitochondria have what is called the **respiratory chain** or **electron transport chain,** and it is the flow of electrons and **redox (electron exchange) reactions** along this chain through a series of protein complexes that extracts the energy in food and then traps it in ATP for use by our cells. The graphic is of a cross-section of a human cell, and this shows the mitochondria sitting in the cytoplasm of the cell along with some other cellular organelles as they are known, such as the Golgi apparatus or Lysosomes with each organelle having a particular function in a cell. Remember, mitochondria in individual cells could number thousands.

Free Radicals & Reactive Oxygen Species (ROS)

In the process of extracting energy from food to produce ATP, both free radicals and reactive oxygen species (ROS) are produced in the mitochondrial electron transport chain within some 'leaky' areas in this chain. Free radicals are released in copious numbers predominantly at Complex-1 and Complex-III in the electron transport chain (respiratory chain) and this free-radical leakiness is now widely accepted (Guarente 2008, Pamplona and Barja 2006). Ubiquinone (CoQ10) is also a major site of free radical generation within the chain (Scientific American 2006).

If these free radicals are not quenched (neutralised), they can damage the mitochondria themselves and cellular structures like the other organelles shown in the previous graphic around them.

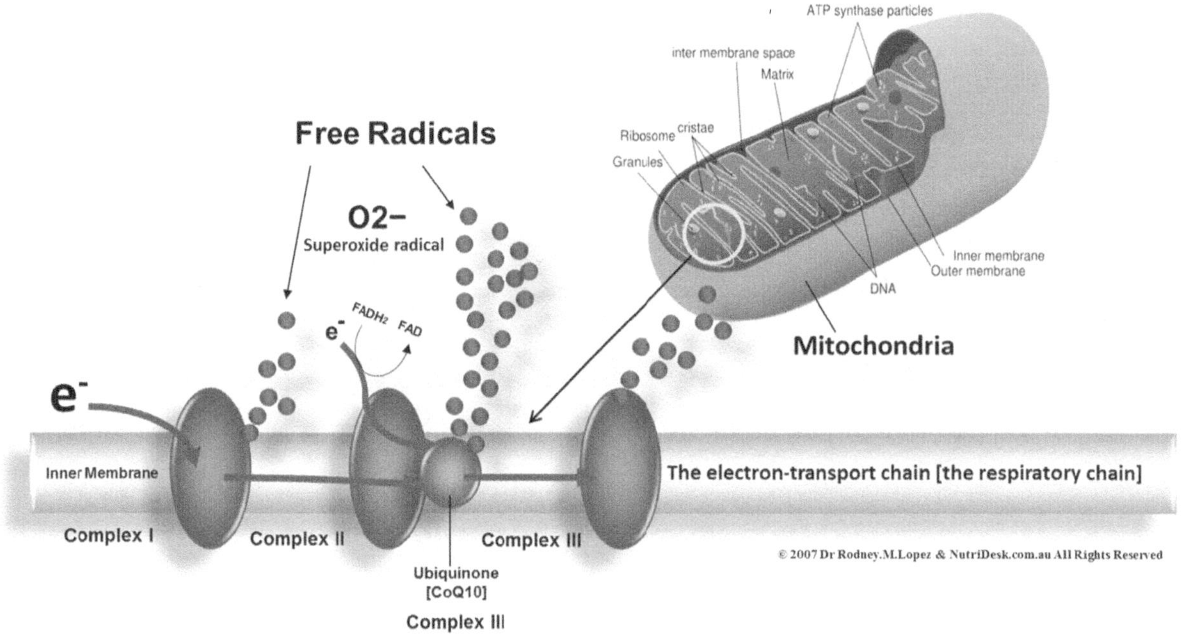

www.a8h.com.au

Many other toxic Reactive Oxygen Species (ROS) are also produced during this energy extraction and capture process and mostly produced by the reactions in the electron transport chain shown above in its partial form. These damaging compounds include the **Superoxide Anion, Hydrogen Peroxide, Hydroxyl Ion and Hydroxyl Radical and Peroxide.** These compounds are damaging to biological tissues, and for this reason, your body generates enzymes like Superoxide Dismutase (SOD) that can convert two Superoxide Anions to hydrogen peroxide and oxygen, and Catalase an enzyme that can convert Hydrogen Peroxide to water and oxygen.

Glutathione: Priming intrinsic antioxidant systems

Glutathione is a selenium-containing antioxidant enzyme that requires the Sulphur group attached to cysteine an amino acid. Whey interestingly is a protein rich in cysteine. Glutathione is arguably the most important antioxidant in the human body and is generated in vast quantities as required by human cells to quench all those free radicals and reactive oxygen species and helps your body get rid of heavy metals. An excellent way to prime your body to dampen down these damaging compounds is to ensure you have enough glutathione in your body by supplying the Sulphur containing amino acid cysteine through the use of N-Acetyl Cysteine (NAC) twice daily (See Appendix-7).

It is hard to change a toxic world to a non-toxic one but what you can do is ensure your body has all the micronutrients including Cysteine to help fight off damaging compounds through the biotransformation processes in the liver and at the level of the cell in various organs.

Let's take a look at the rates of production of various free radicals and reactive oxygen species (ROS's). Table 1.3 in the text 'Molecular Basis of Oxidative Stress: Chemistry, Mechanisms and Disease Pathogenesis (Villamena, 2013), these rates show the amazingly high production of free radicals (rate constants) per second for over 50 reactive species at normal conditions. Many of these had rates in the 10^{10} range **per second** which is 10 billion free radicals produced per second, and this is just one free radical. About hydrogen peroxide, a free radical in the body there is an amazing fact. According to the text 'Robbins Basic Pathology' describing the action of catalase an enzyme that breaks down hydrogen peroxide, the author states:

> *"It is one of the most active enzymes known, capable of degrading millions of molecules of H2O2 per second (Kumar, Abbas, & Aster, 2012)."*

So we can see that the production of free radicals and reactive oxygen species is produced and degraded at a staggering rate per second let alone per minute, per hour or per day. Over your lifetime, this load of free radicals and ROS achieves astronomical proportions and takes its deadly toll on your cells, tissues and the organ systems housing those cells and tissues to produce a range of age-related illnesses.

These free radicals also have to be dealt with by the body's intrinsic antioxidant systems which include enzymes like catalase, glutathione generating enzymes, superoxide dismutase (SOD) and others. **A total load of these toxic particles depends on the quantity and quality of the food you eat and how much free radical and ROS relief you give your cells through fasting periods.**

Keeping portion sizes of food small means far less postprandial and metabolic activity thus decreasing your load of free electrons and ROS with each smaller meal. Adding antioxidant-rich foods such as multi-coloured vegetables and fruits to each meal also means you can quench far more of these damaging compounds simply through your food choices. Smaller nutrient-dense meals versus nutrient-poor, energy-dense meals will mean far less cellular damage through decreased free radical and ROS production.

Your mitochondria are an absolute hive of intense activity that waxes and wanes with every meal you have. In the postprandial (after-eating) state, free radicals are produced in vast amounts. Without the right nutritional resources to support your body's own (innate) antioxidant systems, the damage will occur to the mitochondria themselves and all the cellular organelles, tissues and organs. Charged electrons cause a cascade of reactions throughout the cells and tissues in your body.

Meal composition determines how great a free-radical 'hit' you experience

What you put on your plate determines how massive a postprandial (after-eating) load you are placing in your body regarding oxidative stress created by free electrons and charged molecules like ROS as a result of what you have just eaten. Each meal produces an oxidative stress 'hit' to a lesser or greater extent depending on what you consume regarding quality and quantity of food.

The higher the spikes of blood glucose, triglycerides and amino acids in the blood after eating, the higher the number of free radicals generated due to the extraction of energy from food and all the metabolic processes that are stimulated after eating such as protein synthesis.

Decrease free radical and ROS damage by keeping protein levels down to RDI as discussed. Do not have a high dietary carbohydrate or fat load per meal. Ensure each meal you are consuming is rich in plant-based phytochemicals, antioxidants and micronutrients that support intrinsic antioxidant systems. Glutathione production is supported by N-Acetyl Cysteine (NAC) and high cysteine foods like whey or other sulphur donors. Ensuring omega-3 and micronutrient adequacy will limit inflammatory processes caused by food. A quality multivitamin is an insurance policy that will help support antioxidant synthesis and biotransformation pathways. An efficient biotransformation (detoxification) system rids yourself of endogenous and exogenous toxicities that could otherwise generate copious amounts of free radicals and ROS.

Having a phytochemical-rich juice post-meal or even a small amount of whey protein before a meal can be helpful to increase phytochemical and antioxidant availability when the body is trying to deal with an onslaught of damaging metabolic end-products like the free radicals and ROS's that are killing you incrementally and in a cumulative way over your lifetime.

Intraday fasting helps by keeping this cumulative meal-induced oxidative stress load lower in your lifetime by simply decreasing the number of meal 'hits'. I share with you what I think is a wonderful phytochemical blend in Appendix-4 that is practical in that the components are readily available in many juicing outlets in any city or suburb around the world.

Please ensure you keep damaging fructose levels as low as possible in these blends as I have discussed in Appendix-4. This is essentially a vegetable juice blend with a very small amount of low-fructose fruit NOT the other way around.

Are free-radicals good or bad or both?

Free radicals are indeed associated with many pathologies such as cancer or cardiovascular disease but may also stimulate repair mechanisms in the body. I am hoping you see that a lack of any given micronutrient in the body pretty well interferes with a chain of metabolic events to create significant collateral damage in biochemical pathways because oxidative stress cannot be dealt with effectively. That clinical medicine pays such scant attention to micronutrient deficiencies in acute and chronic disease states stuns me as any acute or chronic illness requires far more nutritional resources for repair processes in healing. Outcomes could be many times better if physicians gave this some thought from the outset in treating all patients in an outpatient or hospital setting.

A simple multivitamin and multimineral capsule with an advanced formulation of mineral chelates and active B-Complex vitamins may be all it would take along with a nice tasting phytochemical blend on a daily basis to produce positive clinical outcomes. Such a cheap solution could save countless millions of lives over the years. The simplicity of this approach supports the tremendous complexity of biochemical and molecular systems that depend on these micronutrients to function. It would be highly unlikely for a physician to provide a highly detailed biochemical or molecular picture of action of even one vitamin or mineral. What is seen as a simple solution has unimaginable complexity!

In the chapter on micronutrients in this book, I discussed the emerging concerns of soil degradation, crop micronutrient insufficiencies, climate change concerns on micronutrients and the fact that Western populations have large numbers of people that are overweight or obese, and this seems to sit at around 6 in 10 individuals in Western populations with increasing obesity rates in developing nations. The concept of being overfed and yet undernourished is important and Western diets are supplying a tremendous amount of energy in food but little in the way of nutrient, fibre and phytochemical density. Free radical and ROS production in these overweight/obese individuals may create significant cellular and tissue damage and this damage to proteins and organ systems, in turn, elicit further free-radical responses creating a vicious cycle of damaging effects.

All of this due to vast quantities of energy eaten with poor antioxidant support caused by micronutrient deficiencies that impair antioxidant systems in the body.

Some flawed studies on antioxidants

An article in Scientific American titled 'The Myth of Antioxidants' (Moyer, 2013) used Beta-Carotene, Vitamin-A and E studies to back up the notion that antioxidants are a myth. Two influential studies were:

1. The 1996 Beta-Carotene and Retinol Efficacy Trial (CARET), showed a significantly increased incidence of lung cancers in smokers with Beta-Carotene supplementation.

2. The Alpha-Tocopherol Beta-Carotene (ATBC) Cancer prevention trial

In both the ATBC and CARET trials, the use of Beta-Carotene supplements increased lung cancer risk by 16% after 6 years in the ATBC trial and by 28% after 4 years in the CARET trial. However, it is important to point out the age groups in these two trials were from 50 – 74 years of age and in the CARET trial, there were heavy smokers included, with asbestos exposure. Thus these were very high-risk individuals for lung cancer, and often there are precancerous lesions or even overt cancers that are being attacked and suppressed by the body's intrinsic immune system locked in a precarious existential balance on a knife-edge in the body.

These immune system attacks on existing abnormal cells involve an attack on these atypical cells through increased oxidative stress and free radical generation used as a weapon against these cells. Thus giving an antioxidant such as Beta-Carotene in high doses is essentially pulling the rug from under the body's defence mechanism at the wrong time in high-risk individuals. Another instance of a timing flaw. Could Beta-Carotene prove protective if given long before the heavy exposures of smoking took their cellular toll over decades and where those changes were allowed to reach a point of no return? (Qiao, Dawsey et al. 2009)

In fact, the Linxian, China study which had a younger cohort than the ATBC/CARET studies found that 'Factor D' which was a combination of 50 µ g selenium, 30 mg vitamin E, and 15 mg Beta-Carotene, given to 29,584 adult participants:

> "*...led to decreased mortality from all causes, cancer overall, and gastric cancer.*"
>
> In fact, Qiao et al. stated: *"The beneficial effects of selenium, vitamin E, and Beta-Carotene on mortality were still evident up to 10 years after the cessation of supplementation and were consistently greater in younger participants." (Qiao, Dawsey et al. 2009)*

The timing of treatments is one huge missing link in such research projects, but the naïve in the medical and dietetics world jump on these findings blindly by reading the punchlines without truly appreciating that nutritional modalities of treatment are not the same as instantaneous pharmacological responses. Nutritional interventions require well-timed interventions (hopefully lifelong) that are long-term preventative strategies and not acute sledgehammer pharmaceutical interventions that target single or multiple molecular mechanisms. We need to keep in mind that such highly targeted drug interventions often have upstream or downstream damaging molecular effects that can lead to serious side-effects because the molecular consequences are like the grid analogy I mentioned in the chapter under 'Micronutrients in health and disease'. If you affect one track, you can have an impact on multiple tracks in the grid that intersects the affected one perhaps leading to gridlock. The term 'gridlock' being a metaphor for cellular or organ failure.

Even today, 'experts' still use this flawed Beta-Carotene trial to hammer home the 'dangers' of supplementation preventing individuals from using effective nutraceuticals that are 62,000 times less dangerous than pharmaceutical interventions and yet hold great promise regarding preventative health benefits.

Even in the CARET study, in the placebo arm where no Beta-Carotene was given in supplement form, those with the highest intake of fruit and vegetables had the lowest risk of lung cancer (Neuhouser, Patterson et al. 2003).

So why did the Beta-Carotene supplemented group fare badly?

As indicated, free-radical damage can also be beneficial when the body is trying to attack a pathogen like a virus or bacteria invading you or to get rid of defective cells or cancerous cells. It is why Oncologists do not like cancer sufferers taking any antioxidants before radiation therapy as the radiation causes inflammation and oxidative (free radical) stress to tumours and the antioxidants can diminish this inflammatory response, thus decreasing the therapeutic effect.

Importantly, Beta-Carotene belongs to a class of carotenoids that includes over 750 pigment compounds. Many of these carotenoids obviously work in synergy, and by using a heavy dose of one carotenoid, you will saturate the carotenoid receptors and signalling pathways by this one carotenoid when supplemented in high doses thus excluding the effects of other synergistic carotenoids that may be important for end-target effects and positive outcomes.

So trying to apply nutrients in a pharmacological sense to highly advanced disease in aged populations with a naturally high risk of cancer is doomed to failure but perhaps they were hoping for a miracle because fruit and vegetables have time and again shown how protective they are in preventing (not treating) cancer. These nutritional effects work if they are started young enough and carried through to your senior years. Nutritional surveys in Western populations have consistently shown that vegetable and fruit intake is dreadfully low in those populations. The diet proposed in this book focuses on vegetables mainly and some fruit to ensure your body has high levels of a wide range of phytochemicals.

Phytochemicals and hormesis

A clinical review published in the British Medical Journal (BMJ) titled 'Diet and the prevention of cancer', stated that up to 80% of bowel and breast cancer could be prevented by dietary measures (Cummings & Bingham, 1998). Isn't this a staggering figure and yet if a pharmaceutical could provide even a fraction of this effect, it would make headline news! These are the two most common cancers in a society that everyone fears as they age and yet, it is in his or her power to control through dietary measures.

There are thousands of phytochemicals produced by plants and incorporated in the leaves, stems, seeds, grains, pseudo-grains and nuts for functional purposes. Some of these phytochemicals are defensive compounds that protect the plant from ultraviolet light; others are virucides (protection against viruses) or bactericides (protection against bacteria). Other compounds like phytates bind to minerals so that animals (like us) or insects and microbes cannot use the minerals for their benefit as I have discussed earlier.

These plant chemicals are bioactive but not essential. In saying this, it is difficult to tease out the exact nature of how these phytochemicals act in protecting the body from harm, as the synergistic action and multiple signalling molecules generated by these chemicals are tremendously complex to evaluate, and yet we know how important they are in preventing disease in our bodies.

What we have discovered from the CARET and ATBC trials, is that thousands of plant chemicals are consumed through our diets and these chemicals have an action at the level of DNA through epigenetic mechanisms that turn genes on or off or through secondary messengers, or stimulation of **Antioxidant Response Elements (ARE's)** in the DNA.

Plant chemicals in high doses may produce toxic results as in the Beta-Carotene trials, but smaller doses may produce desirable actions through hormesis.

What is Hormesis?

Hormesis is essentially a cellular stress response to toxic plant chemical compounds (phytochemicals) that may be either beneficial or harmful in a dose-dependent way.

Our bodies have adapted to these plant chemical 'insults' over our evolutionary development. In the graph that follows, you can see that there is a 'sweet-spot' of phytochemical benefit and to go just beyond this peak, produces a dramatic drop in health value to the body. It can then rapidly dip to harmful levels.

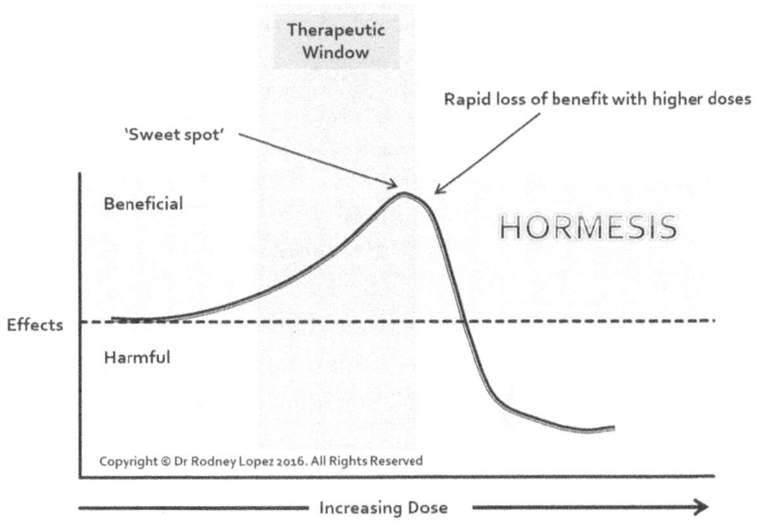

What does this have to do with meal composition and how can this hormesis effect cause harm to you from your dietary choices? From this graph, it tells you that having large amounts of any single plant food could have detrimental effects. The problem with people is that they stick to the same foods day-in and day-out rarely changing them. They may also like one type of food and then have this in large amounts on a daily basis. Such eating habits could easily result in harmful phytochemical effects because there is no **wash-out phase** where that food is avoided for a day or two. Being able to wash-out accumulating phytochemicals that may have an adverse effect in the body is one reason why you are also told to eat seasonal foods.

Signalling molecules have been established for hormesis

The cellular signalling mechanisms for hormesis is now understood, and these involve enzymes such as kinases, deacetylases, Nrf-2 and NF-kB. What distinguishes the hormetic effect of phytochemicals versus pharmaceuticals or high dose nutraceuticals is the strength of the action.

With hormesis, the effect is a 'gentle tap' on the DNA to produce an effect and not a sledgehammer coming down on a relatively small number of genetic determinants. You are constantly taking in a wide range of these phytochemicals daily (hopefully) allowing the multitudinous number of plant chemicals to produce a constant gentle coaxing of the DNA to trigger beneficial gene interactions.

Hormesis is a stress response, and the cell adapts to this stress by producing antioxidants, protein chaperones, growth factors and Phase-II biotransformation responses along with a myriad number of other cellular repair mechanisms like dampening down mTOR signalling or ramping up FoxO.

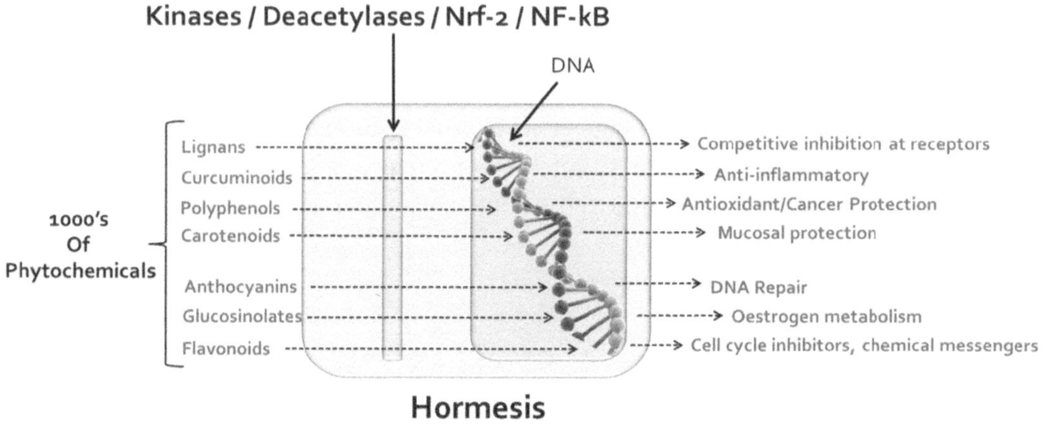

Hopefully, you can see now how you can ensure your body is in a constant healing state by dramatically reducing the energy signal (high AMP, the spent 'bullets' keeping AMPK high) and by keeping protein intakes optimal and not high thus decreasing mTOR signalling and to this you can add consuming a large number of phytochemicals through vegetables and low-fructose fruit through juices, salads, phytochemical blends, soups but remembering to rotate those foods and include more exotic and seasonal varieties to add great diversity to your diet. It is important to remember that diversity of foods not only provides a wash-out strategy by constantly changing the foods consumed, they also increase the bowel microbiome diversity which strengthens your immune system, and this diversity of foods has the added advantage of introducing a range of beneficial phytochemicals to your cells and organ systems. Poor phytochemical intake and diversity adds to the burden of disease and hastens the deterioration and demise of an individual.

Meal planning is at the centre of these wonderful dietary effects and well within your power to control. Having high-energy foods that are nutrient and phytochemical poor is a recipe for disaster. In the intraday fasting intervals when you are not eating, you can always have a vegetable and low-fructose fruit juice with an emphasis on the vegetable component (Appendix 4) to top-up your phytochemical intake and eat low-calorie vegetables mainly and some fruit as a crudité plate.

Even though juicing does not have the fibre of a blend, it has great phytochemical complexity and hormesis boosting power during your working day. I have no idea why this is regarded as a poor choice by dietetic experts because we are after the phytochemicals from these fruits and vegetables for their hormetic effects. With the Activ8Health diets, you are getting a wealth of fibre from blends, salads and vegetables, nuts and seeds. Juicing (or blending) also has the benefit of disrupting the plant matrix to release the carotenoids and improve nutrient bioavailability (Yeum & Russell, 2002).

The Cytochrome-P450 (Cyp450) detoxification enzyme system

The major detoxification (biotransformation) system in our bodies is through the cytochrome-p450 (CYP450) enzyme system, and these clever and amazingly versatile enzymes are found abundantly in the liver but also in the gastrointestinal tract (GIT). These are a family of enzymes that number just 57 (Redlich et al., 2008). Thus these small number of enzymes have to biotransform (detoxify) a huge number of endogenous toxic compounds, i.e. compounds generated by your own body and they need to biotransform every exogenous compound your body comes across from the environment. Just think of the countless thousands of chemicals that exist and the new ones emerging that your body has to deal with every second of the day.

Think of those colourings, food additives, herbicides or pesticides in or on your food and those plastic materials that leach from food packing into what you consume especially if you heat food in plastic containers, that whiff of petrol as you pour petrol into your car at the bowser and all those toxic fumes some inhale in those road tunnels as they drive through with their car windows wide open. All these toxicities have to be dealt with by these 57 CYP450 enzymes.

We are also surrounded by a haze of pollution in cities every day and your home can be highly toxic from insect sprays, artificial leather lounges, polyester carpets and household fragrances or perfumes (phthalates). Let's not forget toxic work exposures and heavy metals in our food such as mercury or cadmium in large fish like tuna. These are just a few of the enormous number of toxic exposures we encounter every day of our lives that have to be detoxified by our CYP450 enzyme system and our antioxidant systems.

CYP450 Enzymes - Versatile but Slow

These 57 enzymes are amazingly versatile but very slow. They ironically convert these toxic compounds into even more toxic compounds in Phase-I reactions that can accumulate in your liver. It is the next phase (the Phase-II part of biotransformation) that will whisk away these Phase-1 'hyper-toxic' compounds to more benign compounds and then excrete them through your kidneys, faeces or biliary system. Unless Phase-II reactions are fast and effective, your body suffers the effects of these toxic Phase-1 compounds accumulating.

It is like a race where the baton is transferred from one runner to another or one phase to the next. If the baton fails to be passed effectively, the race is hindered or lost. Losing means long-term chronic ill health or cancer.

Meal composition is so vital to this CYP450 system. Making sure an adequate intake of micronutrients and phytochemicals enables an efficient Phase-II detoxification system because a Vitamin-B6, B12 or Folic Acid deficiency could result in lower levels of glutathione that can affect this system or very low protein intakes could affect the supply of amino acids like cysteine or glycine that are important in Phase-II reactions.

Accumulation of toxic compounds in this system generates a huge oxidative stress load with all those free radicals and ROS being produced by the Phase-I and II processes to damage not only the liver but the body as a whole – think multiple tracks in the grid being affected leading to 'gridlock' and liver failure or cancer. This imbalance in the Phase-I and Phase-II biotransformation system is how your liver suffers damage and progresses through a fatty liver stage to cirrhosis of the liver due to a chronic poor supply of micronutrients and antioxidants that include Choline from lecithin, necessary to make this system efficient and to rid your body of toxic compounds effectively. A low intake of choline accelerates liver damage, and choline was discussed under the chapter on micronutrients.

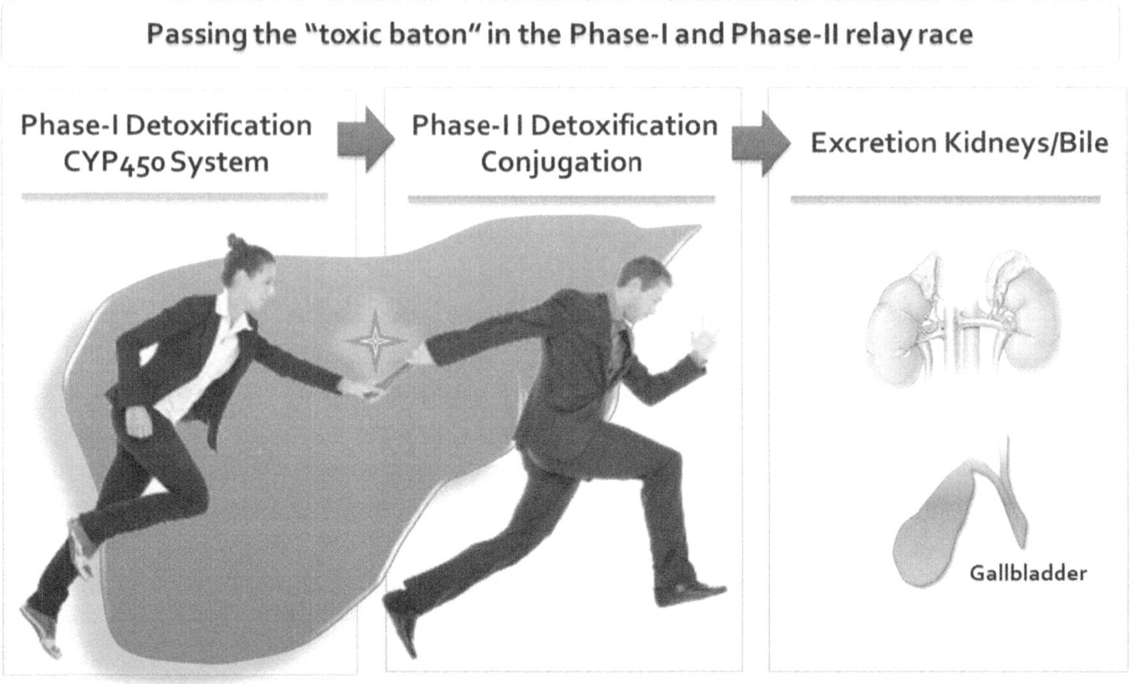

Phytochemicals can powerfully affect the CYP450 enzyme systems by either stimulating (inducing) these enzymes or inhibiting them. These powerful effects are evident when you consider the interactions of certain plant chemicals and drug interactions. One such powerful interaction is that of the furanocoumarins in grapefruit that inhibit CYP34A a particular isoform of the CYP450 system. This interaction is stated in drug information leaflets for particular pharmaceuticals if there is a known interaction of the drug with grapefruit. See Appendix-6 for a more detailed presentation of this system.

That this phytochemical compound in grapefruit can so powerfully affect the CYP450 system to the point of creating dangerous pharmaceutical effects should be proof enough of the powerful and amazing effects of phytochemicals and hormesis in general to your health. As long as we do not overdo it with any particular phytochemical compound by varying our food and not letting them accumulate to toxic levels in our bodies you can enjoy the health benefits of these amazing plant chemicals.

The important point with this system and phytochemicals is that we all have numerous mutations of these CYP450 enzymes and as a result, we may not be able to convert some of these toxic hormetic compounds efficiently, and so they may accumulate rapidly in our bodies. Some of these mutations are discovered in nutrigenomic (genetic) testing. See Appendix-22.

So rotate, rotate, and rotate your foods

As I have mentioned, you may easily dismiss these toxic effects. You may just think you are stressed or getting older or any other excuse for why you do not feel quite right. Such toxic build-ups may affect your mood or make you feel lethargic. By ensuring you take the time to add diversity of vegetables and fruit in every meal to maximise phytochemical intake, and then ensure that if you have certain plant foods on a particular day that you avoid those plants on the next 1 - 2 days, you should be able to enjoy the amazing hormesis benefits of phytochemicals, but avoid the toxicities by not allowing accumulation to occur.

There are around 10 million Single Nucleotide Polymorphisms (SNPs) in the human genome (NLM 2017), so this means you have every likelihood of having multiple SNPs in the CYP450 system that may put you at risk. With such a tremendous variety of vegetables and fruit available all year round, and all those wonderful seasonal foods out there, why would anyone have the same things day-in and day-out? The diversity of food intake is key!

10 Servings of Fruit and Vegetables Ideal

A large and impressive study undertaken by the Department of Epidemiology and Biostatistics at the Imperial College London conducted a systematic review and meta-analysis of 95 studies and 142 publications. This study was published in the International Journal of Epidemiology in 2017 and looked at the association of fruit and vegetable intake and the risk of cardiovascular disease, cancer and all-cause mortality (Aune, Giovannucci et al. 2016).

The findings are vitally important for public and global health outcomes. Reductions in risk for cardiovascular disease and all-cause mortality were seen in a dose-dependent manner, and the lowest risk for these clinical endpoints was seen at 800 grams of fruit and vegetables (10 servings), and for cancer, it was 600 grams (6 servings) with no greater benefit in terms of cancer reduction beyond 6 servings. The reduction in risk was simply staggering with the authors stating that:

> *"There was a 8–16% reduction in the RR of coronary heart disease, 13–18% reduction in the RR of stroke, 8–13% reduction in the RR of cardiovascular disease, 3–4% reduction in the RR of total cancer and 10–15% reduction in the RR of all-cause mortality for each 200 g/day increment in intake of fruit, vegetables, and fruit and vegetables combined." RR = Relative Risk*

If you look at this statement, those percentage reductions are for every 2.5 servings of vegetables, and this is so achievable through juicing, blending, salads, soups and every dish that can incorporate fruit and vegetables. It was also estimated that 5.6 and 7.8 million premature deaths worldwide in 2013 were attributable to fruit and vegetable intakes below 500 g/day and 800 g/day respectively (Aune, Giovannucci et al. 2016).

Have that low fructose juice mentioned in Appendix 4 or that Activ8Health Plan-A Blended Meal in Appendix 13 for breakfast and ensure you pile on the multi-coloured salad on your plate and not the starchy carbs for the phytochemical content.

Excess Fructose: Fructose > Glucose	**High Fructose Load > 3g/Serving**	**Balanced Glucose/Fructose (Less likely to cause symptoms)**
Apple, pear, guava,, mango, nashi fruit, honeydew melon, pawpaw/papaya, quince, star fruit (carambola), Fructose powder Corn Syrup High fructose corn syrup Fruit concentrates	Dried fruit, fruit pastes such as tomato paste, chutney, sauces, fruit juices, fruits with a high sugar content (apple, pear, lychee, grapes, persimmon, cherries). Also coconut cream or milk, fruit bars, honey, agave syrup If wanting to have a low fructose load, have the equivalent of 1 serving of fruit at any time including blends, solid meals (1 medium sized piece of fruit or 2 small sized pieces of fruit such as an apricot)	**Berries:** Blueberry, blackberry, strawberry, raspberry, boysenberry, cranberry **Stone Fruit:** Peach, plum, nectarines, apricot (sorbitol in these may create symptoms in those with irritable bowel syndrome – IBS) **Citrus fruit:** Lemon, lime, mandarin, grapefruit, tangelo, orange, kumquat **Others:** Kiwi, passionfruit, pineapple, tamarillo, rhubarb, jackfruit, ripe banana **Low fructose vegetables:** Avocado, cucumber, Chinese cabbage, green pea, common lettuce, mushroom, parsnip, broccoli, celeriac, pumpkin (butternut), spinach, zucchini, snowpea, zucchini, endive, asparagus

Important: Fructose intolerance can cause irritable bowel symptoms (IBS) and this occurs when there is an imbalance in the concentration of fructose over glucose. However, keeping fructose levels at a low intake is wise due to the glycating effects and uric acid increasing effect of fructose and its association with insulin resistance.
Reference: (Shepherd and Gibson 2006); (Women's and Children's Health Network 2012)

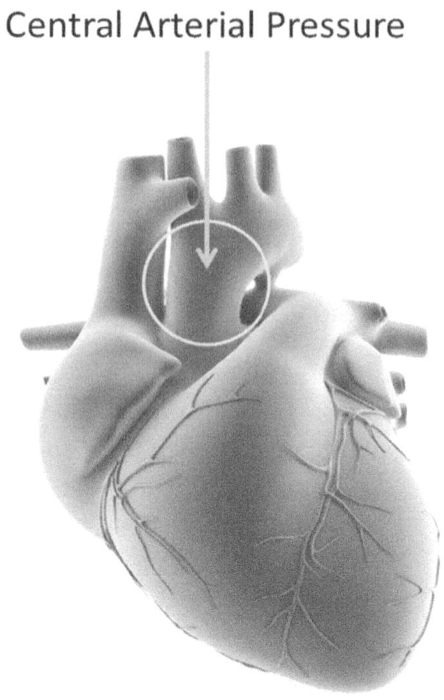

The authors mentioned fruit juice in these associations but a word of caution. Fruit juice is rich in fructose, and this can be counterproductive, and the findings may have been even more impressive if fructose was kept to a minimum.

Fructose is around 7-times more glycating (protein-damaging) than glucose and just one (x1) glass of fruit juice increased the risk of central hypertension as shown in an Australian study at Swinburne University (Pase, Grima et al. 2015). The authors stated:

> *"Central systolic BP was 3–4 mmHg higher for those who consumed fruit juice daily rather than rarely or occasionally. In conclusion, more frequent fruit juice consumption was associated with higher central BPs." (Pase, Grima et al. 2015)* ***BP = Blood Pressure***

What the researchers found was that regular fruit juice consumption was associated with higher central blood pressures and this central blood pressure is that measured in the very large artery called the aorta near the heart. Central blood pressure is a better predictor of cardiovascular and renal (kidney) outcomes than brachial (arm) blood pressure which is the usual type of blood pressure measured in a doctor's office or using electronic home blood pressure machines.

So the greatest benefit of high servings of fruit and vegetables will come from a high intake of vegetables and not fruit.

Keeping fruit intake down to around three servings and 7 – 10 servings of vegetables is prudent in light of the Swinburne University findings. People have a very sweet tooth, and when you see someone ordering a fruit and vegetable juice it is always packed with pineapple, apples, oranges and anything else sweet they can throw in and yet they think that what they are doing is healthy.

Watermelon is a great exception as this has a high-glycemic-index of around 70 which makes it sound very bad but it has a low carbohydrate (fructose) level and so this is an excellent watery choice that will give your juice a nice taste without the damaging effect of fructose and watermelon is high in Citrulline which can be converted to L-Arginine an amino acid that is used for the production of nitric oxide (NO) which causes blood vessel dilation and a good NO level is correlated with good vascular health.

Like anything, do not overdo it on the watermelon but keep this down to around ½ a cup in quantity in your juice. Appendix-4 provides good choices that are commonly available in juicing outlets. See Appendix-21 for additional concerns about fructose.

Fruit (100g)	Fructose (g)	Total Carbs (g)
Watermelon	3.36	7.55
Apple	6.03	12.76
Pear	6.23	15.46
Pineapple	2.12	13.12
Orange	3.17	11.75
USDA Nutrient Database		

So you can see that out of the common fruits available for juicing in many outlets, watermelon has a low fructose load in comparison to the total carbohydrate load. Pineapples and oranges may look good regarding free fructose but look at the higher total carbs per 100g of fruit.

CHAPTER 13

The Human Microbiome

The amazing complexity and importance of all the microorganisms that live in or on you

The human microbiome consists of all the organisms that are in or on your body, and these include bacteria, viruses, fungi, parasites and bacteriophages. The organisms that reside only within your bowel are called the bowel microbiota or gut microbiome. We, as humans can consider us to be 'Superorganisms' as we essentially have two genomes (two sets of genes) with one human genome and the other genome coming from all your associated and environmentally acquired microorganisms.

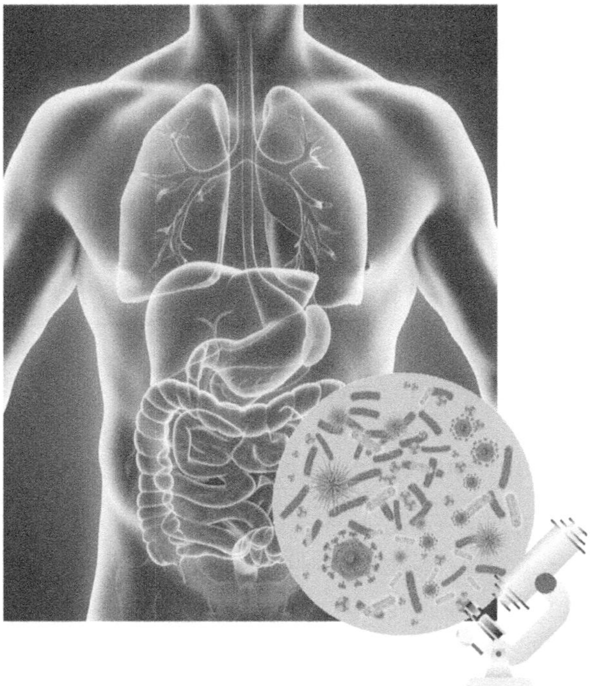

The concept of the **optimally functional hologenome** then, is that these two (human & microbe) genomes have to work together in a harmonious and tightly integrated way to ensure we stay healthy throughout our lives.

The term ***holobiont*** is used to describe different species of organisms living together in synergy as **one ecological unit.**

The human genome numbers around 25,000 genes and yet the environmentally acquired human microbiome numbers around 1 million genes or over (Lal 2011). An amazing 40 times more microorganism genes than human genes.

We have always considered microbial 'bugs' as being bad, but we are essentially a hybrid of human cells and microorganisms that are living in symbiotic harmony for the most part. We need to view these organisms not as a threat but as allies and to consider the host-microbe relationship as a whole to work out how best to manipulate these organisms to provide optimal health outcomes and the best way to repair microbial colonies damaged by the use of antibiotics, poor dietary habits or environmental toxicities.

These organisms start to colonise your skin and bowel from birth drawing mainly from the vaginal microflora of the mother including any faecal matter present at the time of delivery. The anus being anatomically so close to the vagina is perhaps designed for such microbial transfer to a newborn during, and soon after delivery. These early infant gut microbial colonisers are nourished by complex **Human Milk Oligosaccharides (HMO's)** in breast milk, that are not digested by the infant but by the infant's gut bacteria. So mother nature has evolved to ensure these organisms have a firm foothold in the bowel soon after birth, with special compounds secreted in breast milk, that have also evolved to support them nutritionally. If this is not an evolutionary statement of how important these gut microbiotas are, then what is?

There are an estimated 100 trillion organisms just in the bowel (Spector, 2015). The number of human cells has just been calculated and revised to be 37.2 trillion (Bianconi et al., 2013), meaning that there are 3 times the number of bowel microorganisms than there are human cells. The figure was once thought to be more like 10 gut bacteria to 1 human cell, but the number of human cells earlier was thought to be 10 trillion until the recent revision by Bianconi et al. in 2013. Irrespective, of the absolute number, one thing for certain is that we are outnumbered by 'bugs' and that the effect these organisms have on our well-being is of a magnitude far greater than the absolute numbers present.

The race is on to look for tell-tale biomarkers of ill-health of the gut microbiome through genetic fingerprinting of faecal samples or metabolites in blood or urine, or both and to compare these changes with known metabolic signatures of disease states. ***The gut microbiome can dramatically influence how any particular individual responds to any particular meal and that there are huge variations in blood metabolites such as blood glucose depending on the makeup of your gut microbiome so that two people having the same meal may have markedly different effects on subsequent blood glucose and blood fat levels.***

It thus makes it very hard to predict food responses without knowing the makeup of the gut microbiome. This gap in knowledge is fast being filled-in. Israeli researchers, for example, have made magnificent strides in predicting how high blood glucose levels rise with any given food by analysing gut microbial species and testing the responses in hundreds of volunteers (Zeevi, Korem et al. 2015).

Gone are the days where you have to plate out faecal matter and grow the organism on media in Petri dishes or study their metabolic action on sugars in tubes which then change colour. We can find out the composition of the faecal microbes through DNA assessments now as many organisms are nearly impossible to grow easily in Petri dishes within laboratories. Indeed vast numbers of organisms have never been cultured in laboratories, and we only know of their existence through genetic markers. Such testing is revolutionary with the future looking very bright for personalised whole-body approaches to treatment modalities.

Signalling Hub, Quorum Sensing, Autoinducers & Dysbiosis

The gut microbiome acts like a signalling hub to shape our health and future health. These organisms are constantly receiving and sending signals and collectively integrating information from the host and from the environment with data inputs that include diet and lifestyle choices. The microbiome helps to regulate the immune system both near and far in the body. What is emerging from mice and human studies is that if this signalling system is interrupted it can lead to a **dysbiosis** which is essentially an abnormal gut microbiome caused by the colonisation and overgrowth of harmful bowel microorganisms. **If you suffer from bloating, abdominal discomfort, soft stools regularly or foul-smelling stools or wind, then you may well have a dysbiosis which may put your immune system at risk and increase your risk for bowel cancer.**

You can imagine that with a new set of abnormal (dysbiotic) organisms comes a new set of microbiome (dysbiotic) signalling, that affects organ systems systemically, and also affects gut permeability locally – triggers affecting both local and systemic inflammatory changes through the immune system.

Such signalling disruptions could be due to grossly abnormal dietary patterns, FODMAP sensitivities or toxicities coming from medications, antibiotics or even food contaminated with antibiotics, hormones or chemicals. Poor lifestyle choices such as leading a sedentary life, consuming too much alcohol, taking drugs or becoming overweight or obese, can lead to significant changes in the gut microbiome.

Gut dysbiosis has a role in the pathophysiology of irritable bowel syndrome (IBS) (Cremon, Carini et al. 2010). It is the reason why antibiotics such as Rifaximin can have such a powerful short-term effect on IBS, a troublesome gut disease that really should be seen as a **relapsing-and-remitting** disease state that never completely goes away after treatment, but may need episodic treatment for the dysbiosis now becoming a hallmark for this common bowel disease state.

This episodic treatment of dysbiosis in diseases like IBS or inflammatory bowel diseases may include antibiotics, prebiotics or probiotics with or without phages or a combination of all of these. Combination treatments as an integrative approach using antibiotics such as Rifaximin + Targeted Probiotics + Targeted Phages are powerful tools for dysbiosis. Gut microbiome genetic analysis enables targeted probiotic and phage treatments.

Vast quantities of food consumed on a daily basis made up of high-calorie foods that are nutrient-poor and importantly very restricted in food diversity; you can guess the dysbiotic state of the microbiomes in individuals consuming a Western diet.

Restrict food diversity, and you restrict bowel microorganism diversity.

Fixing this dysbiosis is the focus now in research using prebiotics and probiotics and perhaps even vaccinations or medications designed to try to get the microbiomes back to a normal state. Sometimes this takes a poo transplant to set things right again. Coming to your local pharmacy in the not too distant future is the poo capsule (the 'Crapsule') containing faecal matter or perhaps concentrated microorganisms from people who have healthy gut microbiomes to help correct all the damage of 21st Century living and food overconsumption in many individuals who suffer gut problems.

We are witnessing Darwinian evolution in action where a small number of people have such robust bowel microorganisms that it enables them to simply brush off all the hazardous influences on the gut microbiome that modern life throws at them. If we were not so clever, we would allow these people to inherit the Earth, but we want what they have, and we have the intelligence to make it happen! We have the intellectual power to make Darwinian evolutionary principles go and take a hike!

What's all this cross-talk noise?

Cross-talk occurs between the bowel microorganisms, pathogens and host cells through the production of **autoinducers.** You can think of autoinducers as hormones which are used in the process of **quorum sensing** a term used for cell-to-cell signalling by the bacteria as a way of them determining bacterial population numbers. Quorum sensing allows them to adjust genetic expression to help them establish a niche in the bowel population or to trigger the production of virulence factors when numbers are high enough to cause harm.

Quorum sensing is a system of knowing 'troop' numbers and through autoinducers allows control over the 'troops', so they act like one – they act in synchrony like an army of 'zombies' controlled by these microorganism-induced chemicals. So autoinducers are like a General of an army shouting orders like 'troops do this' or 'troops do that' providing an organisational capability as if those groups of organisms have a mind. How clever is that?

We have greatly underestimated the immense importance of bowel organisms historically in medicine. To be fair though, we only now have the technological means to analyse and understand this highly complex ecosystem. We are now mining these organisms for compounds like **bacteriocins** that produced by bowel bacterial strains such as *Bifidobacterium* or *Lactobacillus* which can inhibit or harm other pathogenic bacterial species and we can use them like antibiotics in future.

How much of the microbiome is genetically or environmentally determined?

This question was an unknown quantity until chance collaboration occurred between Professor Tim Spector of Kings College, London and Professor Ruth Ley from Cornell University in America. Professor Spector had been studying countless genetic traits in his large cohort of twins, and he is also the director of the crowd-funded, British Gut Microbiome Project. The age-old argument about nature vs nurture or genes vs environment was also applied to this nascent study of the human microbiome and in particular the gut microbiome.

On hearing Prof Ruth Ley talk about unravelling this particular mystery, he knew her study was underpowered and offered her the opportunity to benefit from the 11,000 twins in his study (Spector, 2015). Stool samples from the twins were sent to Professor Ley at Cornell University, and the stool bacteria DNA was analysed through the use of the **16S ribosomal RNA** marker. 16S is a particular protein that, like a fingerprint, identifies particular strains of bacteria. Using the 16S marker, a range of bacterial species were discovered that have never been cultured in a laboratory.

This analysis revealed that the environment predominated for large bacterial groups like the Bacteroides species in the bowel, but even when divided into other major groups (phyla), over 60 percent of the effects on these bowel microorganisms came from the environment. So this puts a tremendous amount of power into your hands. You have the control to determine how healthy your Gut microbiota is through dietary measures. Meal composition is thus critical to producing a healthy gut microbiome. The diversity of the food you eat produces an equally diverse gut microbiome critical to your long-term health.

This study also showed how amazingly dissimilar we are regarding our microbial friends within us. We only share about 10 – 20 percent of these microbe types, and yet we share around 99.9 percent of our DNA between us. So we all have our microbial signature that we have inherited from our mother, the people around you as you were born and then all the dietary and environmental factors that have resulted in the gut microbiome you now have. However, as has just been stated, this microbiome can be altered for the better by ensuring that you provide the Gut bacteria with a wealth of fibre and phytochemicals allowing them to thrive.

The Gut microbiota: An endocrine organ

An endocrine organ is one that produces hormones that can have a powerful effect on near and distant cells in the body. Many compounds produced by Gut bacteria are designed for cross-talk between the bacteria and the cells lining the bowel wall but also to 'talk' amongst themselves through autoinducers.

Of great interest is the production of short-chain fatty acids (SCFA's) that include **acetate, butyrate and propionate** which can be absorbed by the body and which have an impact on distant immune system cells reaching parts of your body at great distances from your bowel.

One way this happens as discovered by researchers at the Garvan Institute in Sydney, Australia is via the GPR43 receptor also knows as the FFAR2 receptor (free fatty acid receptor 2), which can positively influence immune system responses to protect us against inflammatory diseases. It has been demonstrated by these pioneering Australian researchers how bowel organisms that are seemingly isolated from the rest of the body can have a profound chemically mediated impact on distant sites in the body. In their paper the researchers stated that SCFA's interaction with GPR43 receptors on cells, can:

"profoundly affect inflammatory responses." (Maslowski, Vieira et al. 2009)

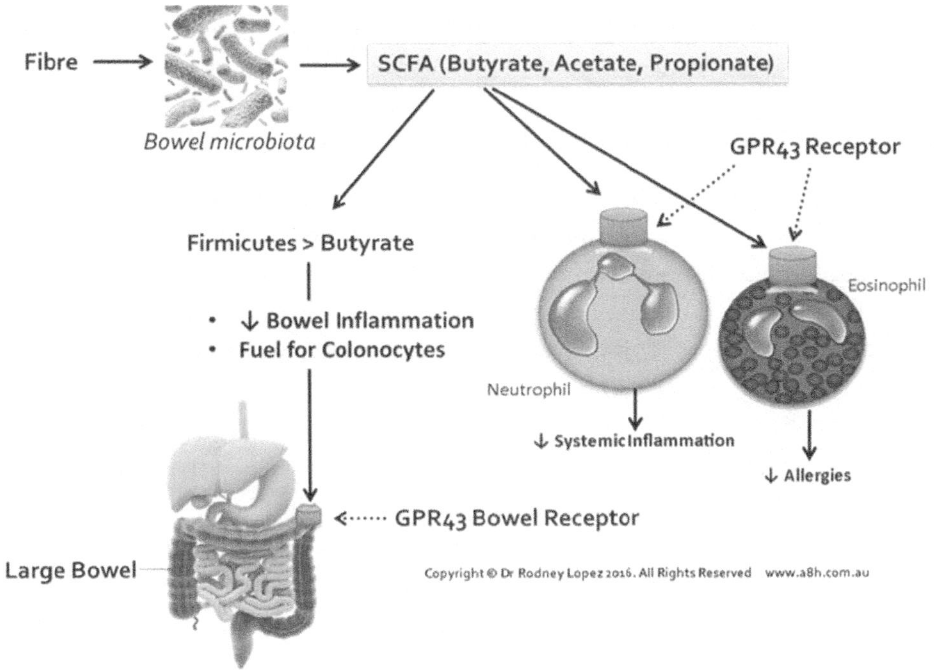

SCFA's - Anti-inflammatory, Anti-Cancer

Your bowel microbiota can be divided into essentially two large groups:

1. Bacteroidetes
2. Firmicutes

The Firmicutes group produce large amounts of butyrate from dietary fibre, and the Bacteroidetes produce significant amounts of acetate and propionate from dietary fibre (Maslowski et al., 2009). Butyrate is a major source of energy for the bowel cells themselves and helps modify cellular proliferation of the bowel lining and ensures bowel integrity thus keeping highly toxic compounds like lipopolysaccharide (LPS) away from the rest of your body.

LPS is highly inflammatory. This will be discussed in more detail shortly. The GPR43 receptors are found throughout the large bowel as well as immune system cells throughout your body this is how your gut bacteria can **affect and influence immune system cells both near and far**. Butyrate has been shown to decrease the risk of bowel cancer and acetate added to the drinking water of mice can lead to a:

"marked suppression of allergic airways disease" (Thorburn et al., 2015)

This knowledge shows how critical fibre is to your health. When you are considering meal composition, it is important not to look at this simply as a source of energy and macronutrient (fat, carbs, protein) composition. Fibre is the magic bullet you need to ensure the highly influential gut microbiome acts in your favour. Food diversity ensures gut microbiome diversity and in turn a robust immune system. Constantly change the fruits and vegetables you are consuming not only seasonally but on a weekly basis. A high vegetable and small fruit intake provide a rich supply of soluble and insoluble fibre, gums and mucilage required for an optimal gut microbiome as these compounds nourish healthy bacterial colonies in your bowel.

It is important not to compartmentalise any organ in the body as this is an outdated view of the human body. Each organ can affect every other organ and no organ functions in isolation including your bowel.

T-Regulatory Cells (Tregs)
A vital link between bowel organisms, your body & fat cells

The immune cells that communicate most with your bowel organisms are a subset of T-cells called T-regulatory cells shortened to Tregs. These were formerly known as suppressor T-cells, and they have an extremely important role in your immune system defence network. They are responsible for determining tolerance to your proteins, preventing your immune system from attacking itself (autoimmunity) and are essentially immunosuppressive cells, acting as a calming agent for the immune system which, if not kept on a tight leash, can be highly dangerous to your survival.

Your health is dependent on these Tregs, and the interesting fact with these cells is that your body's fat cells are covered in these Tregs (Spector, 2015). So what are they doing there in all that fat? We know that not only does your bowel microbiota act like an endocrine (hormone/chemical signal generating) organ which as you remember, produces chemical signals that affect near and distant cells, so do your fat cells function as an endocrine organ producing a vast array of fat hormones called adipokines. The fat deep in your abdomen called deep visceral fat is highly active tissue that can produce inflammation throughout your body and increase the risk of insulin resistance and cancer. So we regard deep visceral fat as an endocrine organ as well because of the chemical signalling compounds these fat cells produce affect other cells both near and far. Visceral fat is associated with prediabetes, diabetes, non-alcoholic fatty liver disease (NAFLD), many cancers and cardiovascular disease.

So, let's get back to what the Treg cells are doing amongst all those fat cells of your body. As indicated, the Tregs have a great deal to do with your gut microbiota. These Tregs act like a go-between forming a communication link between your gut microbiota and the fat cells either dampening down the inflammatory processes of the fat cells (remember, these Tregs are suppressor T-cells), or if you happen to be overweight or obese, these Tregs start to disappear and your highly active and toxic fat cells now go wild, releasing inflammatory chemicals that affect the rest of the body which increases your risk of a wide number of chronic diseases or a devastating illness.

With an abundance of Tregs acting as the immune system police, suppressing inflammation and modulating fat cell toxicities, you remain healthy. If these cells decrease in number and other T-cell populations like the Th1/Th2 and Th17 cells increase, you may move into a disease state (Round & Mazmanian, 2009).

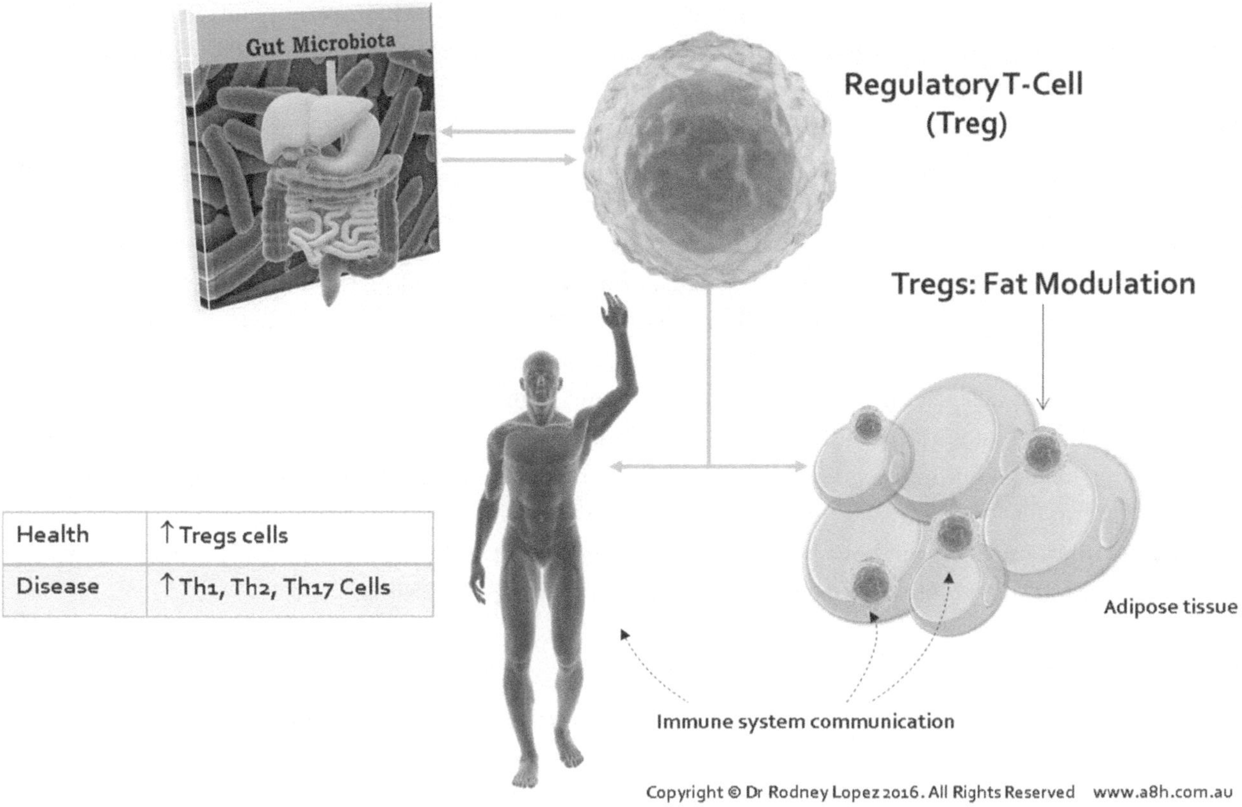

Fat regulation - the duality of human existence, a conflict of interest

There is obviously a tight link between your bowel microorganisms and fat storage in the body due to the symbiotic relationship that exists between us as human beings and the organisms in and on our bodies that depend on us to nourish them. It is an interesting phenomenon that the over-consumption of food can be so deleterious to our health, and yet humans seem compelled to keep on consuming damaging high energy foods that are absolutely micronutrient poor. It is a situation where over-nutrition paradoxically runs in parallel with under-nutrition (the overfed yet undernourished).

That the Western diet leads to overweight and obesity is beyond doubt to anyone that is not visually impaired. People who eat these energy-dense foods and gain weight can suffer debilitating problems but yet cannot stop eating foods that condemn them to a poor quality of life. Even if you have not gained weight, the triage system discussed earlier in the book, ensures your bones and organs suffer from micronutrient deficiencies over your lifetime.

Excessive body weight and micronutrient deficiencies or insufficiencies can lead to numerous chronic illnesses. The excessive weight itself leads to premature joint damage of the knees and hips because for every kilogram carried on the trunk, leads to 4 kilograms of added stress on the joints with every step taken (Messier, Gutekunst, Davis, & DeVita, 2005).

Such joint damage and pain limit activity and the limited activity leads to weight gain and muscle loss. You are caught up in a vicious cycle that shortens lifespan considerably.

Many who are overweight or obese suffer sleep apnoea (US apnea) and wake up feeling flat and lethargic as if they have run a marathon in their sleep. They are simply not well. So why do humans eat to the point of feeling like this? Why aren't there evolutionary systems to put a brake on all of this? The answer is clear when you consider the duality of human existence where we are essentially two distinct organisms in one corporeal form - holobionts. Each entity, human and microorganism have their own evolutionary imperative. When you eat the type of foods that are energy dense, rich in bad fats, refined sugars and low in plant foods and fibre, you set up a distinctly unhealthy colony of microorganisms in your bowels. **You set yourself up for gut dysbiosis.** These particular 'bad' pathogenic microorganisms thrive on this high-energy, nutrient-poor type of diet and as a result, these bad guys send out signals to your body and brain to keep on eating more of the same. The bad guys like it, want it and then demand it by pressuring you to keep on eating these damaging foods through your command centre, your brain! You produce a dysbiosis that lingers and damages your health in the short and long-term. These organisms are essentially calling the shots, and your human behaviour complies with their demands. You have a conflict of interest pure and simple that results in human ill health.

From animal studies using germ-free mice, feeding them a high-fat diet does not result in weight gain. You need the bowel microbiota intact to affect weight gain (Spector, 2015).

So regarding meal planning, keeping your microbiota foremost in your mind, is vital to long-term health. Ensure you eat for 'bugs' and not just for your human self. Eating the right type of foods ensures a diverse group of good microorganisms in your bowel that stops demanding all that junk food that the bad bacteria thrive on, and as a result, you live a long life, illness-free for as long as possible.

Fat intake and Lipopolysaccharide (LPS)

So eating foods that are energy and sugar-rich are perceived by the body as a threat. I have discussed how these foods produce a postprandial (after-eating) response seen as a threat to the body by the innate immune system. Authors of a paper titled, 'Fatty acids and postprandial inflammation' (Margioris, 2009) stated:

> *"Indeed it now appears that our organism perceives each meal as an exogenous 'threat' stressful enough to mobilise homeostatic mechanisms to adjust to the stress of the postprandial state." (Margioris 2009)*

What was pointed out by these authors is that:

> *". triglycerides and saturated fatty acids induce a soaring postprandial inflammatory response." (Margioris 2009)*

Notice the superlative word 'soaring'. The consumption of dietary saturated fats is a hotly debated topic. A small intake of saturated fat may have a neutral effect on blood lipids and cardiovascular risk, but this is not the same as having a high intake of saturated fatty acids found in meat and dairy (milk, meat, butter and ice-cream). The fact that a high intake of saturated fats can produce a "soaring" inflammatory response in the blood after eating is a cause for great concern.

Taking diet to the extremes only results in negative outcomes and cardiovascular risk. There seems to be a high-fat intake movement that, long-term can cause harm. There are around twelve different saturated fats, and palmitate is the most abundant saturated fatty acid found in foods. This saturated fat makes up about one-third of beef and butterfat and is likely to cause an inflammatory response through toll-like receptor 4 (TLR4).

The toll-like receptors play a key role in the innate immune system response to microbial and chemical threats, and palmitic acid which is abundant in diets that include meat and dairy is a natural compound that binds to the TLR4 receptor. As the scientists say, palmitate is a natural ligand of the TLR4 receptor. Once the Palmitate stimulates the TLR4 receptor, this sends downstream signals to stimulate TNF-a and NFkB that are stimulants of inflammation in the body. So palmitate a common saturated fat is more likely to cause inflammation, particularly in obese individuals. Interestingly, if palmitate consumption occurs with olive oil or fish oil, it is not inflammatory (Maedler, Oberholzer, Bucher, Spinas, & Donath, 2003).

Myristate is a saturated fat found in coconut oil, palm oil and butterfat and is the most potent cholesterol-raising fatty acid (Temme, Mensink, & Hornstra, 1997). Lauric acid also raises cholesterol, and yet stearate does not (Hunter, Zhang, & Kris-Etherton, 2010).

So you can see that consumption of saturated fats depends on the type of fat consumed and in the dietary circumstance, i.e. what are you consuming with the saturated fatty acids as we saw with palmitic acid and the decreased inflammatory effect by consuming olive oil or fish oil at the same time. Again, this highlights the importance of meal composition to add fish in the diet or use olive oil say on your salad or for cooking.

As a bonus remember, adding oil to your salad enables you to effectively absorb the fat-soluble vitamins (Vitamins A, D, E, K). Adding the chosen oil to vinegar (vinaigrette) also helps to decrease the glycemic index of the whole meal through the vinegar component. Replacing saturated fats with polyunsaturated and monounsaturated fats may be a better option to improve cardiovascular risk but substituting saturated fats with carbohydrates is a disaster with increases in small-dense lipoproteins and blood triglycerides. Blood triglycerides as you now know can produce that 'soaring' inflammatory response after eating, making carb substitutions a very bad choice.

Nutrigenomic testing can point the way regarding whether you should use polyunsaturates (PUFAs) or monounsaturated fats (MUFAs). Having the right type of oil that is personalised to your genetics helps lower your cardiovascular risk the best and can keep the threat of LPS induced damage to a minimum. See Appendix-22.

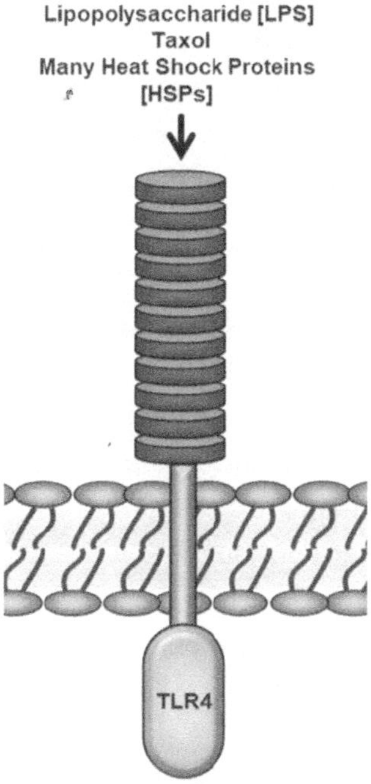

Getting back to lipopolysaccharide (LPS): Endotoxemia

There seems to be a significant push to high-fat diets touted by many nutrition gurus stating that it is not the fat that is the problem, it is the carbohydrate content of food and processed carbs that are evil. Indeed, a high carb diet is problematic as discussed with raised Insulin/IGF-1 levels and glycation of proteins and increased triglycerides, but a high-fat diet is not benign.

High energy intakes and in particular, high-fat intakes may be associated with endotoxemia which is the release of a toxin (lipopolysaccharide or LPS), into the systemic circulation, the toxicity of which affects all tissues of the body. Endotoxins can have a toxic and powerful effect both near and far like a hormone. Endotoxin is a general term used for bacterial toxins, but now the term is more commonly used to describe lipopolysaccharide (LPS) located in the outer membrane of gram-negative rods (they appear red on a Grams Stain). Bacterial LPS are extremely strong stimulators of the innate immune system. Interestingly, it is the toll-like receptor 4 (TLR4) that is the major LPS sensing complex of the innate immune system (Wang and Quinn 2010). Remember, the common dietary fat palmitate attaches to TLR4 to stimulate inflammatory processes in the body.

So with high animal fat foods, you not only have the palmitate targeting the TLR4, but you now have the LPS also targeting this same toll-like receptor driving downstream inflammatory signalling. A double-whammy!

High-fat diets and LPS endotoxemia

In animal studies, just a 4-week high-fat diet led to a 2x – 3x increase in LPS beyond the threshold used to define metabolic endotoxemia (Cani et al., 2007). High-fat diets changed the bowel microbiota to one where there were more LPS gram-negative bacterial types present. **Can LPS endotoxemia occur with a single fatty meal? Yes indeed!** Once again each meal you consume contributes to an inflammatory effect in your body leading to small, incremental and cumulative damage over time. Just one fatty meal can increase LPS in your bloodstream by 50% (Erridge, Attina, Spickett, & Webb, 2007). These same authors stated that low-grade LPS endotoxemia contributes to the development of atherosclerosis through TLR4 activation and downstream inflammatory mechanisms. High-energy, high-fat diets produced the greatest increase in LPS in contrast to a high-carb intake (Amar et al., 2008).

Once again, this shows how critical meal composition is to your long-term health. Just consider a high-fat meal such as a large hamburger or pizza or any number of fat laden, carbohydrate-rich foods in any food court that can simultaneously stimulate both the Insulin/IGF-1/mTOR pathway or induce LPS endotoxemia in your bloodstream meal-after-meal due to the high-energy, high-fat content. You simply need to recognise that each meal is a threat to your body and each meal damages your body one meal at a time.

Each meal is an external threat, perceived by your body and as a result, your immune system is called in to react to this threat through the innate immune system. So your body is just seeing poorly composed meals as a danger to its existence and is rallying the troops, i.e. your immune system to deal with this danger through mechanisms that result in collateral damage to your blood vessels, cells, tissues and organs.

These immune system responses are perhaps an overkill because they have been designed to deal with deadly pathogens (bad bugs) or chemical threats and not so much the modern and unusual threat produced by fast-foods which are a relatively new phenomenon for human bodies to contend likewise.

So it is a sobering thought that the human system reacts so significantly to dietary threats in the same way as it does to deadly microorganisms or environmental toxins. How amazing is it that the 'primitive' arm of the body's immunity, the innate immune system designed over millions of years, can deal with the modern phenomenon of highly processed foods and abnormal macronutrient intakes!

LPS and insulin resistance, fatty liver and obesity

One of the deadliest problems in society is prediabetes, as I have previously discussed. This condition is often symptom-free. It is where an individual has an elevated insulin level due to insulin resistance. What distinguishes prediabetes and diabetes is a cut-off point in blood glucose but this is very deceptive in that prediabetes is just as deadly, and should be treated in the same way as diabetes. Remember as I have stated that in Australia it is estimated that around 16.4% have prediabetes over 25 years of age (Twigg, Kamp, Davis, Neylon, & Flack, 2007). This means that a large number of you reading this book have this condition. A very large number of people have abnormal liver function tests when routine blood tests are done to investigate clinical problems. Often these changes in liver enzymes are deemed 'mild', and a patient is tapped on the shoulder and told 'do not worry about this'. If you have had liver function tests (LFTs) done, look at the ALT level. This ALT level, is often raised in fatty liver disease.

If this ALT level is raised, you just need to have a look at your waist in the mirror. If you have abdominal adiposity (a large floppy belly or muffin top), then this high ALT will almost certainly indicate that you have fatty liver as a result of a pre-diabetic or perhaps an undiagnosed diabetic state.

However, there is a distinct risk that fatty liver disease could progress to cirrhosis of the liver and this may happen when other risk factors are present such as a high alcohol intake or high level of abdominal fat or perhaps the iron storage disease haemochromatosis.

Non-alcoholic fatty liver disease (NAFLD) is often the hallmark of prediabetes. I often see this in general practice where the seriousness of this problem is totally underestimated. By not identifying prediabetes as the culprit of NAFLD, that particular individual may be condemned to a life of cardiovascular disease or deadly cirrhosis of the liver and an early demise when this could easily have been prevented.

LPS and endotoxemia can lead to insulin resistance, and insulin resistance can lead to non-alcoholic fatty liver disease. Underlying chronic disease and obesity is a chronic low-grade inflammation (Cani et al., 2007). The downstream effect of LPS (endotoxin) produces numerous inflammatory chemicals and tumour necrosis factor alpha (TNF-a), has been shown to alter the insulin receptor found on cell membranes thus inactivating this receptor (Cani et al., 2007). Inactivation of the insulin receptor, in turn, prevents insulin from doing its job and that is to allow glucose to enter the cell for energy production or fat storage as triglycerides.

Insulin also does many other jobs. Insulin receptor inactivation thus sends a signal to the body that there is not enough insulin available when in fact there is a large amount of insulin floating around in the bloodstream but simply not recognised at the level of the receptor. Your pancreas in response tries to overcome this block by sending in, even more, insulin 'troops' to try to overcome this obstacle. This can result in beta-cell burnout where the pancreas simply has no more insulin to give.

You put yourself at significant risk every time you consume high-energy, high-fat diets. The adverse effect of the Western diet is undeniable and trying to overcome the massively damaging effect of diet through pharmaceuticals is a stop-gap measure. We need to look at the underlying cause of prediabetes, diabetes and non-alcoholic fatty liver disease which are due to the Western diet and lifestyles.

LPS and increased membrane permeability

Many studies have shown that the LPS endotoxin increases in the bowel with high-energy, high-fat diets, and results in damage to the lining of the bowel itself allowing LPS to enter the portal circulation, then to the liver to wreak inflammatory havoc there and to induce fatty liver changes.

Tight Junctions serve as a 'molecular fence' that stops large molecules, bacteria and viruses from crossing the bowel lining cell barrier preventing these elements from entering the lymphatics and blood. LPS has been shown to damage the tight junctions between the cells lining the bowel (Park, Thomson, & Clandinin, 2010), allowing not only LPS but also bacterial fragments and food proteins to enter your circulation.

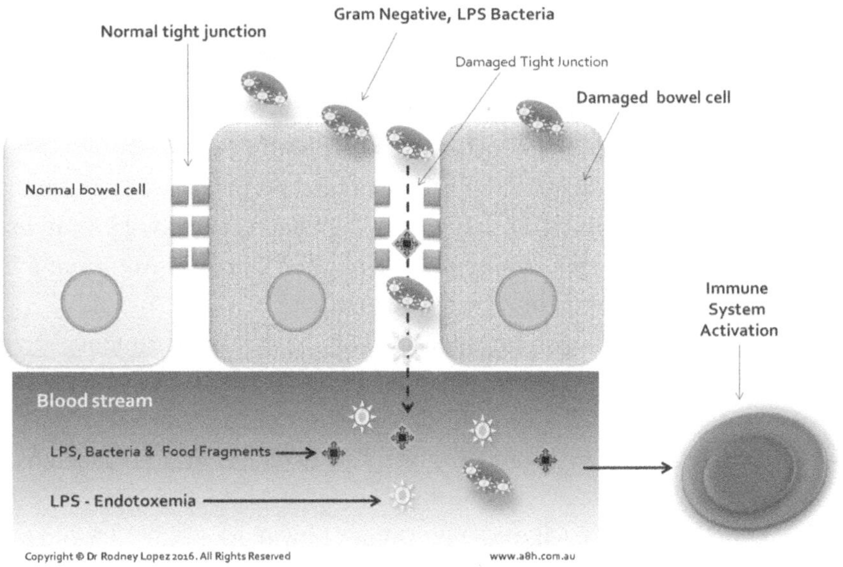

These unwanted proteins and toxins circulate in your blood to create inflammatory processes and immune cell activation. Generalised inflammation after eating can damage all your organs. LPS induced inflammation in the postprandial (after-eating) state contributes to the damage of the lining of your blood vessels predisposing you to atherosclerosis (blockages of the arteries of the heart and arterial vessels of the body).

It is known that blood glucose and triglycerides rise after eating to cause after-eating inflammation, but one study showed for the first time that LPS was also a powerful contributor to this after eating inflammatory surge (Erridge, Attina, Spickett, & Webb, 2007), and that high-energy, high-fat meals are toxic to the body, meal-by-meal.

The bacterial fragments, whole bacteria and potential whole food proteins that can also cross the intestinal barrier due to tight junction damage, may have other consequences. Autoimmunity is where your body attacks organs or healthy tissues in the body. Some common autoimmune diseases include Hashimoto's Disease of the thyroid, Systemic Lupus Erythematosus (SLE), Rheumatoid Arthritis or Type-1 Diabetes Mellitus to name a few. There may be many mechanisms involved in triggering off autoimmunity (Oldstone, 1998).

- Molecular mimicry is where amino acid sequences on food proteins or bacteria and viruses, that escape the tight junctions into the lymphatics and bloodstream, may be very similar to amino acid (protein) sequences in your organs or tissues. The immune system by recognising these fragments as foreign and mounting an attack results in the similar sequence in organs or tissues also being attacked. Resultant collateral and ongoing damage to your body.
- The gut organisms themselves may damage your body cells causing the release of cell and tissue proteins that are seen as foreign and then attacked by the immune system resulting in autoimmunity
- Autoimmune disorders can also occur with micronutrient deficiencies. I discussed how Hashimoto's disease can occur when iodine and selenium are deficient and where the antibodies directed by the immune system towards the thyroid can clear when these micronutrient deficiencies are corrected (Nordio & Pajalich, 2013)

The important thing to remember is how interconnected all of this is. Meal composition can have a profound impact on your body through the following mechanisms that interact and mutually drive each other:

- Postprandial inflammation – driven by glucose and triglyceride surges can worsen inflammatory joint disease caused by rheumatoid arthritis or SLE
- Postprandial inflammation and intestinal permeability (tight junction damage) also known as 'leaky gut' – driven by high-energy, high-fat meals caused by LPS can leads to numerous autoimmune disorders and may also be involved in the 'March of Autoimmunity' where if you have one autoimmune disease, you may be prone to others
- The release of lipopolysaccharide (LPS), bacterial fragments or viruses into the bloodstream then stimulates the innate and adaptive immune systems to worsen any existing chronic illness and perhaps create new diseases and autoimmune states.
- Inflammation drives and magnifies any immune attack caused by these factors

The composition of each meal determines how marked the LPS and the after-eating inflammatory response is. LPS, glucose and triglyceride surges after eating, also damage your vascular system leading to premature vascular disease. It is the inflammation that makes plaque unstable, and this can rupture an unstable plaque blocking an artery in your heart, brain or peripheral circulation. Inflammatory autoimmune disease may double the risk of cardiovascular disease due to the inflammatory state affecting the whole body.

- Immune system activation after eating plays a part in damage to your blood vessels over your lifetime leading to premature heart disease.
- Once you develop an autoimmune disease state or vascular or heart disease, each meal will drive further these disease states to produce even more cumulative and devastating effects on the body. It is imperative if you have a chronic illness of any kind that you adopt an optimal diet based on sound scientific principles such as the Activ8Health Plan-A or Plan-B diets provided freely in this book but personalisation is highly advisable.

Your gut microbiome and weight loss

Professor Liping Zhao is a Chinese professor and pioneer in the bowel microbiome. His interest is to look at causal links between the bowel bacteria and certain disease states. He visited Sydney University in 2016 and jointly presented this topic with Professor Andrew Holmes from the Charles Perkins Gut Microbiome node at Sydney University, Australia. He has helped many obese people in China through his WTP diet which consists of a high-fibre gruel which has components rich in prebiotics and some traditional herbs. Through this diet, he has had great success in reversing the obesity of numerous people who have presented to him for help.

That the bowel microbiota can become drastically changed and abnormal is beyond doubt. One of the Professor's early cases was that of a Chinese man who weighed 174.8 kg. Professor Zhao found that DNA analysis of this patient's stool contained a highly dominant bacterial species called Enterobacter and one strain, in particular, was Enterobacter B29 which had a particularly toxic lipopolysaccharide (LPS). This strain made up 35% of the bowel bacteria which was astounding and was crowding out the other bacterial strains in this man's bowel driving his obesity. This man had a profound gut dysbiosis. On the high fibre WTP diet with concentrated prebiotics, this man lost 51.4 kg after 23 weeks with the highly toxic LPS becoming undetectable at this time interval as well. His markers of inflammation, diabetes and hypertension also improved dramatically.

During his visit to Sydney University, Prof Zhao who was once overweight was looking lean and fit. He stated that this weight loss was due to dietary measures only and that he lost 20 kg on this diet.

How inflammatory disease states can affect your microbiome

In future, treatment of inflammatory states such as Rheumatoid Arthritis (RA) will focus on the bowel microbiome, and the reason is that this microbiome can change dramatically with an inflammatory disease process at play. Changes in the diversity of bowel microflora can be altered not just through medications or dietary factors but by the inflammatory process itself that feeds back to the microbial colonies in the bowel. One species, in particular, Prevotella copri increases and can crowd out other species. Prevotella is a gram-negative species implicated in many diseases including periodontal (gum) disease.

Prevotella can produce a lipopolysaccharide (LPS) and this can stimulate periodontal (gum, mouth) macrophages (an immune system cell) to produce pro-inflammatory chemicals.

Studies show that docosahexaenoic acid (DHA) from fish and krill oil or microalgae sources can counteract these inflammatory mediators. Increasing fish or krill oil consumption when someone is suffering from inflammatory disease states is prudent, and there is a plethora of research articles on the inflammatory dampening effects of omega-3 essential fatty acids.

No doubt, highly specific probiotic or prebiotic preparations can be devised for the various chronic disease states in future ensuring that pharmaceutical approaches which can damage the microbiomes of the body are not the only treatment modalities on offer.

How can you practically increase probiotic consumption?

How you do this depends on your food preferences and food avoidance tactics. Many people 'do not do dairy' and this is fine as there are so many probiotic-rich options out there that can act as substitutes. For those who want to avoid dairy, you now have coconut-based kefir or coconut yoghurt and no doubt other forms of non-dairy kefirs, non-dairy yoghurts and many nut-based, non-dairy kinds of cheese now available with new versions coming out. Kefir is a fermented drink created by a large number of microorganisms such as yeast and bacteria (kefir grains) that can be used as a 'starter' again and again to ferment not only milk but other forms of milk made from nuts or coconut.

Kimchi a traditional Korean side-dish is made up of fermented vegetables. It usually contains 10^{7-9} colony forming units (CFU) per ml with high levels of lactic acid bacteria (Shi, Shahidi et al. 2005). Having kimchi every second day along with prebiotic foods such as leeks, figs, high fibre foods (vegetables, fruits, seeds), Jerusalem artichokes, onions, green banana helps probiotics thrive in your bowel.

In the Activ8Health Plan-B diet where starchy grains are applied in a particular circumstance, I recommend well-chosen carbs like Teff a very small Ethiopian grain that contains a lot of resistant starch beneficial for the bowel. In fact, around 40% of Teff may have this resistant type of starch which is brilliant for the bowel organisms which thrive on this fibre. This will have a tremendously beneficial effect on your immune system through the fibre and resistant starch and can help you lose weight or maintain a healthy weight. Always start off with very small amounts of fibre of any kind, including resistant starch like Teff or Green Banana Powder, and build up slowly perhaps ½ to 1 teaspoon initially and increasing every 2nd or 3rd day by ½ to 1 teaspoon if tolerated. Unless you have a food or chemical sensitivity, you should be able to tolerate kimchi. Those with histamine intolerance should take care with fermented foods.

The Activ8Health dietary plans have a high focus on prebiotic fibres and probiotics to promote optimal health and immune system function.

Bacteriophages

Probiotics + Bacteriophages = the new frontier of bowel microbiome treatments

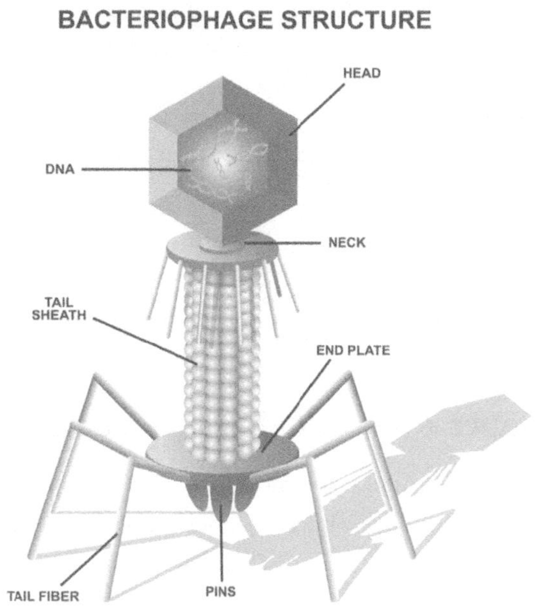

Even microbes have their enemies, and bacteria have their nemesis called a bacteriophage. Collectively, they are also known as phages. These are viruses that look like a NASA landing module. They attach to specific receptors on the surface of a bacterium and can thus enter a bacterial cell and destroy them. The fact that they need **specific bacterial receptors** means that they can be used to attack **specific bacterial species** which is advantageous in a therapeutic sense as a new form of targeted 'antibiotic' treatment or phage treatment for bacterial infections. The name bacteriophage means 'bacteria-eating'. They have either DNA or RNA in their head.

The role of bacteriophages in the creation of disease in the bowel is probably greatly underestimated and that phage infection can cause a **'rupture of eubiosis'** (De Paepe, Leclerc et al. 2014), which then creates a dysbiosis in the bowel that can lead to short-term and long-term health consequences.

Eubiosis is the normal, healthy microbiome and dysbiosis is the unhealthy, diseased state and such phage infection may be the cause of irritable bowel syndrome (IBS) where someone may one day have a totally healthy bowel and can eat anything they like and the next day suffer a debilitating and chronic gastrointestinal problem where they may become frustratingly sensitive to a vast number of foods for life. Are bacteriophages the trigger for inflammatory bowel diseases such as Crohn's or Ulcerative Colitis? If so, can we create a vaccine for the phage pathogens and hence prevent these diseases in future?

Bacteriophages were discovered pre-World War 1 (WW1) in Eastern Europe and the potential for treatment was known for over a century, but use in the treatment of bacterial infections was overshadowed by the discovery of penicillin in 1928. Alexander Fleming (Scottish), Howard Florey (Australian) and Ernst Boris Chain (German) all got the Nobel Prize in Medicine for this discovery that has saved 100's of millions of lives since1928.

New and novel antibiotics have emerged since then, and bacteriophages were essentially forgotten. With increasing resistance by bacteria to a variety of antibiotics and multiple resistance strains emerging putting all of humanity at risk, bacteriophages are now being looked at in detail as a tool to treat pathogenic strains and severe sepsis not responding to standard antibiotic treatments.

Dysbiosis can have significant impacts on inflammation in the body and can lead to fatty liver and insulin resistance. Dysbiosis is essentially associated with a wide array of disease states from cancer to Alzheimer's disease (Carding, Verbeke et al. 2015).

What is emerging from animal and human studies is how close the relationship is between gut microbiota and psychological disorders. Carding et al. pointed out:

> *"Coupled with evidence that probiotic interventions may alter psychological endpoints in both humans and in rodent models, these data suggest that CNS-related co-morbidities frequently associated with GI disease may originate in the intestine as a result of microbial dysbiosis." (Carding, Verbeke et al. 2015) CNS = Central Nervous System.*

Many people feel fatigued all the time or have clouded minds as if they are walking around in a fog. Dysbiosis could be the cause of this mental fog. Psychological consequences differ between individuals and the result of an interplay between the types of organisms causing the dysbiosis and the genetic makeup of an individual.

Neurogastroenterology is a new term used to describe a link between your bowel microbiota and the psychological states they can create. This new discipline in medicine is described as a 21st-century paradigm shift. The gut-brain axis is a real entity and psychological and psychiatric treatments in future will no doubt target this axis. Learning which bacterial species are linked to various types of mental health issues will be hotly researched, and this is where phage treatment may become a tool in the treatment of psychological disorders.

Probiotics + Bacteriophages = A powerful antibacterial combination

Of interest are new probiotic and bacteriophage blends now being produced that can attack pathogenic bacteria while replenishing beneficial ones. Right now there are commercial blends that may impact intestinal disorders like irritable bowel syndrome (IBS), inflammatory bowel diseases (IBD) such as Crohn's Disease or Ulcerative Colitis and coeliac disease. They may also have a beneficial impact on extra-intestinal problems like allergies or asthma or a range of metabolic disorders such as insulin resistance, diabetes and cardiovascular disease.

Personalising bowel microbiome treatments

A huge area of medicine is emerging under the umbrella of 'personalised medicine'. In the not too distant future, your faecal matter can be assessed through DNA markers to evaluate your gut microbiome regarding bacterial composition. Pathogenic bacteria can then be identified and the appropriate bacteriophage or bacteriophage combination can be used to attack and kill harmful organisms in your bowel. This kind of targeted treatment has potential to be a game-changer for a huge number of individuals suffering from chronic bowel problems. Host-microbiome interactions can be altered to restore balance, and this journey has already begun.

E-coli organisms exist in the bowel, and most are harmless, but some E-coli strains are quite pathogenic. Haemolytic uraemic syndrome (HUS) for example may be caused by certain strains, for example, the E-coli strain 0157. These pathogenic E-coli organisms release toxins that damage the bowels leading to blood in diarrhoea and leads to mild chronic kidney disease in around 50% of individuals who have suffered HUS. Renal failure and death can occur in cases not treated early. Studies done on phages that attack E-coli have produced some staggering results in animal studies.

Results in hours, not days or weeks

If you take probiotics on their own, you may be disappointed with the slow progress. This is not to say that probiotics do not have a role to play in treating bowel-related conditions. What you are trying to do with probiotics is to take them in large numbers that work by a surge action where these beneficial organisms overcrowd the 'bad guys' and take over their territory.

However, bacteriophages in combination with probiotics have a dual action. These combinations work by attaching to and killing troublesome organisms like E-coli strain H10407 and other pathogenic organisms, by the bacteriophages in the blend and then seed the bowel with the good probiotic organisms as well in a kill-and-replace or 'weed and seed' strategy.

These phage 'cocktails' can work within 24 hours not days or weeks (Sulakvelidze, Alavidze et al. 2001), and only small doses are required in the blend or probiotic-phage cocktail. Some commercially available blends can be purchased that include bacteriophages labelled LH01-Myoviridae or LL5-Siphorviridae.

No doubt researchers are working on how to ascertain the makeup of the bowel microbiota best and then create algorithms where dysbiosis caused by specific bacterial strains results in a custom-made blend of probiotics and bacteriophages to specifically destroy pathogenic bacteria in a particular individual. Research is well underway to highly individualise (personalise) probiotic-phage blends, and this is an exciting time in medical history for all those people suffering from bowel problems they thought they would have to bear for the rest of their lives. Technology is moving at a rapid pace to help these individuals.

70 - 80 of all your immune cells are in your bowel at any given moment in time!

Your overall health depends on your bowel health, and this is undeniable. Your immune system depends on the interaction of immune system cells with the bowel microbiota. It is an amazing statistic that 70% of all your immune system cells are in your bowel within the gut-associated lymphoid tissue (GALT) at any given moment in time. Even more amazing to know that 80% of all your plasma cells that produce all the antibodies that fight off infection are also located in the GALT (Vighi, Marcucci et al. 2008).

This gut-immunity association should not be underestimated. You can only enhance this link through the healthy dietary practices as outlined in this book and this includes an optimal exercise regimen that does not have to be strenuous or time-consuming. An optimal diet that focuses on meal composition and an effective exercise strategy goes a long way to helping you increase your healthspan.

Supercharge your fibre intake through the Chia pudding described next that has a whopping 35 grams of protein if created as suggested but this can be modified and the components rotated in the spirit of washout periods. This pudding has an amazing blend of fibres, prebiotics and probiotics and mucilage to keep the healthy organisms in your bowel well fed and contented. Your weight and well-being depend on these organisms.

The Activ8Health Super-Fibre Chia or Basil Seed Pudding

A vital component in bowel health is providing your bowel organisms with the fibre they need as food thus enabling them to thrive. Your good bacteria respond to the prebiotics by vigorously multiplying and crowding out any bad organisms that could harm your health. The adequate intake (AI) for fibre intake is 25 grams/day for females and 30 grams per day for males. However, this is an absolute minimum.

The Activ8Health Plan-A and Plan-B diets are rich in vegetable and fruit fibres, but we want to make sure we have a high intake of fibre like our hunter-gatherer counterparts. Typically, their fibre intakes may have been around 100g/day (Eaton 2006).

Fibre intake should comprise a wide range of soluble and insoluble fibres, gums like guar gum that increases the viscosity of food to slow down gastrointestinal transit. Lignans found in many seeds like flaxseed and sesame seeds can be converted to compounds that antagonise the effects of oestrogen thus protecting glandular tissues like the breast and prostate. Inulin is made up of long chains of fructose found in many foods and can effectively increase bifidobacteria counts in your bowels, and you can now purchase Inulin powder but remember to start off with a very small amount initially. Resistant starch found in high concentration in green bananas and other foods like Teff are protective of the bowel and pectins are a valuable fibre component that is rich in galacturonic acid. Pectins are found in fruits and berries. Add citrus rind to your pudding to benefit from the bioflavonoids and pectin.

The benefits of fibre would take another book to explain but we all know how important this is and yet vast numbers of people in Western populations get a fraction of the fibre they need for bowel health. According to the Australian Bureau of Statistics (www.abs.gov.au), only 4% of Australians were consuming enough vegetables, and most Australians were below the recommended intake for fibre daily which is often set at 30 grams of fibre a day. This fibre intake compared to a hunter-gatherer is very low indeed.

With traditionally low fruit and vegetable intakes far below the 5 & 2 (5 servings of vegetables and two servings of fruit) recommended by governments, it is no wonder that fibre intakes are so shockingly low. According to the Cancer Council, bowel cancer is the second most common form of cancer in Australia low fibre intakes contribute to this tally. Always start low and increase gradually as your bowels will love the extra fibre you are consuming. The trick is to find something that is easy, quick and tasty enough to do on a regular basis with variations thrown in.

Chia (*Salvia hispanica*) seeds Packed with goodness

Rich in extractable oil that makes up 25-30% of the seed and can comprise up to 55% of the short-chain essential omega-3 fat called alpha-linolenic acid (ALA) makes this seed the richest source of vegan omega-3. Remember, that ALA is a short-chain omega-3 that has to be elongated to EPA and DHA, and humans do this very poorly. Thus fish and algal forms of DHA and EPA are a better source of these important long-chain essential omega-3 fatty acids. You can always add a serving of high-quality fish oil to the chia. Chia is rich in B-group vitamins and minerals such as iron and magnesium with a high level of zinc important for the function of over 300 enzyme systems in the body. According to the USDA food nutrient database, 100 grams of Chia contains 37.7 grams of fibre.

The dieter's dream - weight loss through a high fibre intake

A study published in the journal Nature no less showed that food rich in Chia decreased the after-eating glucose elevations and also increased satiety (decreased hunger). It has been known that Chia has cardioprotective effects in diabetics and this paper set out to find out reasons for this vascular protective effect (Vuksan, Jenkins et al. 2010). Prediabetes and diabetes are very prevalent with many people not even knowing they have this problem. One quick glance at your belly can indicate an abnormal waist-to-hip ratio, and this is a good indication of possible visceral fat associated with insulin resistance and systemic inflammation.

Under the microbiome chapter in this book, I discussed fascinating work by Chinese Professor Liping Zhao and the amazing weight reductions he was getting with a high fibre diet in obese patients in China through the so-called WTP diet. In a paper co-written by Prof Zhao the authors stated:

> *"A diet rich in non-digestible but fermentable carbohydrates significantly promoted beneficial groups of bacteria and reduced toxin-producers, which contributes to the alleviation of metabolic deteriorations in obesity regardless of the primary driving forces" (Zhang, Yin et al. 2015).*

It is not the bad bacteria that benefit from prebiotics (fibre) but the good bacteria (Enders 2015). The good bacteria numbers 'explode' when you provide the right combination of fibres for a healthy microbiota.

As Giulia Enders says in her wonderful book on the gut, that if you are not producing wind, you are not keeping your bowel organisms happy. Acidophilus and Bifidobacteria according to Enders, do not produce foul smelling wind, and if you have this unpleasant problem, you need to consider you have a bacterial dysbiosis.

Chia is a nutritional powerhouse

It is a gluten-free seed that swells due to its ability to absorb 12x its weight in water. Building up to 2 – 4 heaped tablespoons helps you lose weight and help improve metabolic parameters like blood glucose levels and keep you satisfied, so you are not constantly snacking. The gel-like consistency of Chia after contact with water could work by preventing enzymes from breaking down carbohydrates thus keeping blood glucose levels down. This gel is known as Chia mucilage formed from diverse neutral sugars (Felisberto, Wahanik et al. 2015) and mucilage from food often lacks in Western diets. Flaxseed is another form of mucilage we can take advantage of in this pudding.

The Activ8Health Super Fibre Pudding

Here is a fibre-packed food that is easy enough to make within minutes. If you have all the components ready to go, it does not take long to prepare. Beginning slowly is wise. Each tablespoon of Chia provides around 5 grams of fibre, and you can always begin with 1 teaspoon of Chia and 1 teaspoon of flaxseed meal and increase this gradually to 2 – 4 tablespoons of each. Add a nut milk to the chia component blend such as Macadamia, Almond or Coconut milk (all unsweetened and low-carb, i.e. less than 5 grams per serving), and you can mix in probiotic-rich Kefir or yoghurt.

For those who 'do not do dairy', you can use non-dairy products like coconut kefir or coconut yoghurt. Some kefirs may have milk products so choose 'dairy-free' labelled kefirs or yoghurts. Do not fill it right up because there are other components you can add to increase the complexity and fibre content and fibre variety in one hit.

You can also vary the components such as the type of berry used or switch the prune spread to a date spread and even a teaspoon of high quality, low-sugar marmalade that is rich in citrus rind for those wonderful pectins. To rotate foods as suggested, you could have chia only one day, basil seed and flaxseed the next and then just flaxseed meal or flaxseed seeds only with a mix of the other components adding or leaving out some of them to fit in with the rotation and wash-out period idea. Add some nuts for extra fibre and micronutrients. Black sesame seeds are a great addition with a high calcium content, lignans and anthocyanins. Basil seeds can be a great alternative to chia for mucilage as these seeds also swell significantly and can thus add variety to your puddings.

Prepare and leave in the fridge to set for 20 - 30 minutes – do not swallow chia or basil seeds without soaking first!

Allow the seeds to absorb the fluid in the fridge. This should take ½ an hour usually but can also be left overnight as a great high-fibre breakfast. Simply add protein like the Activ8Health Whey (See Appendix 10) in the portion for your weight if you need to make up a protein portion missed in the intraday fast and the rest of the protein can be eaten as a meal.

Chia needs to be soaked because the Chia seeds have a tremendous capacity to absorb water and you do not want this happening in your oesophagus or stomach. The same for Basil Seeds. So never swallow raw chia or Basil seeds! The mixture sets due to the gel or mucilage which fully forms with soaking, allowing you to have a pudding-like, fibre-rich dessert to enjoy. Drink fluids afterwards.

This fibre mix is very gentle on the bowel and should be tolerated well even by those who suffer from irritable bowel syndrome IBS as long as high FODMAP foods are avoided such as a lot of fructose or lactose. The key point is to increase fibre slowly and not to regard increased wind or flatulence as a bad thing. You should view increased gas in your bowel as the bowel microbiota having the time of their lives gorging on foods they enjoy (fibre and resistant starch), thus joyously releasing gas as they enjoy the high concentration of prebiotic foods you have just given them.

Some people make an issue out of phytate in Chia, but this is negligible compared to phytate in vegetables, nuts seeds and other foods. Phytate also has anticancer properties. Many studies have shown the enormous benefit of Chia on cardiovascular and metabolic health and these problems are common causes of mortality in society. Soaking for long periods of time can help break down phytate, but you do not depend on this one super-fibre source for all your minerals. The Activ8Health Plan-A and Plan-B diets along with appropriate supplementation for reasons discussed provide most of the nutrients necessary for optimal health with some supplementation.

Add complexity to this super fibre pudding

You could also add organic sultanas or Sulphur-free organic black currants and frozen blueberries as mentioned. Blueberries and blackcurrants are sources of high levels of anthocyanins and have been shown to help with short-term memory and stimulating neurogenesis and providing protection to the brain and hippocampus against inflammatory threats (Pojer, Mattivi et al. 2013).

You could certainly have more than one pudding a day before or just after main meals to offset the metabolic shifts of that meal greatly and to have an impact on your waistline. I often add a small amount of a premium olive oil in the mix and a comprehensive omega-3 liquid to the mix that provides me with ALA/DHA/EPA and GLA in this one food.

Adding probiotics to the chia pudding

You could easily add some probiotic powder/s to this mix to create a highly complementary probiotic/prebiotic mix. If you are using Kefir or yoghurt, then you have a perfect medium for the added probiotics.

You have now created an amazingly complex and tasty chia pudding that is incredibly rich in soluble and insoluble fibre and also rich in gums and mucilage and pectin if you add the citrus peel or small amount of Marmalade. If you have added either kefir or yoghurt to this mix and a probiotic powder and prebiotics like inulin or green banana powder, you now have a very powerful blend of prebiotics and probiotics in one small high-fibre meal.

Avoid	Why
Agave Syrup	Up to 70% may be fructose a highly glycating compound that can raise uric acid levels and increase the risk of fatty liver and insulin resistance
Artificial sweeteners	Try to avoid chemical sweeteners. Add a little bit of Stevia or natural vanilla. Adding prune paste, prune juice or just a little Pomegranate or Sour Cherry juice
Fruit	Add low fructose fruits like blueberries, blackberries, raspberries, strawberries or small amounts of seasonal fruits. It is the quantity that matters. Fruit can be rich in fructose. Avoid a lot of dry fruit.
Honey	50% fructose (see Agave Syrup)
Maple Syrup	Glucose, fructose – empty calories
Molasses	Glucose, sucrose, fructose --- avoid
Polyols	Such as Xylitol, Sorbitol as these can increase symptoms in those with irritable bowel syndrome (IBS)
Table Sugar (Sucrose)	50:50 Glucose and Fructose. Glycating effects, energy dense, calorie poor

Suggested components that can be rotated to make this a versatile, fibre-packed daily routine are shown on the next page.

Food	Amount	Fibre – Max Dose (grams)	Comment
Chia Seeds	1 teaspoon initially increased gradually to 4 – 5 tablespoons	20 grams	Rich in antioxidants, minerals, vitamins, fibre, mucilage (gel). High in alpha linolenic acid (ALA) – Never swallow without first soaking allowing the seed to swell naturally.
Basil Seeds	1 teaspoon building up to 2 tablespoons	Alternate with Chia to provide that mucilage and fibre	Swells like chia after soaking. Also known as Sweet Basil Seeds or Subja. These are small black seeds that are used in Indian sweet drinks like Falooda. Found in Asian stores and Indian food supermarkets. Never swallow without first soaking allowing the seed to swell naturally.
Flaxseed Meal (or seeds)	1 teaspoon initially mixed with the Chia increasing gradually in line with the Chia to 2 tablespoons	3.8 grams	Rich in mucilage and flaxseed lignans. High in fibre and alpha linolenic acid (ALA)
Black Currants (Dried or fresh) Preservative, free of added sulphites	1 tablespoon	~ 1.4 grams	Rich in anthocyanins and blackcurrant phytochemicals like proanthocyanidins, quercetin, phenolic acids. Offers neuroprotection (nerve cell protection) by decreasing oxidative stress (Karjalainen, Anttonen et al. 2008)
Berry compote	½ cup	~ 2 grams	Vary say 2 different types of berries and crush them into a fresh berry compote and pour on the surface after mixing the components. Black berries are rich in anthocyanins and all berries are rich in antioxidants and low in sugar.
Prune spread	1 Tablespoon	~ 1.4 grams	Prunes are simply the dried version of plums. They are rich in antioxidant phenols and in soluble and insoluble fibre and sorbitol. This spread can add some natural sweetness. Prunes are rich in Boron found to significantly reduce the risk of prostate cancer. 6 prunes is all that is necessary (Zhang, Winton et al. 2001).
Green Banana Powder Or Teff Powder	1 – 2 teaspoons	~ 1 – 2 grams	The fibre component is not the focus of green bananas or powder. It is the amazing resistant starch. This is a particular type of carb that is not digested in the small bowel but goes into the large bowel where the good bacteria love this food. They reward you by converting resistant starch to short chain fatty acids so important for bowel and systemic health. Teff is composed of around 40% resistant starch.
Inulin Powder	1 teaspoon (5 grams)	4.5 grams	Start off with a very small amount initially
Kefir or Yoghurt	1 – 2 tablespoons	Negligible	Adding probiotics to this powerful prebiotic mix makes sense. Small amounts of dairy can be added or if you 'don't do dairy' then there are many non-dairy kefir's or yoghurts.
Total		~ 35.1 grams	

CHAPTER 14

The 'S' word: Supplementation

Ignoring potential micronutrient insufficiencies or overt deficiencies would have to be one of the most negligent and dangerous oversights by any medical practitioner, dietitian or nutritionist that is involved in the care of a patient. Never allow yourself to become insufficient or overtly deficient in any of the essential micronutrients otherwise you face a bleak future in your health.

Chronic diseases will kill far more people than any acute presentation to a medical clinic. There is a plethora of research to show how individuals in the 21st century are suffering from long-latency micronutrient insufficiencies or overt deficiencies and I think that medical practitioners and dietitians are putting themselves in harm's way from legal action if the paradigm of treatment does not change. Long-latency disease as the term suggests will occur over a long period to unmask disease states caused by micronutrient insufficiencies or deficiencies but which take a long time to manifest. An insufficiency is a micronutrient depletion, not as severe as an overt deficiency – it may progress to an overt deficiency if not treated in time.

People are becoming more and more aware and highly knowledgeable about nutritional concepts and have a great deal of understanding in this regard from a huge range of books and websites that are highly reputable with information provided by Ivy League universities and professors at the cutting-edge of nutrition research. What hope does a general practitioner, dietitian or nutritionist have against this powerhouse of knowledge that is most likely coming from the very same universities they received their qualifications.

Most people have a far greater understanding of clinical nutritional concepts than the vast majority of doctors or dietitians and all because these professionals are trained with limited knowledge about clinical nutrition. Cutting-edge knowledge in medical science is essentially passed down to the general practice level by a trickle-down effect that may take up to 2 decades to become established as a therapeutic norm (Sanders 2010).

Knowledge has shifted to the lay public who have access to a wealth of information but also need guidance due to their limitations in understanding. What I find in clinical practice is that people now want guidance about integrative healthcare from trained professionals where treatment is not skewed towards purely pharmaceutical approaches because many diseases have their basis in diet and lifestyle inadequacies that cannot be fixed by a magic bullet that comes in the form of a pill, capsule or injection.

If we just look at the epidemic that is prediabetes or diabetes, how can any pharmaceutical pill, capsule or injection negate all of the effects of a bad diet? It is absurd.

The pace of a snail: The slow embrace of aspirin

As Dr Lisa Sanders states in her excellent book - 'Every Patient Tells a Story':

"Doctors are not known for their rapid embrace of the new ...... Physicians are so reluctant to change the way they practice medicine that it takes on average seventeen years for techniques well established by research ---such as giving aspirin to a patient having a heart attack --- to be adopted by even half of those in practice."

Aspirin is regarded as the sine qua non of antiplatelet (anti-clotting) treatment. It has a striking effect on preventing occlusive and embolic (clot-related) stroke or a heart attack in those at high risk, i.e. those that have had an occlusive stroke or heart attack. This aspirin-related research was published in every major journal you can think of, and yet this was adopted at a snail's pace in general practice.

Yet practitioners love loftily state that they practice a superior model of medical care due to an evidence-based approach, and yet, when an undeniable, incontrovertible medical approach hits them in the face like a sledgehammer , they do not even recognize or embrace the most exalted and revered double-blind, placebo-controlled trials published by the gurus of medicine trying to guide them. Why?

How many GPs get their 'evidence-based' knowledge in a staff room provided by pharmaceutical reps with a vested interest in the products they promote? The vast majority of GPs will never read a research article or have such research presented to them in a way free of commercial interest by the profession itself. At least this is rare in comparison to an industry-based liaison that land on the doorsteps of medical practices.

If this is the case for an in-your-face pharmaceutical approach to treatment then what chance does a nutraceutical have even though a great deal of research has already been carried out to validate their use in a clinical setting.

If we consider that one-sixth of vascular death is prevented by antiplatelet therapy (Trialists' Collaboration 2002), then the following statistics are chilling. The Australian Heart Foundation stated that there were 45,392 deaths from cardiovascular disease in 2015. If we used this figure and extrapolated this to the 17 year period where nothing eventuated from all that aspirin research, we would have had 771,664 deaths over this period. If aspirin treatment could have avoided one-sixth of these deaths, then we would have had 128,610 deaths prevented with some variation in this number if early adopters were included, but these numbers would have been few and far between.

So many people could have survived for many more years after their acute vascular event and lived fruitful lives with their families for so much longer if this undisputed research was implemented in clinical practice. Isn't this tragic and where do you hear about this wasteful loss of life? Who condemns this? Is this acceptable?

According to the CDC, there are 610,000 deaths from heart disease in the USA every year, and this accounts for 1 in 4 deaths (https://www.cdc.gov/heartdisease/facts.htm). This is an unbelievable 10,370,000 people that died in that 17 years of inaction. If aspirin was adopted early in the piece, then one-sixth of these people may have lived that much longer in the embrace of their families and loved ones, and this makes up 1,728,333 people whose lives could have been saved!

This is simply a lack of strong leadership to guide the profession, and this is the same case with the use of dietary and nutraceutical supplements that have a strong evidence-base and simply being ignored because of conceited attitudes and ignorance of the huge amount of research done on supplements.

Nutrition as important to Psychiatry as it is to Cardiology, Endocrinology and Gastroenterology

This important message was published in Lancet Psychiatry (2015) and outlines some cutting-edge ideas on the link between poor diets and psychiatric health (Sarris, Logan et al. 2015). How long will it take for this to sink into the minds of medical practitioners who rely on quick-fix drug solutions? We can only look at the aspirin story to see how this will pan out!

That anyone can doubt that a link exists between suboptimal dietary intakes and mental ill health astounds me as no doubt many in the medical profession will simply blame genetics, personal circumstance and factors in the 'ether' that contribute to psychiatric ill health.

For those in the medical profession that have a very poor understanding of how important dietary factors are to the human brain, it is important to look at some statistics of the fatty composition of our brains. The brain is 60% fat (Chang, Ke et al. 2009) and **Docosahexaenoic acid (DHA)** a 22 carbon long-chain essential fatty acid, is the predominant structural omega-3 in the brain making up 40% of brain **polyunsaturated fatty acids (PUFAs)** and 60% of the PUFAs in the retina (Singh 2005). This is a staggering compositional level for a single molecule (i.e. DHA) in incredibly important organs in our bodies.

DHA cannot be manufactured directly in our bodies --- it is essential, and this means we cannot produce this and need to either consume DHA in our diets or consume Alpha Linolenic Acid (ALA) the parent omega-3 compound and then convert this ALA very inefficiently by human beings to EPA and DHA. Marine algae do a far better job of this conversion to EPA/DHA and fish that consume these marine algae, concentrate the EPA/DHA in their flesh. Consuming fatty fish which most people in Western worlds avoid or by simply consuming practitioner-only, high-quality omega-3 supplements that truly have the concentration of DHA/EPA stated on the labels, will ensure we meet our needs for DHA and brain integrity and function. See Appendix-2 & Appendix-18. I think it is important to get the full gamut of Omega's – DHA/EPA/ALA/GLA from diet and supplementation. Unlikely you will meet your needs simply from the diet.

How many professionals even know that neurotransmitters to a very large extent are dependent upon amino acids from protein sources as the foundation molecules to derive neurotransmitters. Amino acids such as glycine are neurotransmitters in themselves. So you can see how absurd it is to keep nutritional factors like protein and amino acids out of the equation as if they are peripheral to the brain and central nervous system health and function. They are not peripheral but indeed absolutely central!

Amino Acid	Neurotransmitter/s
Arginine, Citrulline (Preferable)	Nitric Oxide
Glutamine	Glutamate, Gamma Aminobutyric Acid (GABA)
Glycine	Glycine (inhibitory)
Histidine	Histamine
Phenylalanine/Tyrosine	Dopamine, Noradrenaline, Adrenaline
Tryptophan	Serotonin, Melatonin

Many in the medical and dietetic professions are enlightened people who see beyond the vested interests of their associations and training, but there are some who gloat when they read that omega-3's fail in certain clinical trials as if to think that omega-3's are of no use in a multitude of other clinical states. This is the same as throwing away the much-beloved statin drugs for cholesterol control because they failed to fix ingrown toenails or fungal skin infections. Such rigidity of thought of some within these professions.

Statins have fantastic effects in those with high-risk cardiovascular disease and should be used in this context! There is no question that drugs have a powerful role to play in established disease, and as a corollary, there is no question that diet and nutritional factors likewise have a powerful role in disease prevention and treatment. This statement about dietary interventions is not arguable, it is an absolute incontrovertible fact!

There is no room for right-wing views as this will only result in the loss of countless lives. It is important to remember that dietary management that includes the use of judicious supplementation is NOT mutually exclusive to pharmaceutical treatment but highly synergistic!

The Lancet Psychiatry paper titled '**Nutritional medicine as mainstream in psychiatry**' (Sarris, Logan et al. 2015), should be a compulsory read for anyone practising medicine at the primary care level or in psychiatry. This paper has a great deal of wisdom. This viewpoint is from the perspective of an international collaboration of academics no less, who are members of the International Society for Nutritional Psychiatry Research.

This group of academics should be lauded in promoting what is a glaring hole in the treatment of individuals with mental health disorders who are fed a concoction of toxic compounds to control their mental health problems where these pharmaceutical interventions can have devastating metabolic effects on that individual such as triggering off a pre-diabetic or diabetic state, or increasing body weight and hence push those individuals towards cardiovascular risk. Is this acceptable when other non-toxic possibilities exist that may have a profound impact on their mental state? Why adopt these pharmaceutical approaches when far cheaper possibilities exist and should be trialled first where possible before drug approaches are used?

This Lancet paper points out some potential nutraceutical treatments and how they can benefit mental health states. The references to back up these treatments can be found in the paper mentioned above, and this can be downloaded free through a Google search.

Nutrient	Mental Health Concern
B-Group Vitamins/Folate	Needed for neuronal function. Folate deficiency is associated with depression in certain populations and may be a factor for a poor response to antidepressants. High dose L-Methylfolate (Neurofolin®) at 15mg daily was found to have significant synergistic antidepressant effects with SSRI's used to treat the depression. Lower doses of L-Methylfolate did not work. So dose is a critical factor.
N-Acetyl Cysteine (NAC) (See Appendix-7)	Bi-Polar Depression, Schizophrenia, Compulsive and Addictive Behaviours, Trichotillomania, Modulates Glutamate effects, Anti-Inflammatory.
Omega-3's	Bi-Polar Disorder, PTSD, Depression, Prevention of psychosis, Neurogenesis via BDNF upregulation, Neurotransmitter modulation (Noradrenaline, Dopamine, Serotonin), Anti-Inflammatory effects, Cell membrane fluidity

SAMe	Effective antidepressant, Synergistic augmentation with other antidepressants,
Vitamin-D	Vitamin-D is a neurosteroid. Low maternal levels are associated with Schizophrenia in the offspring, Low levels linked to increased depressive symptoms
Zinc	Cytokine modulation, Hippocampal neurogenesis by BDNF upregulation, Modifies N-Methyl D Aspartate and Glutamate Activity, An important adjunctive factor with antidepressants
Phytochemicals	As the Sarris et al paper states that phytochemicals are a part of the overall antioxidant system important for mental health disorders but also for general health. Many mental health disorders such as depression are thought to be triggered by inflammatory processes. In Appendix-4 I have described a vegetable juice with a small amount of fruit to keep fructose levels low but to increase carotenoids, Vitamin-C through the addition of lemons or limes and Nitrates along with a huge number of other phytochemicals. Appendix-27 shows how you can increase phytochemical complexity. How certain phytochemicals can help with brain health is yet to be ascertained, but Hormesis is an important concept not only for brain health but your body in general.

This important paper goes on to state:

"Diet and nutrition offer key modifiable targets for the prevention of mental disorders, having a fundamental role in the promotion of mental health. Now is time for the recognition of the importance of nutrition and nutrient supplementation in psychiatry. Nutritional medicine should now be considered as a mainstream element of psychiatric practice, with research, education, policy, and health promotion supporting this new framework." (Sarris, Logan et al. 2015)

Nutritional medicine needs to be put into clinical context by medical practitioners who have a vast knowledge of disease states and pathophysiological processes. If the risk is the argument for not using a supplement, then practitioners medical or dietetic need to view the Alliance of Natural Health Analysis on the comparison of adverse events between pharmaceuticals and supplements that soon follows in this chapter. Governments should make access to the compounds mentioned above on the Pharmaceutical Benefits Scheme (PBS), as these compounds are incredibly cheap in comparison to pharmaceutical agents used as first-line treatments.

To try and separate diet and nutrients from someone's mental state or indeed their state of health, in general, is now an incredibly anachronistic way of thinking. This way of thinking is an absolute relic of time that has no place in modern medicine.

Lumping all supplements together

The controversy surrounding supplement use is often confused where all supplements are lumped into a useless basket, and this is illogical, inherently untrue and misleading. This lack of distinction can be downright dangerous if someone who is suffering a nutrient deficiency is left undiagnosed and untreated. Such a deficiency could easily trigger off an acute event. You can easily imagine a lack of magnesium or calcium causing an abnormal rhythm of the heart. This does not have to be an overt deficiency it can just be an insufficiency waiting for the right set of factors to fall into place and these could be a severe flu, significant trauma, weight gain or sleep apnoea for that deadly abnormal heart rhythm to appear and all because of diminishing magnesium and/or calcium levels in the body that put organ systems like the heart in jeopardy.

Osteoporosis, for example, is a thinning of the bones which can be caused by chronic (long-term) Vitamin-D deficiency or a lack of a large number of synergistic minerals that act to keep bones strong over your life. The way we should view supplements is that we need to distinguish:

- Supplements found on a shelf for self-treatment versus practitioner-guided
- Supplements that have an evidence-base for their use versus those concocted with very little scientific understanding and then promoted to have a specific therapeutic benefit.
- Supplements that have a well-established and incontrovertible scientific basis for use in clinical treatment and I have listed some of these in the table below.
- Supplements like multivitamins and minerals that may fill in a gap in nutritional insufficiency states to prevent long-term, long-latency diseases caused through the many 'holes' in agriculture and food production and all the other factors in-between trying to get food from the paddock to the plate.

The Triage-Theory of nutrition shines some light on this insufficiency mechanism. A plethora of factors including dietary insufficiency due to poor food choices, nutrient-poor soils, nutrient loss in storage, or transport and cooking, genetics, environment, lifestyle, illness and medications can profoundly impact on an individual's nutrient needs and nutrient sufficiency.

To blindly label all supplements as being of no use is a blatant disregard of the well-established medical use of many vitamins or minerals in clinical deficiency states. Having an optimal intake of all nutrients during pregnancy can prevent malnutrition of the foetus and future adult ill health (Barker Hypothesis). Ensuring micronutrient sufficiency in pregnancy may prevent the early onset of a chronic illness in that child or to even prevent the development of major anatomical problems like spina bifida and other neural tube defects in the developing foetus.

Many individuals show no interest in pharmaceutical interventions due to the significant risk of side-effects, and this is a great opportunity for doctors to become knowledgeable in a range of nutraceutical products such as L-Citrulline that may provide highly significant benefits to men suffering from erectile dysfunction. L-Citrulline can be used in a highly synergistic way with Cialis® or Viagra® or as adjunctive treatment in those suffering other vascular diseases to help boost nitric oxide (NO) levels.

It is truly sad that such promising adjunctive treatments are not even considered. The history of medicine is riddled with such stories of ignorance and resistance when new concepts present to them and challenge the rigidity of thought and the irrational fight against change.

Commonplace micronutrient deficiencies

Iron, Magnesium, Vitamins-A, B1, B6, Folate, B12 and Zinc are commonplace deficiencies (Ames, 2006), that can slowly impair and slowly kill. Chronic illness kills over 35 million people worldwide, and these are largely preventable deaths (Strong, Mathers, Leeder, & Beaglehole, 2005). Chronic micronutrient deficiencies add to this toll. To ignore these common micronutrient deficiencies in general practice to me is simply astounding in an age where no one in their right mind can argue that dietary practices in Western populations are ideal. Ignorance of the importance of these micronutrient deficiencies or insufficiencies is no excuse as these are bona fide causes of increased morbidity and mortality with a huge weight of research to back up their importance. Just think of the magnesium deficiency state I mentioned and how this may be contributing to the huge numbers of people who suffer sudden death due to an arrhythmia.

We now have a compelling mechanism in the Triage Theory of nutrient allocation to understand how deaths in chronic illness are hastened. Metabolic shifts in chronic disease and genetic mutations demand individualised (personalised) nutrition assessments and intervention, but medical care for these illnesses is far from optimal and far from best practice!

Classical reductionist and interventionist medicine has no place in treating the subtle and long-term effects of a micronutrient insufficiency/deficiency. Allowing micronutrient shortcomings to complicate matters and slowly worsen any chronic illness is not good clinical management. More often than not, nutritional care is an afterthought and usually only considered when disease manifests itself overtly.

Supplements commonly used in general practice

Supplement	Uses	Comment
Vitamin-A	Mucosal immune system function, skin disorders Roaccutane (Isotretinoin) is a retinoid used for severe acne and is related to Vitamin-A	Vitamin-A deficiency is regarded as a nutritionally acquired immunodeficiency disorder
B12	Key role in the nervous system and red blood cell formation. Treating megaloblastic anaemia due to B12 deficiency	A deficiency of Vitamin-B12 may cause devastating central nervous system damage and megaloblastic anaemia
Vitamin-D	Bone health, prevention of osteomalacia and osteoporosis	Often checked by Psychiatrists now because of a growing body of evidence of low Vit-D levels in depression and other psychiatric illnesses like Schizophrenia
Folic Acid	Prevents neural tube defects in pregnancy	Found in many pre-natal supplements
Iron	Common anaemia in women	Menstrual loss commonly causes iron deficiency in females but can be due to cancer of the gastrointestinal tract. This supplement is often infused intravenously for significant iron deficiency states.
Magnesium	Atrial Fibrillation, heart ectopic beats, muscle cramping	A common deficiency with poor diets. Anyone with atrial fibrillation (AF) or ectopic heart beats should strongly consider checking their RBC-Magnesium level and supplementing with magnesium at RDA
Omega-3's	High triglyceride levels. Post Myocardial Infarction Product Omacor, medical grade omega-3 acid ethyl esters.	TGA approved for the two indications mentioned (TGA 2010). May decrease the risk of sudden arrhythmias (abnormal heart rhythms)
Thiamine (Thiamin)	Vitamin-B1. Used to prevent Wernicke–Korsakoff syndrome (WKS)	Vitamin-B1 should be used in heavy alcohol drinkers

Scurvy in the 21st Century

I have mentioned that scurvy has raised its ugly head in Western societies in the 21st Century. The Portuguese recognised that citrus could prevent scurvy in 1497, but it took a few centuries after this for this to be proven. This particular micronutrient deficiency was recognised by Westmead Hospital in Sydney, Australia in 2016 as the reason chronic ulcers in people with diabetes were not healing. I will discuss this shortly, but one can see that this is a bona fide medical problem being caused by a micronutrient deficiency and not recognised because of a lack of knowledge about such problems and also because testing for micronutrient deficiencies as a complicating factor of chronic illness is not common practice.

This could easily be seen at best as poor medical practice but at worst, malpractice where chronic leg ulcers are treated with every lotion, potion and paste and given antibiotic after antibiotic trying to coax an ulcer to heal, without treating the trophic (nutrient-related) causes for that ulcer to manifest and persist in the first place? Sure a lack of blood supply to the tissues caused by vascular disease over years of dietary neglect or venous insufficiency is contributing to the problem. Venous insufficiency occurs in many individuals that are overweight or obese and again the cause of many years of dietary neglect and sedentary lifestyles. So these underlying conditions can all be taken back to diet and underlying genetics predisposing that individual to such fates. Remember, genetic predispositions are not the cause. Genes are the loaded gun but we need an environmental trigger, and dietary factors make up a huge range of triggers for a large number of genetic determinants.

Human tissue simply cannot repair, heal or survive without all the nutritional elements in place. It is absolutely unacceptable not to consider that damaged tissue needs nutrients to heal and that the Western diet is devoid of nutrients. Just look at the food that patients are given in hospitals or nursing homes where carb-rich foods and even desserts are given to people with diabetes and where the nutrient density of hospital food is greatly lacking. This should be foremost in the minds of physicians and hospitals, but often these issues of poor nutrition are at the bottom of their considerations.

Just think of the damage to the microbiome by all the antibiotics often given to these people with non-healing ulcers. An antibiotic damaged dysbiotic microbiome will in turn damage the immune system which in turn affects the healing of the ulcer. **A vicious cycle indeed!**

The use of topical antiseptics increases the possibility of inducing antibiotic or antiseptic-resistant strains of organisms that could make matters worse from those lotions, potions or pastes. Just think of all the suffering and hardship that could be saved by using a simple Multivitamin, multimineral and Vitamin-C tablet costing just cents a day as an adjunct to medical treatment modalities that support healing. Countless millions of dollars are wasted on ineffective treatments all because the absolute and incontrovertible foundation of healing is being ignored, i.e. ***Human tissue simply cannot repair, heal or survive without all the nutritional elements in place.***

Humans, primates and guinea pigs cannot synthesise L-Ascorbic Acid and thus require this in their diet. When we consider that around 90% of people in a Western population do not get anywhere near their 5 servings of vegetables or 2 servings of fruit on a daily basis, it should be absolutely obvious that there could be a Vitamin-C deficiency in a vast number of people in a Western population and especially if the patient is elderly with a poor diet due to infirmity. That scurvy can exist in a wealthy country like Australia in the 21st Century is not an arguable point, it is a scientific fact!

"Scurvy causing poor wound healing in diabetes"| 21st November 2016

As mentioned here is the story on scurvy in Sydney, Australia. I find this an amazing title in a major medical newspaper, the Australian Doctor distributed to all general practitioners in Australia keeping them abreast of developments in medicine.

Professor Jenny Gunton is the director of the Centre for Diabetes, Obesity and Endocrinology at the Westmead Institute for Medical Research in Sydney, Australia. She studied 11 people with poorly healing ulcers and tested them for Vitamin-C levels. Seven of these patients had Vitamin-C levels of 19umol/L. On Douglass Hanly Moir's website, SonicEdu, available to medical practitioners, the reference range for fasting Vitamin-C is 26 – 85 umol/L and so you can see that the levels found in the study subjects showed quite a significant deficiency.

As a medical practitioner who saw a tremendous number of people with chronic ulcers coming into the medical centre where I worked over my medical career, I always thought nutritional deficiencies or insufficiencies would, without doubt, be at the heart of many of these poorly healing ulcers that sometimes required months of treatment using pastes, lotions and potions and perhaps antibiotic after antibiotic to persuade them to heal.

Checking Vitamin-C along with Zinc, Vitamin-A, Vitamin-B12, Omega-3, Omega-6, haptoglobin (HP-2) and Folate levels along with a range of minerals should be standard, and there should be a Medicare rebate for all nutrient status testing in patients with chronic non-healing ulcers, with doctors educated about these nutritional concerns. Ensuring a rich intake of Omega-3's and phytochemicals even in the form of concentrated powders or capsules would greatly enhance healing times and save our cash-strapped health system a huge sum of money in the process. This is enlightened medicine and not one limited to pharmaceutical or surgical approaches.

Haptoglobin (HP-2) and Vitamin-C Deficiency

This fascinating genetic mutation crushes the often stated concept that people can get all the necessary nutrients they need from that mythical 'optimal diet'.

The HP-2 mutation also highlights the potential of personalised dietary management through genetic testing and guidance. We know that individuals with a genetic polymorphism (mutation) of the haptoglobin (HP-2) gene may trigger Vitamin-C deficiency by ineffective inhibition of haemoglobin-driven oxidative stress (free radicals, ROS), which leads to Vitamin-C depletion. It is not so important to understand the underlying mechanism but just to know that this mutation results in the **overconsumption** of Vitamin-C in the body in someone who has this mutation putting them at risk for a Vitamin-C insufficiency at the least and at worst, Vitamin-C deficiency (Scurvy).

Vitamin-C comes from fruits and vegetables, and so if over 90% of the population does not get anywhere near the minimum intake of fruits and vegetables a day and if this genetic mutation is quite common, it should be clear that these individuals are at great risk for scurvy.

This genetic variation is very common and present in **35% of the white population** and **50% of South and East Asians**. (Delanghe, Langlois et al. 2007) The authors of this paper stated:

"The classical view of vitamin C and scurvy being a pure nutritional condition needs to be updated."

This genetic mutation of haptoglobin beautifully highlights the fact that a nutritional resource like Vitamin-C can be depleted not simply due to a lack of nutrient intake. The mythical 'balanced diet' propaganda needs to simply vanish as this common HP-2 genetic mutation is showing us the reality of gene-nutrient interactions and where genetically guided dietary advice comes into play.

Haptoglobin (HP-2) is one of many genetic factors that can conspire against an individual in a nutritional sense. Thousands of other mutations can have similar effects, and there is a huge number that are yet to be discovered and their mechanisms ascertained.

Suffice it to say that in the modern world of suboptimal agricultural practices and nutrient-poor foods commercially produced along with a potential 10 million single nucleotide polymorphisms (SNPs) in the human body, it is safe to assume we are primed for micronutrient deficiencies. We are just scientifically unaware of a multitude of these gene-nutrient interactions.

There is a simple insurance policy and that is to ensure micronutrient adequacy through the best diet you can muster along with targeted supplementation such as a good multivitamin/mineral most days + Omega-3's most days along with some extra Vitamin-C daily and additional help in antioxidant capacity through N-Acetyl Cysteine on a daily basis, plus choline daily. This regimen is a minimum number of basic supplements one should strongly consider in a less than perfect world.

Suboptimal diets the rule, not the exception: Overfed yet Undernourished

So why should this happen in a wealthy country like Australia, one of the 20 major economies in the world (a G20 country)? Almost all the patients in Professor Gunton's study above were obese and had a low intake of fruit and vegetables.

Grains contain no Vitamin-A, Vitamin-C, or Vitamin-B12 and apart from yellow maize, cereal grains contain no Vitamin-A precursors like beta-carotene (Cordain, 1999). Moreover, grains, are the focus of dietetic organisations and governments around the world. Fruit and vegetable intakes are precariously low in every nutrition survey. The 2014 -2015 National Health Survey published by the Australian Bureau of Statistics, showing only 1 in 20 Australians met the recommended guidelines of at least five servings of vegetables and two servings of fruit consumed daily, and this is a staggeringly low 95% of Australians not meeting these minimum guidelines.

Fruit and vegetables do not have the economic clout of grains that can be stored and exported in vast quantities adding to the economy regarding export dollar returns to a country. According to a study published in the Archives of Pediatrics & Adolescent Medicine on fruit and vegetable intakes in children and adolescents in the USA: *"Nearly one-quarter of all vegetables consumed by children and adolescents were French fries."* (Krebs-Smith, Cook et al. 1996)

On the Centers for Disease Control and Prevention (CDC) website a report was titled **'Adults Meeting Fruit and Vegetable Intake Recommendations — United States, 2013'** - It stated: *"However, during 2007–2010, half of the total U.S. population consumed <1 cup of fruit and <1.5 cups of vegetables daily; 76% did not meet fruit intake recommendations, and 87% did not meet vegetable intake recommendations."* https://www.cdc.gov

When have you ever analysed the food you consume on a daily basis to ensure you are getting all the micronutrients you need? Do you even know which foods to consume to meet your RDI's for the large range of essential nutrients? The vast majority of people simply throw food on a plate and hope for the best!

So the agricultural machine turns to ensure grains are the focus of dietetic guidelines not the consumption of fruit and vegetables. See Appendix-28.

From this understanding, it would be safe to assume numerous insufficiencies exist in many people and these are exacerbated by underlying genetic traits and lifestyle factors such as excessive exercise or alcohol consumption or drug use both recreational and pharmaceutical.

Those that have undergone bariatric (obesity) surgery, and those who are chronically ill or elderly, may need far greater nutritional resources.

Tryptophan, the building block of Serotonin

Many micronutrient insufficiencies or deficiencies including protein-energy malnutrition (PEM), present as lethargy. A multitude of neurotransmitters including Serotonin are produced from amino acids derived from protein. Serotonin is manufactured in the body from the amino acid tryptophan provided by protein in the diet. So instead of treating the cause, i.e. a deficiency of protein and amino acids, we treat the result – decreased serotonin. We use Selective Serotonin Reuptake Inhibitors (SSRI's) to increase serotonin in the nerve synapse by trying to artificially elevate this neurotransmitter by blocking the reuptake in the synapse by these SSRI antidepressants. Why not ensure there is enough serotonin, to begin with by making sure an individual has enough protein and hence tryptophan to make serotonin?

How many people for various reasons may have protein-energy malnutrition and how many of these would be on antidepressants?

The misguided reluctance to use a supplement

I have no problem prescribing a raft of medications to people if I feel the benefits far outweigh the risks and if those medications have an evidence-base to back their use in a particular clinical circumstance. I also understand that there could potentially be life-threatening complications from the use of a particular medication that clashes with the genetic makeup of an individual. Pharmacogenetics will go a long way toward finding this risk where genetic mutations can be discovered as markers of adverse reactions to certain medications and thus avoided in those individuals. It will save many lives in future.

Drugs as dangerous as war! Looking at relative risk of adverse outcomes

There are figures of around 58,000 US military fatalities in the Vietnam War and around 417,000 US military casualties in WWII. Keep these figures in mind when reading the following on lethal adverse drug reactions.

Should we fear an adverse supplement reaction (ASR) in comparison to a fatal adverse drug reaction (ADR)? Such a thought beggars belief when hard data is taken into consideration in particular when we compare adverse events caused by a supplement in comparison to those caused by pharmaceuticals.

A study published in the prestigious Journal of the American Medical Association (JAMA) indicated that around 100,000 deaths in the United States of America every year are due to lethal Adverse Drug Reactions (ADR's) (Lazarou, Pomeranz, & Corey, 1998). This astonishing figure was disbelieved by many experts who criticised the data, and this was understandable as the figure was so high and frightening. ***The figure is equivalent to the casualties of two Vietnam wars every year and equivalent to the US military casualties of WWII every four years due to pharmaceutical related deaths!***

The authors estimated ADRs ranked from the fourth to sixth leading cause of death depending on whether the lower or higher mortality rate was considered.

The figure reflected a 0.13% incidence of fatal ADR's. This figure was vindicated when a British study published in the equally prestigious British Medical Journal (BMJ), looked at 18,820 hospital admissions in the United Kingdom (Pirmohamed et al., 2004). This UK research group found a higher 0.15% incidence of fatal ADR's which when adjusted for population number differences between the UK and USA. The study produced a similar or even greater number of deaths due to lethal adverse pharmaceutical drug reactions.

A study from Sweden, one of the richest countries in the world and published in the British Journal of Clinical Pharmacology in 2007, found that fatal adverse drug reactions accounted for 3% of all deaths in the general population and fatal adverse drug reactions were estimated to be the seventh most common cause of death in Sweden (Wester, Jönsson et al. 2008). Simply staggering! Moreover, just one supplement associated with an adverse event will make headline news in a medical newspaper or magazine and even in the mainstream press. How ridiculous!

I would like to state from the outset that as a bona fide medical practitioner, I use pharmaceuticals regularly in clinical practice from treating potentially life-threatening infections to preventing stroke through optimal treatment of high blood pressure or trying to prevent a heart attack by using Statins in a high-risk individual. We also need to take into consideration that pharmaceuticals can save lives or prevent a clinical condition. It is important not to have a right-wing view about anything in science and to accept that there are pros and cons to using both pharmaceuticals or nutraceuticals and both should be used after considering the benefits versus the risks and if these are clinically relevant. However, in the light of extremely high incidence of fatal drug reactions, it seems absolutely absurd to talk about supplement reactions that are often mild and rarely fatal.

To put this into context, the chance of an adverse event is 62,000 (that is right – sixty-two thousand) times higher with the use of a pharmaceutical than a supplement (see below).

Valuable and potentially life-saving interventions through diet and supplements as adjunctive measures to medical treatments are disregarded, all because of an extremely remote possibility of a reaction to a supplement.

People do not have a few lifetimes to wait for every skerrick of information to come through before implementing treatment. **When has this ever stopped a drug from being used? Most drugs are released after limited trial times, in restricted trial demographics that avoid high-risk individuals and the real trial then begins in real-time when released for use by populations** - a glaring double-standard.

It is also an established and incontrovertible fact that research-based clinical guidelines may fall far short of being exact and that implementation of treatment in the clinical setting will be based on the individual in front of the physician and not imperfect algorithms of management created from imperfect and incomplete research.

That medicine is an art and not a perfect science seems to be an accepted fact among practitioners. If this is the case, then why is this same principle not being applied to nutritional science where we do not have all the answers? We do however have a significant body of evidence to implement nutritional strategies in conjunction with medical treatment!

The Alliance for Natural Health Analysis

The Alliance for Natural Health (ANH) undertook a large analysis and collected hard data from an extensive list of official sources. You can find and download these graphs as bar charts or an impressive bubble chart to see the relative risk in various individual circumstances in comparison to the potential adverse reaction to a vitamin, mineral or food supplement from their website (ANH, 2012). The huge difference in relative risk is just staggering.

Remember, I am not anti-drug as this would be absolute folly as the pharmaceutical industry to a very large extent is made up of well-intentioned people trying to unlock the cellular complexities in their endeavour to work out how to best treat disease. These are not mad scientists trying to kill us, so this is also absurd to have a right-wing mindset against pharmaceuticals.

Countless millions would die every year without the pharmaceutical tools we have from a huge range of disease states. My point is that we need to use both pharmaceuticals and nutraceuticals in a clinical context weighing up all the pros and cons and not excluding supplements based on outdated and biased views.

Researchers in the nutritional science industry are also trying to unravel the mysteries of nutrient-molecular actions and interactions at many esteemed universities around the world. Please do not forget that nutritional science is all about the complex biochemistry, hormonal and molecular signalling mechanisms driven by nutrient intake and that there is a great overlap with the biochemical and molecular targets of the pharmaceutical industry.

So synergistic approaches abound because these molecular targets intersect.

The adage that a 'picture paints a thousand words' is self-evident from the graph adapted from the ANH research data:

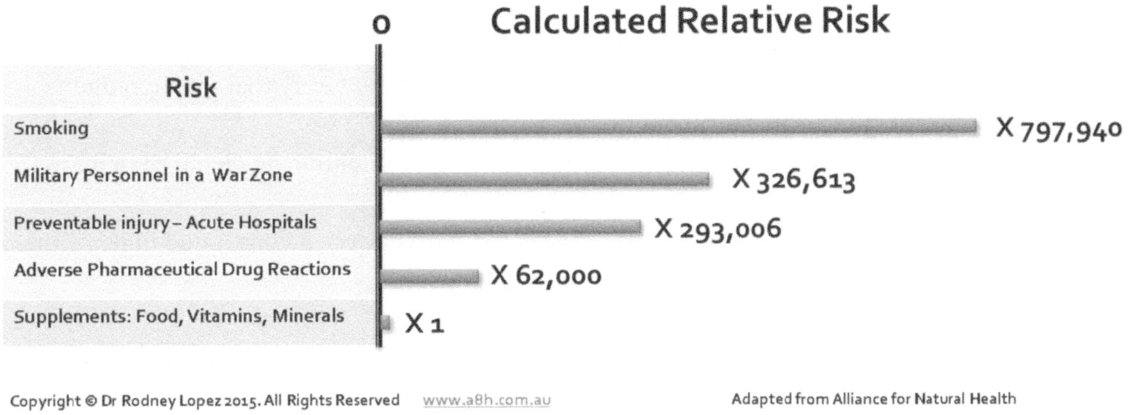

We shouldn't think that diet, exercise and lifestyle are fixing everything as well. We must remember that poor nutrition does not cause all disease. **However, optimal dietary management is relevant in all disease states.** We have diseases caused by cancer producing viruses or environmental and occupational hazards and genetic time-bombs to contend with that no amount of supplementation will fix.

We all need to understand that pharmaceutical interventions create many down-stream effects and can impact on a huge number of intersecting metabolic processes. Micronutrients can also do the same thing but are so much tamer in effect in comparison to a pharmaceutical which is highly targeted, and highly specific in a molecular, hormonal and biochemical sense.

Using vitamins, minerals and trace elements or whole food supplements would have to be the safest treatment option you could think of and yet so underused because of irrational concerns of an adverse event that we can easily see from the Alliance for Natural Health (ANH) data on safety is extremely low.

It is up to you, as an individual to make your mind up about diets and supplements and it is interesting that people spend over one billion dollars on complementary medications in Australia alone. According to the Australian Bureau of Statistics under a search for 'Complementary Medications', 26% - 44% of people had recently taken a vitamin or mineral supplement (www.abs.gov.au).

With such a large number of people using supplements in Australia or for that matter in the USA or UK, doctors will be preaching to the converted and will have a very receptive audience who would love to hear highly trained doctors discuss supplementation. Most people trust their doctors and would like to have such knowledge come from professionals that understand risk and know how to monitor such risk. It is up to the medical profession to wake up and start to educate doctors and move away from trying to solve complex problems by the use of simple magic-bullet pharmaceutical approaches.

Shonky business - the other side of the coin

It is just as important to understand that there are many manufacturers of dubious integrity that produce products that fall far short of what they should be. Reliable supplements with stringent quality control mechanisms in place are mandatory if this industry wants to move forward with credibility in the medical world and credibility in the eyes of consumers.

What makes a supplement worthwhile?

- ✓ An evidence-based approach for their recommendation
- ✓ Recommended doses need to provide therapeutic levels that reflect the dosages showing benefit in research
- ✓ Supplements need to be of pharmaceutical grade
- ✓ They should undergo quality assessments and third-party testing to verify that the ingredients per capsule or tablet reflect the stated strength on the packaging
- ✓ They need use well-researched fillers or excipients to minimise or eliminate chemical or allergic reactions to non-therapeutic components
- ✓ They need to be guaranteed to be free of toxic elements such as heavy metals found in poor quality fish oils
- ✓ Organically sourced, if these are whole foods
- ✓ They need to be packaged appropriately to ensure no spoilage or deterioration occurs within the use-by date as long as they are stored appropriately after opening
- ✓ They need to be reformulated regularly to reflect new findings in dose and to incorporate new and improved nutrient compounds
- ✓ Multi-nutrient components need to be used in synergistic ratios formulated using chelates or other bonded compounds that provide the highest bioavailability and the lowest interference regarding the absorption of other nutrient compounds
- ✓ Information on nutrient-nutrient and drug-nutrient interactions and side-effects should be available in each product as per a pharmaceutical compound. Even better a searchable database that is kept up-to-date for medical practitioners to use freely to check drug-nutrient interactions will be greatly appreciated by the medical profession
- ✓ Any adverse outcomes should be displayed warts-and-all as per any pharmaceutical
- ✓ Products produced by a company should try to avoid the risk of additive exposures. For example, a company may produce numerous products and recommend their use in combination. Many of the products may have perhaps Vitamin-B6 known to be neurotoxic if given in high doses or given to a susceptible individual even in moderately high doses. It would be far better to manufacture synergistic compounds and ask an individual to use a multivitamin rather than add a load of vitamins or minerals in separate preparations thus increasing the risk of toxicities by the use of multiple products with the same ingredients.

Practitioners need to ensure:

- ✓ That mono or poly-supplementation should only be recommended if they are clinically necessary
- ✓ That supplements are used in the right amounts and at the right intervals
- ✓ That there is no additive effect with other supplements in use concomitantly– polypharmacy (the use of multiple medications) can cause significant serious adverse side-effects and poly-supplementation is no different, where multiple products containing herbs, vitamins, minerals and trace elements may lead to toxic overdoses of individual compounds
- ✓ That interaction with current pharmaceutical medications are assessed before recommendation and use

- ✓ That there is no interference between compounds where one compound can affect the absorption or action of another
- ✓ That a wash-out period is recommended
- ✓ That there is no history of allergy to the compound or excipients used in the tablet or capsule
- ✓ That the supplement will not exacerbate any underlying clinical problem
- ✓ That synergistic effects of two or more compounds used will not cause harm
- ✓ That, just like pharmaceutical interventions with a tremendous possible risk of adverse events, use of any nutraceutical is followed-up to assess efficacy and usefulness and that no harm is being done.
- ✓ Practitioners should not oversell the virtues of supplementation and should never neglect the fact that an individual should see a medical practitioner before commencing any supplement regimen
- ✓ Ensure monitoring of blood pressure or blood markers where appropriate in conjunction with a medical practitioner

Why practitioner-only products?

A study published in a Nature research journal called 'Scientific Reports' by a New Zealand group which looked at fish oil supplements. 32 fish oil supplements were analysed for eicosapentaenoic acid (EPA) and docosahexaenoic acid (DHA) which are the clinically valuable long-chain, omega-3 compounds in fish oil supplements and the reason why one would take these supplements. What these researchers found was startling! The researchers stated;

> *"Only 3 of 32 fish oil supplements contained quantities of eicosapentaenoic acid (EPA) and docosahexaenoic acid (DHA) that were equal or higher than labelled content, with most products tested (69%) containing < (less than) 67% (Albert et al., 2015)."*

Even more concerning was the fact that many of the fish oil supplements were rancid, i.e. they had gone off. The researchers went on to state:

> *"The vast majority of supplements exceeded recommended levels of oxidation markers. 83% products exceeded the recommended PV levels, 25% exceeded AV thresholds, and 50% exceeded recommended Totox levels. Only 8% met the international recommendations, not exceeding any of these indices." (Albert, Derraik et al. 2015)*

The initials PV stand for peroxide values, AV for anisidine values and Totox, total oxidation values. These are all markers for oxidation of the fish oil making these products rancid and unfit for consumption.

What this does not mean is that fish oils and omega-3 essential fatty acid supplementation are of no value. Omega-3's can be obtained on a script written by doctors for the right reason such as raised triglyceride levels. What it does mean is that gold-standard manufacturing, storage and third-party testing is vital to produce a worthwhile product that is safe and effective.

The problem with detractors and skeptics is that they see these findings as an excuse to blemish all supplements and undermine the need for any supplementation which is simple-minded and downright idiotic. This does not take away the fact that omega-3's are critical for health and that these are essential fatty acids that the body cannot make efficiently – remembering that the term 'essential' means you need this from dietary sources.

The notoriously poor Western diet lacks meaningful levels of Omega-3's and those in Western populations shun the cold water fish types that provide an abundance of omega-3's for optimal health such as sardines, herring, mackerel, salmon and trout because these fish are too 'fishy' for their tastes. Try getting these types of fish into a child's mouth or for that matter, try to get a pregnant woman to eat these types of fish when they are nauseous and sensitive to smells that could make them vomit. How important do you think omega-3's are to a developing brain in a child, let along one in utero as a foetus? Critical is the answer. In these circumstances, supplementation is the answer and easily tolerated by children or pregnant women.

Remember what I have stated regarding statins that if they fail to fix ingrown toenails does not mean they are clinically useless and will not have a powerful effect on cardiovascular disease. We need to keep this in mind with omega-3's that fail in some research end-points and shine in others.

The changing face of micronutrient supplementation

In the chapter on antioxidants, I mentioned the research findings in the CARET and the ATBC trials where either beta-carotene or alpha-tocopherol (a component of Vitamin-E) was used in trials to see if these supplements could be protective against lung and other cancers. There were significant flaws in these studies, and I have outlined the 'holes' in the research in the antioxidant chapter. The point I want to make here is that beta-carotene is but one carotenoid from a family of 600 known carotenoids. Thus pointing the finger at one of them (beta-carotene) and then providing this in a pharmacological dose is not a prudent approach. It is doomed to fail.

We are family!

Why would the use of one component create any problems? Because in a diet rich in whole foods, you will get a wide array of the 600 members of the known family of dietary carotenoids. These carotenoids work synergistically, and if you saturate the receptors and carotenoid signalling mechanisms with one dominating component, you will block the effects of the others. Also, dietary approaches do not work in an acute pharmacological sense. They do not exert their effects rapidly but ply their benefits over a long period over your lifespan.

Research has often looked at nutrient components in research through this pharmacological lens. This is why teaching your children how to eat well is critical to their healthspan and why you should start as soon as possible with an optimal diet rich in plant-based foods with the greatest of food diversity and colour that you can muster. It is the bright orange and red colours that are rich in carotenoids some of which can be converted to Vitamin-A. Remember, as I have stated in postprandial disorders, that cardiovascular disease begins in childhood and a diet that has all the components necessary for health mentioned above, will ensure you give that child the best chance in life to prevent all the dreadful diseases baby boomers and subsequent generations suffer.

Companies now manufacturing supplements have also analysed these studies and have learnt from them. Many supplements whether they are powders, liquids or multivitamins, now have mixed carotenoids in them so not singling out one 'star' component like beta-carotene. We know that these stars nutrients may not shine brightly on their own and that they need to be in a team to exert that hormetic effect and work as a family of compounds in synergy.

I have discussed in this book under antioxidants. Lutein and zeaxanthin are xanthophyll carotenoids, and these have been shown to be of benefit in protecting the macula of the eye from Age-Related Macular Degeneration (ARMD) in many studies. Many good supplements are being developed that include not only mixed carotenoids but lutein and zeaxanthin as well in synergistic blends as one big family of compounds.

The Vitamin-E Family of Compounds

As far as Vitamin-E goes, there are eight (8) isomers. We have alpha, beta, delta and gamma tocopherols and alpha, beta, delta and gamma tocotrienols. The most active form of Vitamin-E is alpha-tocopherol, and this has been the 'star' in a multitude of research studies. Alpha-tocopherol is also the main component used in commercial Vitamin-E supplements.

However, more and more research is finding that this may not be the best therapeutic Vitamin-E isomer choice. Many of the other isomers are showing significant antioxidant and clinical benefit with some of the isomers of Vitamin-E showing quite different mechanisms of action. As with beta-carotene, this Vitamin-E family works in synergy and thus best consumed as a family of compounds in supplement form. In fact, the tocotrienols which are rarely found in Vitamin-E supplements are shaping up to be very important regarding lowering LDL (the 'bad' cholesterol). Now here's another research flaw that taints the minds of doctors and dietitians. That alpha-tocopherol has not shown to be that great in research, and positive outcomes make the skeptics jump for joy.

Alpha & Gamma-Tocopherol

Alpha-tocopherol has been studied in a pharmacological sense in that we use one compound at high doses in a tablet and capsule form to perform double-blind, placebo-controlled studies to show effectiveness but in this scenario, the research had shown no benefit in cardiovascular disease when alpha-tocopherol, as monotherapy, was used in comparison to Vitamin-E, acquired from food. It makes great sense as nutrients in food are made up of families of compounds acting synergistically.

It is gamma-tocopherol that is the more abundant tocopherol in the diet than alpha-tocopherol, but it is the alpha-tocopherol that is related to the daily Vitamin-E requirement (Grilo, Costa et al. 2014). We bump gamma-tocopherol out of the way when we use too much alpha-tocopherol in supplements. It is known that gamma-tocopherol and its metabolites (not alpha-tocopherol) are powerful inhibitors of cyclooxygenases that produce inflammatory eicosanoids from arachidonic acid (Jiang, Yin et al. 2008). So research has been barking up the wrong tree about Vitamin-E.

Of great concern in American populations is that only 8% of men and 2% of women reached the daily requirement for intake of Vitamin-E (Grilo, Costa et al. 2014).

Not having enough of the whole family of Vitamin-E compounds puts you at risk as these are highly effective antioxidants and in fact, gamma-tocopherol is regarded as the most potent free-radical scavenger of nitric oxide species (Grilo, Costa et al. 2014).

Manufacturers of nutraceuticals do listen and learn from research. I suppose there is no such thing as bad research because flaws in the research with negative findings point the way towards a better understanding of how things work and a critical analysis of why it failed then proceeds. In this instance with Vitamin-E and alpha-tocopherol, the findings on cardiovascular benefit did not make sense. Alpha-tocopherol as monotherapy (using one compound only), failed and yet Vitamin-E from whole foods are protective of the cardiovascular system. One study stated that there was:

> *". an inverse association of coronary heart disease with the intake of vitamin E from food (Kushi, Folsom et al. 1996)."*

By 'inverse association' is meant that with higher intakes of Vitamin-E from food, the lower the risk of cardiovascular disease. Nuts are a rich source of Vitamin-E, and like any food matrix, nuts have a mix of the tocopherols and tocotrienols in various concentrations. Nuts have been shown to have an inverse relationship to mortality from cardiovascular disease (Fraser, Sabate et al. 1992). Importantly, nuts are oil rich (the good fat), and this is important about Vitamin-E as this is a fat-soluble vitamin just like Vitamin-A/D & K and the fat-soluble coloured pigments, the carotenoids. Having a little bit of a good oil like olive, avocado or macadamia oil with food is always a good idea to absorb these fat-soluble vitamins. Without oil around, Vitamins A/D/E & K are poorly absorbed. So food provides a synergistic mix of the vitamins but also provides the best delivery mechanism in the form of good oils to help bioavailability after consumption.

This is not to say we cannot learn from nature and create supplementary forms of Vitamin-E for use in disease states or to promote health. We want to use nutritional compounds in a preventative way to promote health and not just depend on drugs that are used after a disease state manifests itself.

So what is emerging is the need to use a whole family of compounds like the carotenoids or the complete family of Vitamin-E isomers in highly bioavailable, supplementary forms and this is happening in many well-formulated, practitioner-only products.

A practitioner should prescribe these products which should be put into clinical context, taking into consideration any interactions with current medications or sensitivities or previous allergies to supplements.

Gamma-tocopherol and prostate cancer prevention

A very large prospective study was carried out on 295,344 men aged 50-71 who were cancer-free at enrollment (Wright, Weinstein et al. 2007). By prospective is meant that these men were observed over time to see who did and didn't get prostate cancer based on their specific dietary intakes. What these researchers wanted to know was what impact did the various forms of the 4 Vitamin-E tocopherols have on prostate cancer risk. The authors stated that gamma-tocopherol levels were *"inversely related to the risk of advanced prostate cancer"* (Wright, Weinstein et al. 2007). In other words, the higher the level of dietary gamma-tocopherol, the lower the risk of advanced prostate cancer. No effect was seen in the supplemental Vitamin-E group which we must remember is almost invariably the alpha-tocopherol type, and consumption of high doses of alpha-tocopherol depletes the gamma-tocopherol component whereas taking gamma-tocopherol will increase both (Jiang, Christen et al. 2001).

Now this decreased risk of advanced prostate cancer is an amazing finding when you consider how many men will suffer from and ultimately succumb to prostate cancer. It is the 3rd most common cause of cancer deaths in Australia with 16,665 new prostate cancer cases in 2017. According to the CDC figures in the USA, in 2014 there were 172,258 men diagnosed with prostate cancer and 28,343 deaths from this disease. To not consider such dietary factors regarding prevention seems unbelievable to me when an inverse relationship to advanced prostate cancer simply by consuming more gamma tocopherol is an amazing dietary effect and an evidence-based finding.

Riboflavin and phototoxic compounds

Riboflavin has always been promoted as being safe. However, this compound can react with light to form compounds like lumiflavin and lumichrome (Misra, Bajpai et al. 2001) leading to photosensitivity and possible DNA damage (Epe 2012). Lower doses of less than 5 mg per day are all that is needed, and yet some formulations have very high doses.

Any formulation should ensure the riboflavin is protected from light to stop photo-induced compounds forming. This problem with riboflavin highlights some of the complexities associated with supplement formulations that can be overcome through rigorous production standards. These issues are just as important with pharmaceuticals that can deteriorate in light or heat. The right packaging and storage conditions are vital in protecting from product deterioration.

Benefits of Multivitamins

That whole argument of creating 'expensive urine' when taking a multivitamin and mineral supplement, meaning that we are simply excreting these compounds in our urine and flushing them down the toilet, suggests we are just wasting our money. This is very short-sighted indeed as many studies have shown benefit. The general population does not seem to buy into this argument because, as I have discussed in this chapter, there is a vast amount of money that is being spent on supplements by the public. Some multivitamin and mineral supplements contain toxic levels of riboflavin at levels many times the safe dose. It is riboflavin that turns your urine yellow after you take one. Steer clear of a multivitamin, mineral formulation that is not in a container that blocks light completely. Well designed, practitioner-only multivitamins are formulated with great care. Search for a multivitamin on www.a8h.com.au if this is of interest to you.

An evidence base for the benefits of multivitamins

Large numbers of studies have shown significant benefit from using multivitamins. These results seem to be ignored or simply forgotten by the medical profession or discarded by skeptics hoping such findings will simply be erased from memories. The irony is that the medical and pharmaceutical professions often quote ad infinitum studies like the Nurses' Health Study by Harvard University, with a gigantic cohort of 88,756 women to back up their arguments and these same studies have shown a significant lowering of bowel cancer in women who took a multivitamin for 15 years or more.

Once again, the timing was a significant factor here as well. The benefit of taking a multivitamin on bowel cancer risk was negligible to small if taken for 4 – 14 years. However, when the group of women who took the multivitamin for 15 years or more, the authors stated that the risk of bowel cancer was "markedly lower" (Giovannucci, Stampfer et al. 1998).

Studies like these show categorically that disease prevention is a long-term process and that the benefits of diet and nutrient interventions occur over an individual's lifespan. So **timing, timing, timing** is the one component in diet-lifestyle interventions that has been poorly understood or assessed in medical research that is more focused on acute interventions and instantaneous results looking for effects over a short time-span. It is this bias that has set back nutritional treatments that offer so much if given enough time to work.

This same Nurses' Health Study showed that the women who took multivitamins with Folate and Vitamin-B6 reduced their risk of heart disease significantly. The study was published in the Journal of the American Medical Association (JAMA) (Rimm, Willett et al. 1998).

A study published in the Scandinavian Journal of Clinical and Laboratory Investigation found that a combination of Folate and Vitamin-B6 could reduce homocysteine by 32% (Mansoor, Kristensen et al. 1999). Why is this important? Because homocysteine is a toxic compound that can lead to long-term complications like cardiovascular disease and stroke. Homocysteine rises when methionine intakes from protein are high and where there are B-Group vitamin deficiencies such as B6, Folate or B12 insufficiencies or deficiencies.

High consumption of grain-based foods such as bread, pasta, pastries may produce an insufficiency of Vitamin-B6 as cereal grains have a particular form of B6 called **pyridoxine glucoside** that inhibits absorption of other B6 forms, decreasing B6 nutritional status in individuals who have high cereal consumption.(Cordain 1999). Damage caused by homocysteine is a long-latency problem that takes two decades or more to manifest. Preventing homocysteine-related damage is thus not a short-term acute pharmacological strategy. It may take two decades for a multivitamin to show benefit regarding homocysteine-related damage to the cardiovascular system and brain.

Biotin

The other concern with cereal grain consumption is low levels of Biotin. Both wheat and sorghum have both low biotin availability and an inhibitor of biotin metabolism (Cordain 1999). The effect of biotin deficiency is to prevent elongation of linoleic acid an omega-3 essential fatty acid to arachidonic acid (See Appendix-2). Biotin deficiency or insufficiency leads to scaly skins, alopecia (hair loss) and seborrhoeic dermatitis. Biotin is also a key regulator of gene expression according to the Linus Pauling Institute's micronutrient information centre. All of these skin problems are very common presentations in general practice. It is unlikely a dietary history will be taken or that a biotin deficiency will be diagnosed as a contributing factor to these skin conditions. A Dietitian would point a person in the direction of a 'balanced diet' and then tell them to eat whole grains that inherently have the same problems with nutrient availability described above

What makes sense is to take a multivitamin supplement a few times a week. Professor Walter Willet, chair of the Harvard School of Public Health says to take a multivitamin as an insurance policy to fill in the nutritional-gaps. In an online article titled 'Multivitamins: Should you buy this insurance?' it stated Professor Willett's views:

> *"taking a multivitamin daily is a form of nutritional insurance. He still says it's a good policy, despite the spate of negative study results." (Willett 2006)*

In keeping with the timing theme discussed above regarding multivitamins showing a significant decrease in bowel cancer after 15 years, Professor Willet stated that even with beta-carotene, studies looking at effects at the 12-year mark were negligible but when viewed at 18 years, positive effects started to emerge. This online article points to the 2005 Dietary Guidelines for Americans which suggests fortified foods or supplementation for Vitamin-B12 for those 50 years and over, and folate for planned pregnancies including iron. As Professor Walter Willett points out, a good multivitamin can provide all of these components.

It is not as if whole foods are totally benign because a high intake of liver, for example, could lead to Vitamin-A toxicity or a high intake of carrots or carrot juice could do the same as pointed out in the NHMRC's guidelines.

Applying research at a population level to an individual is fraught with danger and those studies may have no relevance whatsoever to an individual who presents to a medical practitioner.

The Wild-West frontier of supplements sold across the counter

The concern that medical practitioners and Dietitians have about across-the-counter supplementation as not being on the same level playing field occupied by pharmaceuticals is a valid one. Many reputable companies understand the 'Wild West' mentality out there with unscrupulous companies producing supplements that are way below par and which taint this area of clinical management using nutraceuticals. To this end, many practitioner-only companies are emerging, and these companies produce products for use by ethical and informed practitioners that can put the product into the clinical context of the individual and to ensure the risk of adverse reactions is minimised. These companies are very strict. You cannot purchase their products from a retail outlet or from distributors who flaunt this rule. They will have the products withdrawn from their control, resulting in those companies being blacklisted by the product manufacturer.

In Australia, products produced for the Australian public undergo stringent Therapeutic Goods Administration (TGA) assessment regarding the marketing, quality and safety of supplements or pharmaceuticals used in Australia. The TGA is a part of the Australian Government Department of Health. Any product, for which therapeutic claims are made, needs to be entered into the Australian Register of Therapeutic Goods (ARTG).

So why are these ethical nutraceutical companies so strict about product use? Because they have a strong belief in the therapeutic use of supplements in disease states and they have a desire to see these used in an integrative way with pharmaceuticals as additional tools in the management of diseases. Such an approach is far more enlightened in the management of health and disease.

Integrative medical practitioners want to see diet and lifestyle modification at the heart of any treatment modality being considered whether medical or surgical and really who can argue with this concept when every research finding backs this approach with tremendous benefits found over pure drug or pure surgical treatment approaches.

Nutraceuticals where necessary should be used alongside pharmaceutical interventions. Companies producing practitioner-only products want a very high standard of manufacturing and quality control and want to ensure these products are prescribed in the very same way pharmaceuticals are prescribed to patients with due diligence processes at the heart of every recommendation.

A strict code-of-conduct by manufacturing companies producing practitioner-only products and a strict code-of-conduct by clinical nutrition practitioners will ensure this area of integrative diet/lifestyle medicine will flourish and thrive.

The Activ8Health approach to micronutrient sufficiency

Analysing an individual's diet in-depth using sophisticated smartphone apps and professional software packages that can 'crunch' the numbers, could shed a great deal of light on the nutritional adequacy in an individual's diet. Well-qualified Dietitians do this (See Appendix 19). No practitioner should have any objections to the correction of a nutritional insufficiency or deficiency if this were discovered through direct measurement of dietary intakes, as this is based on sound, solid scientific understanding and well-recognised nutrient databases supporting dietary nutritional analysis. This helps personalise nutritional guidance.

This service is offered on the Activ8Health's web portal (See Appendix 17). If an individual is absolutely precise with the dietary input in terms of the quantity and type of food eaten, including any 'sinful' foods like sweets, pastries, chocolates, then a clear picture emerges of the adequacy of macronutrient intake (protein, carbs, fibre and fat) and micronutrient intake (Vitamins and Minerals, Trace Elements). Correcting these through dietary and supplementary approaches makes sense. The key points below puts into perspective a compelling argument for the use of supplements to maintain ongoing, long-term health.

Key Points

- Perhaps if we lived in an idyllic sustainable world with unlimited renewable resources, where this planet had the richest of topsoils for plant growth worldwide with an abundance of micronutrients in those soils required for optimal plant and animal growth, where plant cultivars were selected for nutrient density and not yield, where climate change was not a factor, where there was no need to use pesticides, herbicides, fertilizers, hormones or growth factors to support yield, and where the time taken from 'paddock to plate' was rapid ensuring no nutrient loss, and no need for nutrient-depleting time in storage, no loss of nutrients in transportation or poor cold-chain practices, plus no nutrient loss during cooking - then maybe, just maybe, we could all be consuming an optimal diet that was sufficient for us, providing a full spectrum of nutrients for optimal health.
- Even if we had the best of practices as stated above, that ensured no nutrient loss; an individual would still need to ensure each meal had the right composition to take advantage of that food!
- Even if our food is rich in micronutrients, adverse environments, chronic disease, genetics, medications and lifestyle factors all conspire against us, as every human needs varying amounts of micronutrients for optimal health. Our food now doesn't come anywhere near the micronutrient density we need to prevent disease.
- Haptoglobin (Hp-2) gene mutations – it was pointed out that this mutation can deplete a nutrient like Vitamin-C irrespective of you consuming an 'optimal diet'. This mutation undermines completely that notion of getting all your nutrients from dietary sources only. Many of these nutrient-depleting genes will no doubt be discovered in future.
- **Personalization is key – this is the paradigm shift in dietary management**
- The 'balanced diet' claim in 21st Century living is just a myth.
- Targeted practitioner-only supplementation provided ethically and professionally may just prevent slow decline (slow-kill) over a lifespan and save or prolong many lives.
- Enlightened medicine needs to acknowledge the elephant in the room causing a huge burden of disease, and this is diet predominantly and lifestyle.
- Integrative health should be the model for modern medical practices

CHAPTER 15

So, how should you proceed?

In point form:

- **DEXA Body Composition:** Get a reliable baseline body composition study done before undertaking dietary or exercise programs. DEXA is a great choice for the assessment and documentation of various body composition parameters. It is safe and reliable. It provides a measurement of your total body fat percentage (BF%), the amount of visceral fat (deep abdominal fat), the amount of lean muscle mass and how strong your bones are (Bone Mineral Density or BMD). Many people love to argue about BMI and state that the figure is not accurate for a range of reasons. But DEXA is not something you can argue with as it is what it is!

- **Waist Circumference and Waist-**To-Hip Ratio – Easily measured and documented

- **Blood Pressure –** It is good to ensure you have a baseline blood pressure measurement as well. Many people have high blood pressure (hypertension) and changes to the diet and weight loss can have profound beneficial effects on lowering blood pressure.

- **Blood Tests –** Important baseline blood tests would be your fasting blood glucose and lipid levels that include Total Cholesterol, Triglycerides, HDL, LDL. Get your fasting insulin levels done and perhaps homocysteine. Your doctor may want to check other parameters in your blood. Even small changes in weight that may be a 5% to 10% weight loss can produce dramatic improvements in blood parameters thus preventing an early vascular event.

- **Liposcan Testing (detailed blood lipid assessment)–** If you have a strong family history of heart disease or a past history of high cholesterol and/or triglyceride levels, you can request a detailed blood lipid study on the www.a8h.com.au website. A far more targeted approach can then be used from a dietary sense and a medical sense. If you know your 'enemy', you can take action!

- **Personal Dietary Assessment:** Technology now allows us to analyse in –depth what you are eating. Most people think they are consuming a 'good' diet but dietary analysis may indicate otherwise. Using an App, you can choose the type of food by name and then the quantity you are consuming and do this for 3 or more days. After you have finished, you send a file to a qualified independent dietitian using the Activ8Health portal to provide this service (www.a8h.com.au). Just contact an **independent practitioner** through the Activ8Health portal to discuss your needs. A dietary analysis provides a far more effective, personalised approach to the Activ8Health Plan-A and Plan-B diets

- **Nutrigenomics:** That you are able to now assess your genetic 'ticking-time-bombs' is a powerful gift of 21st Century technology. What took over 1 billion dollars can be achieved for a few hundred dollars. We have around 10,000,000 genetic mutations called Single Nucleotide Poly-morphisms (SNPs) and we have no idea of what many of these do and it will take many decades of solid research to find out about these mutations, and it will take Quantum Computing to ana-lyse the effects of all of these in a human being. Right now we can assess over 100 SNPs that we know about and how they can affect you and how they can be modified by dietary and lifestyle measures. Activ8Health has a number of dietitians trained in nutrigenomics and can organise this testing for you and provide a report that you can discuss with any health practitioner that looks after your health. This is personalisation in medicine and genetics. Just find a practi-tioner on the Activ8health portal to help you at www.a8h.com.au.

- **Activ8Health Plan-A Meals (for fat loss or weight maintenance):** If you are after fat loss or wanting to maintain weight, then the Activ8Health Plan-A diet will be for you. This is the meal choice for the vast majority of people who exercise in a mild to moderate sense. Appendix-13 and Appendix-14 provide you with an Activ8Health Plan-A Blended and Plan-A Solid version of this diet. A blended meal provides all the phytochemicals; fibre and protein needs for that meal and is an easy choice for breakfast or a quick meal. Do not pour anything out of a box for breakfast in-cluding oats!

- **Activ8Health Plan-B Meals (for rapid glycogen store replenishment)** The Plan-B meal types found in Appendix-15 (Blended) and Appendix-16 (Solid Meal) provide meaningful starchy carbohydrates that are not simply white processed foods devoid of fibre and nutrients. Plan-B meals will be appropriate for anyone who exercises excessively, runs marathons, engages in hard labour for a living, is an elite athlete who rapidly depletes their glycogen stores and ends up 'hitting-the-wall', i.e. becoming lethargic as a result. These individuals may not be able to replace their glycogen stores rapidly enough with a Plan-A type diet. Many individuals who engage in in-tense activities will eat large quantities of worthless carbs just to build up their glycogen stores placing them at great risk for future chronic disease. The body needs far more than carbs and gly-cogen replacement to function effectively.

- **Intraday Fasting:** Plans-A and Plan-B diets can be used with intraday fasting to provide calorie re-striction but optimal nutrition. Intraday fasting is NOT semi-starvation, and thus we want all our protein and micronutrients necessary for optimal health. If you miss out on a protein portion during your fasting period, make up for this at the next meal as protein timing is not important. Your body can shuffle amino acids around throughout the day as I have described irrespective of when you have had your protein. This type of fasting means you will need to increase intake of the fibre and phytochemical component during the meals eaten.

- **Protein intake:** If you are less than 65 years of age keep protein intakes to that recommended as you need lower protein intakes to prevent mTOR overstimulation. If you are over 65 years of age, you do better with more protein but not excessive amounts. Under 65's need to use the RDA of 0.8 grams per kg but to ensure they understand the difference between the visible protein portion on the plate and the hidden protein in many foods like vegetables or fruit that are often ignored in calculations and meal composition. Over 65's should have around 1 gram of protein per kg body weight and ignore the hidden protein. Refresh your memory by reading the chapter on protein and calculate what your protein needs will be. These recommendations are for people who have low exercise regimens. Protein needs for those who exercise moderately to intensely will need their protein intakes personalised. This can be done through an independent practitioner using the Activ8Health portal to contact one that can help you – www.a8h.com.au

- **High Vegetable Intake**: The magic figure seems to be 8-10 servings of vegetables per day and around 2 – 3 servings of fruit. Remember the dangers of fructose regarding glycation, triglyceride generation and increased central (aortic) blood pressure with just one glass of orange juice. The vegetables should be the non-starchy types in the Plan-A diet (Appendix-5), and the fruit should be the low-carb, low-fructose types – See Appendix-21. Increasing vegetable intake through blends, solid meals, soups, juices to increase phytochemical intake can make this relatively easy for you to achieve. See Appendix-28.

- **Multivitamin/Mineral Supplement.** Intense exercise, medications and chronic illness may need far more nutritional resources to stay healthy. This fact is often never discussed. Find a practitioner on this website as the amount of omega-3 that needs to be taken will depend upon any underlying inflammatory clinical condition. Practitioner-only products can be found at www.a8h.com.au. See Appendix-20 as well for a list of supplements.

- **Fat Soluble Vitamins:** Vitamin A, D, E, K are all vital to health. Carotenoids from fruit and vegetables can be converted to Vitamin-A, but some individuals do this poorly. Having preformed Vitamin-A is important along with all 8 isomers of Vitamin-E and both Vitamin-K1 and K2 for bone and vascular health. Have Vitamin-D3 at least 1000 IU per day in non-summer months (adults). Search for fat-soluble vitamins on www.a8h.com.au

- **High-Quality Omega-3's:** Getting the full spectrum of DHA/EPA/ALA and GLA is vital to good health. ALA can be obtained from Chia and Flaxseed. Search for the others at www.a8h.com.au

- **N-Acetyl Cysteine (NAC):** Is a strategy that can be used to prime your biotransformation pathways i.e. the CYP450 system (Phase-1) and Phase-II conjugation pathways to eliminate a range of toxic compounds your body generates itself and importantly, the huge variety of toxic compounds you are exposed to in the environment. It is difficult to change the world to a less toxic one and so it makes more sense to ensure your elimination pathways are functioning as best as they can to decrease your risk. N-Acetyl Cysteine (NAC) provides the sulphur containing amino acid Cysteine to ensure you generate all the glutathione antioxidant you need to help eliminate toxic compounds from within your body. Vitamins and minerals are also involved in the biotransformation (detoxification) processes once again highlighting how prudent it is to ensure you have as optimal an intake of micronutrients as you can. NAC is essentially a low-cost insurance policy to rid your body of toxicities we all find difficult to avoid. NAC will help you recover from exercise and support nitric oxide (NO) formation in your blood vessels. NAC and L-Citrulline are synergistic regarding NO formation. NAC has been shown to have significant beneficial impacts on mental health and this was discussed under the chapter on supplements.

- **Choline:** As adults, just 5 grams (1 teaspoon) may help protect skeletal muscle and the risk of non-alcoholic fatty liver disease (NAFLD) that is so common in Western societies. This is a cheap supplement and consider non-hexane extracted sunflower lecithin as there is a lot of GMO soy out there with cheap chemical extraction of lecithin. Choline is important for any woman considering pregnancy as there is concern that a lack of choline may result in future mental health problems in the child. Review the information on choline in this book.

- **Activ8Health Protein (Organic Whey):** Is an excellent way to add protein to a blend. Whey has many advantages but for those who 'do not do dairy', there is brown rice protein, egg white protein (Paleo) and even essential amino acids (EAAs) that can be used effectively in blended meals. The Activ8Health proteins have been selected based on the quality of manufacturing, reputable companies and country of origin. They avoid all the chemical complexity found in many products on the shelves of various outlets. These proteins also have added amino acids such as L-Citrulline, L-Arginine and L-Glutamine but in lower amounts because the higher the amount of amino acids used, the greater their oxidation or burning off as energy which means they are not being used for the purpose you want which is to support nitric oxide (NO) production or muscle growth.

- **Essential Amino Acids (EAAs):** Are an excellent way for anyone concerned about calorie restriction but still wants to have that protein synthesis drive without the excess caloric or amino acid levels that abnormally drive mTOR stimulation. It is all about quantity and portion size. It is known that 3 to 4 grams of L-Leucine in a serving of EAAs will provide the protein synthesis drive of a whole protein meal. EAAs are a great choice for those going to the gym where the recommended amount can be added to a sports drink mixer in powder form and water added in the gym. Consume 1/3 before exercise, 1/3 during exercise and the remainder immediately after exercise. EAAs have been shown in research to be an effective way to drive protein synthesis during and after exercise.

  Researchers state the absolute importance of EAAs with regard to protein synthesis and muscle growth with exercise and indicate that there is a: ***"central role of EAAs as the principal (and perhaps only!) macronutrients required to optimise anabolic responses in protein turnover to exercise"*** (Atherton and Smith 2012)

  Activ8Health EAAs also have L-Citrulline + L-Arginine + L-Glutamine that help increase muscle blood supply through effective nitric oxide (NO) levels, and this is important to flush out lactate, other metabolic end-products, channel amino acids to the worked muscles to support growth and help support effective EPOC mechanisms. The EAAs in the Activ8Health blend are pharmaceutical grade.

- **Nicotinamide** – To increase NAD^+ levels. You can refresh your memory on this vital compound for energy systems and how this works in with the Sirtuins and longevity. Many factors diminish as we age and we seem to wind down from an energy perspective. This applies to a multitude of other nutrients as absorption and then assimilation of nutrients can be diminished for a variety of physiological reasons from low hydrochloric acid secretion in seniors to diminishing molecular transport, receptor and signalling systems. This makes any bias against supplementation absolutely illogical.

- **L-Citrulline**: A Nitric Oxide booster far more effective than L-Arginine (see Appendix-23). Look for 'Citrulline' at www.a8h.com.au for a pharmaceutical grade product. 1 – 2 grams can be added to water and consumed most days. The Activ8Health pharmaceutical grade EAAs already have L-Citrulline so you do not need to add this if you get this product and use the EAAs for exercise purposes. L-Citrulline may be of help to anyone who has cardiovascular disease, a history of stroke caused by a blood vessel blockage, high blood pressure or erectile dysfunction (ED) and can be purchased for daily use. You only need a small amount on a daily basis which could be as small as 1 – 2 grams twice daily in a small amount of water or a small amount of pomegranate juice.

- **Creatine Monohydrate**: as discussed in Appendix-25 is of benefit to anyone performing exercise and this may be of help in exercise recovery. Decreased production of Creatine may occur in your 20's and seniors should strongly consider using this most days at the recommended dose. This should be a strong consideration in any senior person. Up to 3 grams a day is very safe. Ensure your renal function is normal to begin with. Creatine may assist with increasing muscle mass through exercise and is a source of immediate energy for the powerful muscle fibres.

- **Home-Based Exercise**: Possible routines using inexpensive equipment and body weight exercises can be done 2 x a week. Great if you can throw in a full-body gym routine as well. See Appendix-11, 12

- **Formal Exercise**: A gym session should be strongly considered as the variety of equipment is hard to match at home and you can push higher loads to reach those elusive Type-IIX muscle fibres. You just need one (x1) full-body routine executed well and with perfect form. Otherwise, you could do a split routine where you work one-half of the body one day, rest and then the other half.

- **NEAT**: Non-Exercise Activity Thermogenesis. This is all the non-formal exercise you can muster. As described walking that extra distance, using steps, move around more at work. As mentioned even an HIIT session on a bike for 3, 20 – 30 second fast/slow phases can be done as a brief formal exercise during the day and this can add to the ability to shift glycogen from muscle stores and add to aerobic fitness. Using NEAT exercise during the intraday fast when you haven't eaten is a great way to mobilise fat stores and stay lean.

- **Exercise Physiology Assessment** – It is wise to get a formal assessment by an Exercise Physiologist (EP) before beginning any exercise routine. They can also guide you in regard to progressive exercise training and can also accommodate any injury or illness you have to ensure your exercise program is compatible in your clinical circumstance.

Appendix-1: The glycemic-index (GI)

The glycemic (or glycaemic) index of a food is a ranking system of carbohydrates from 0 to 100. The higher the number, the higher the GI. Carbohydrates that are absorbed rapidly to release their glucose have higher GI's than carbohydrates that are slowly digested. All GI's are calculated against pure glucose. Amylose and amylopectin are two forms of starch that are present in varying amounts in a carbohydrate. The ratio of amylose to amylopectin will essentially determine the glycemic index (GI) of that carbohydrate. The following graphics will explain why. Glycemic-index [GI] is determined by giving someone a load [10 – 50 grams] of a carbohydrate and then collecting their blood at 15 to 30-minute intervals for 2 hours.

Universities such as Sydney University [www.glycemicindex.com] measure the area under the curve [AUC] of the reference food [glucose] and the area under the curve of the test food.

GI then is a comparison of the areas under the curve of the test carbohydrate to the reference carbohydrate [AUC^{Test} / $AUC^{Reference}$ x 100 = GI (%)].

High-GI foods reach a blood glucose peak earlier and then blood glucose levels drop when compared to blood sugar levels of low GI food which maintain stable blood glucose levels for longer with a lower blood glucose peak.

GI's are thus not only a measure of the rate of intestinal absorption but the effect high-GI or low-GI carbohydrates have on the blood glucose level after consumption. Intestinal absorption depends on whether the carbohydrate is predominantly amylose [linear carbohydrate molecules and slowly absorbed] or amylopectin [branched carbohydrate molecules and rapidly absorbed]. As shown, amylopectin has numerous bonds available for enzymes to cleave the glucose molecules off the parent molecule whereas amylose has to be broken down only from the ends which takes longer to release the glucose.

Why is glycemic-index [GI] so important? The Linus Pauling Institute states "By definition, the consumption of high-glycemic-index foods results in higher and more rapid increases in blood glucose levels than the consumption of low-glycemic-index foods. Rapid increases in blood glucose are potent signals to the beta-cells of the pancreas to increase insulin secretion."

High insulin levels after eating can lead to numerous metabolic changes putting you at risk for cardiovascular disease, diabetes, obesity, inflammation and many cancers.

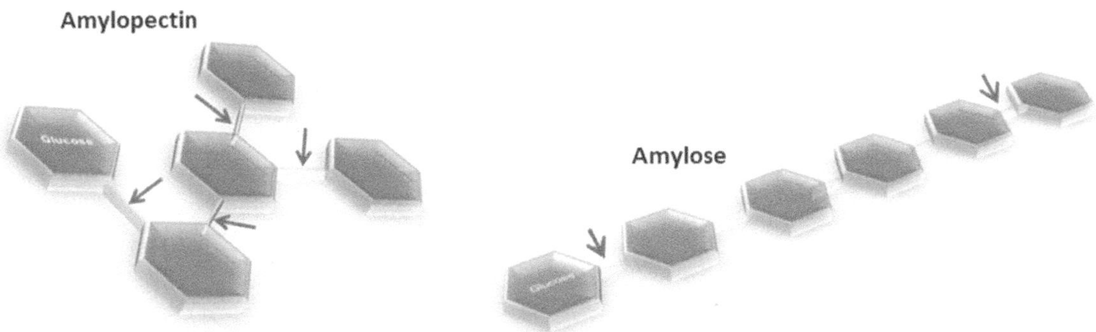

References:

http://lpi.oregonstate.edu/infocenter/foods/grains/gigl.html www.glycemicindex.co

Appendix-2: The Omega-6 to Omega-3 (N6/N3) Ratio

The simplest way to think of omega-6 and omega-3 fatty acids it that they are essential in other words; we cannot synthesise these and thus, need them in our diets. The parent form of the omega-6 family of fatty acids and eicosanoids is linolenic acid (LA) and the parent form of the omega-3 family of fatty acids, is alpha-linolenic acid (ALA). LA and ALA cannot be synthesised in humans (Lee, Lee, Kang, & Park, 2016). LA can be converted to ALA in plants and marine plankton as these organisms have the omega-3 desaturase enzyme that humans lack (Lee, Lee, Kang, & Park, 2016). Plants and plankton can then convert the ALA to the long-chain omega-3's EPA and DHA. Fish eat the plankton and accumulate these important long chain omega-3's that humans benefit from. Humans can convert ALA after consumption to EPA and DHA but some experts think that only 1% of the ALA can be converted in the human body to these valuable longer-chain omega-3's thus consuming enough cold-water fish or using fish oil supplements is vital to good health and to reduce inflammatory processes in the body. The omega-6 family produce inflammatory compounds and the omega-3 family produce anti-inflammatory compounds.

In the diagram below where LA (Omega-6) and ALA (Omega-3) are converted to inflammatory or anti-inflammatory eicosanoids. Notice that the parent compounds for eicosanoid production are **Eicosapentaenoic acid (EPA) and Arachidonic Acid (AA).** The EPA produces series-3 & 5 eicosanoids and the AA produces the inflammatory series 2 & 4 eicosanoids. GLA, although an omega-6 compound, produces anti-inflammatory series-1 eicosanoids through DGLA and these can block leukotriene the inflammatory eicosanoids from arachidonic acid (AA). It is important to see that at each step the same enzymes are used to move the process forward. Thus this is a competitive system. Which one predominates i.e. inflammatory eicosanoids or anti-inflammatory eicosanoids, will depend on how much LA/ ALA or EPA/DHA you consume. The Western diet ensures we all consume about 15 times more omega-6's polyunsaturated fats (PUFA's) than omega-3 polyunsaturated fats. We are thus primed for inflammation and this inflammation drives many diseases of Western societies such as heart disease, cancer, cerebrovascular disease, dementia to name a few.

When you take aspirin or ibuprofen or prednisone, you are targeting the omega-6 inflammatory eicosanoids to dampen arthritic pain or fever or other inflammatory states. **We should aim for a complete intake of essential fatty acids and to ensure we get enough ALA/DHA/EPA and GLA** and supplementation will ensure this as many people avoid fish and have poor diets in the first place. Search the website www.a8h.com.au for possible products recommended and use terms like omega, omega-3, anti-inflammatory in the search box.

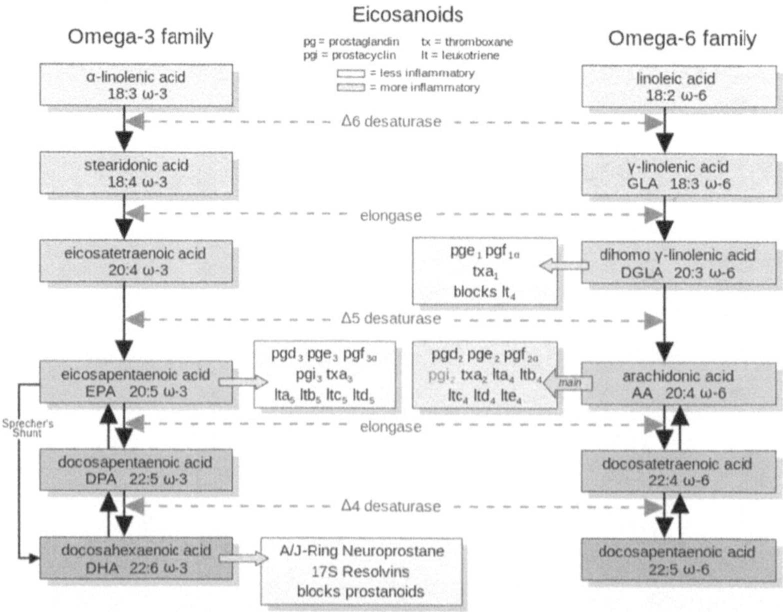

Appendix-3: Comprehensive Blood Tests

Test	Comment
MBA	Multiple Biochemical Analysis. Liver, Kidneys, Electrolytes
Uric Acid	Possible early marker for insulin resistance and heart disease (often done in the MBA)
Albumin	The most abundant protein in plasma. A marker for malnutrition. Often done in the MBA
Fasting Cholesterol	High level may be problematic. Premature heart disease in the family?
Fasting Triglycerides	Early elevation may be a marker for insulin resistance
Fasting HDL	The 'Good Cholesterol' – helps remove cholesterol from tissues
Fasting LDL	The 'Bad Cholesterol' deposits cholesterol in tissues particularly if oxidized
Fasting Glucose	Even high normal may be an indicator for insulin resistance, cancer or heart disease
Fasting Insulin	Levels between 5 – 10 mIU/L may be suspicious but over 10 mIU/L highly suspicious for insulin resistance (pre-diabetes)
GTT with Insulin Levels	A 2 hour GTT with insulin at every stage --- initial, 1 hour and 2 hours after the glucose load. If this is suspected due to a high normal fasting glucose, high fasting insulin, large abdominal girth, raised triglycerides and raised uric acid which are all suspicious of insulin resistance, then this test also called an Insulin Response Test will tell you if you are either normal, have insulin resistance (pre-diabetes) or if you are diabetic.
25-OH-Vit D	Critical for bone health, to prevent many cancers to decrease inflammation and heart disease
RBC Zinc	Zinc is critical for immune function. Over 300 enzymes depend on adequate Zinc levels
RBC Magnesium	Magnesium is involved in over 300 metabolic processes. Most is found within cells.
Random Urine Iodine	Iodine is deficient in large numbers of people on a Western diet
Hormones	This can be discussed with your doctor and may include LH, FSH, Oestrogen (E2), Free and total Testosterone, SHBG and perhaps Prolactin. Each test has to be interpreted expertly. Men can have raised oestrogen levels in their mid years especially if they have large abdomens (visceral fat) that has an enzyme aromatase that can convert testosterone to oestrogen and this could be a risk for prostate disease or in women this process can put their breasts at risk.

See also Appendix-18 to view blood lipid testing.

Appendix-4: Juicing Recommendations

Take advantage of the many juicing outlets near your workplace to benefit from phytochemical intake. Ensure you have a vegetable-rich, phytochemical-diverse drink most days. Your Activ8Health diets are rich in fibre.

This drink is to add phytochemicals to your diet, not the fibre which you get in abundance in your Activ8Health diet. If you can add all of these in a blended drink with the fibre even better, but outlets that provide these as blends are limited.

What should be limited is fructose and these juices should never be sweet and never be made up mainly of fruits with a small stick of celery thrown in for good measure as a token gesture of something green in that toxic fructose blend. Remember, fructose is highly glycating and can raise blood triglycerides and uric acid that can cause gout.

Choose 'Clean-15' fruits and veggies and avoid the 'Dirty Dozen' where possible. Avoid apples, strawberries, peaches, nectarines and celery as these are often very contaminated and make the top of the Environment Working Group's (EWG's) top contaminated list. Choose just one or two of the fruits mentioned below in the quantities stated. Watermelon is low in carb, and so you can be a little more generous with this fruit.

The table provides choices that are commonly available in juicing outlets in Australia; These choices provide an amazing, rich juice of mixed carotenoids, lutein, zeaxanthin, nitrates, potassium, Citrulline, electrolytes, Vitamin-C, magnesium, Vitamin-K, choline, B-group vitamins, magnesium, folate and a wealth of minerals. It is an absolute shame that dietitians or nutrition 'experts' always throw a negative into the mix (pun intended) with regard to juicing by stating 'but you are not having the fibre'. The concept of hormesis through the intake of a vast array of phytochemicals has obviously escaped them. Have the diets recommended in this book and that wonderful Chia or Basil Seed pudding and you will be having a huge hit of fibre every day to keep your gut microbiome happy.

Juice choices	Comment
1 Carrot	Purple carrot if possible. Rich in anthocyanins and carotenoids that can be converted to Vitamin-A
Kale	Rich in Vitamin-K, and Vitamin-A (Carotenoids), Vitamin-C, Manganese and Copper, Folate. Over 45 different flavonoids. Rich in glucosinolates important for detoxification (biotransformation) processes.
Beetroot	Rich in nitrate for vascular health. 1 large piece and this will make the juice blood red. Avoid if you have a history of oxalate kidney stones
Cucumber	Electrolyte rich. Watery and so a good choice to thin down the drink
Spinach	Rich in Magnesium, Potassium, Vitamin-K, Vitamin-A (Carotenoids), Folate, Copper, Choline, B-Group Vitamins
1 Full Lemon or Lime	Citrus. Rich in Vitamin-C and highly alkaline. Ask for the rind to be kept on as this is rich in bioflavonoids and pectin.
Watermelon	A 'Clean' fruit, low in carbohydrate and rich in Citrulline a nitric oxide donor
½ Orange or ½ Pear or Small Mandarin	If you need a small amount of fruit for taste – remember, we want to keep fructose intake low so avoid these if possible and just enjoy a vegetable and watermelon-rich drink
Pomegranate (1/4)	If available. Hard shell and a 'Clean' fruit. Multiple health benefits from cancer protection to attenuating heart disease and inflammation.

Appendix-5: Low-GI Vegetables and Fruit

Glycemic-Index (GI) and Glycemic load (GL) measure the effects of food on blood glucose levels which ultimately will increase insulin demand. Glycemic-index has been studied extensively at Sydney University by Professor Jenny Brand-Miller and Glycemic load was developed by researchers at Harvard University. The glycemic-index does not take into account the amount of carbohydrate in the food and just measures the effect of a standard portion of food on blood glucose, but this is not the best predictor of blood glucose response. For a particular food with a particular GI, the GL is calculated as follows:

Glycemic Index (GI)	Interpretation
55 or Less	Low GI
56-69	Medium GI
> 70	High GI

Glycemic load = GI x grams of carbohydrate/100. Thus if an apple with a GI of 40 and with a carbohydrate content of 15 grams, the GL is 40 x 15/100 = 6. A diet with a high Glycemic load (high carb intake and high GI carbs) is a significant independent predictor of developing type-2 diabetes mellitus (T2DM) and cardiovascular disease. There is evidence of protection against breast cancer, bowel cancer and obesity-related cancers (Foster-Powell, Holt et al. 2002). You can have large amounts of vegetables without affecting the GL but starchy carbs can affect the GL greatly depending on how much you have. Choose low GI options and if you are consuming starchy foods, keep the portion size low. Choices of low-GI fruit and vegetables can be found in the tables on the next page.

Glycemic Load (GL)	Interpretation
10 or Less	Low GL
11 - 19	Medium GL
> 20	High GL
Less than 80 Units	Low daily GL
Over 120 Units	High daily GL

Low Glycaemic Veggies	
Greens	Baby Spinach, Rocket (Arugula), Bok Choy, Lettuce, Kale, Turnip Greens, Swiss Chard, Purslane
Cruciferous Vegetables	Broccoli, Mustard Greens, Watercress, Brussels Sprouts, Cauliflower
Herbs	Coriander (Cilantro), Parsley, Basil, Chives, Bay Leaves, Dill, Lemongrass, Kaffir Lime, Garlic Chives
Low Carb Vegetables	Capsicum, Cucumbers, Celery, Zucchini, Broccoli, Cauliflower, Brussels Sprouts, Raw Carrots, Bamboo Shoots, Radishes, Okra, Green Beans, Snow Peas, Tomatoes, Spaghetti Squash, Artichoke, Bean Sprouts
Root vegetables (small amounts will keep carbs low)	Parsnips, Rutabaga, Pumpkin, Sweet Potato (Australian), Turnips, Low GI Potatoes, Cooked Carrots

Low Glycaemic Fruit	
Berries	Blueberries, Blackberries, Cranberries, Raspberries, Strawberries
Other	Oranges, Grapefruit, Grapes, Kiwifruit, Cherries, Peaches (raw, limit)
Other (small amounts due to higher carb levels)	Mango; Banana, Dates, Dried Figs, Breadfruit, Apricots, Plums, Bananas, Sultanas, Currants and other dried fruit should be eaten in very small amounts.
Special mention	Watermelon with a high GI of 72 but a very low carbohydrate level - excellent in fruit and vegetable drinks due to the watery nature and high Citrulline content which can raise blood L-Arginine levels and hence Nitric Oxide important for blood vessel dilation.

Remember the Israeli study described under postprandial effects. The gut microbiome is a significant determinant of blood glucose responses and a factor that has to be taken into consideration as knowing the GI or GL of a particular food only provides a rough idea of how individuals will respond to the exact same food consumed. A world of personalised medicine is now being developed where genetics and an analysis of your microbiome will determine the best foods for you to limit these toxic elevations in blood glucose after eating.

Appendix-6: Biotransformation Pathways - (Detoxification)

The human body is exposed to thousands of toxic compounds on a daily basis. Toxic elements can come from the environment or are produced by the body itself from a myriad number of cellular metabolic processes. Without a detoxification (biotransformation) system, we would all be slowly poisoned. Keep in mind that what we consider as antioxidants or beneficial plant chemicals (phytochemicals), also have a narrow therapeutic window and levels can become toxic rapidly as discussed under hormesis. The body gets rid of toxic compounds in a two-step process called Phase-I and Phase-II biotransformation reactions and we also know that there is a Phase-III which is an important component for pharmaceutical and xenobiotic biotransformation. The Phase-I component is known as the 'fast-phase' and consists of the CYP450 system made up of around 57 enzymes. These CYP450 enzymes are extremely versatile. They can be hindered by competitive inhibition when 2 or more toxic compounds compete for the action of the same enzyme. This can be a problem with medications where multiple treatments (polypharmacy) occur in treating a patient. This CYP450 system can convert compounds into even more toxic intermediates than the original compound. Unless these intermediate compounds are rapidly removed from the liver by the Phase-II system, they can cause tremendous oxidative damage. This is where an efficient Phase-II is important but this is called the 'slow-phase'. What can overwhelm this system is having too many toxic compounds enter the body competing for the enzymes or where the function of the enzymes is impaired due to genetic mutations. Mutations can affect the enzymes of both phases. Micronutrient and phytochemical deficiencies can have an impact on both phases as well.

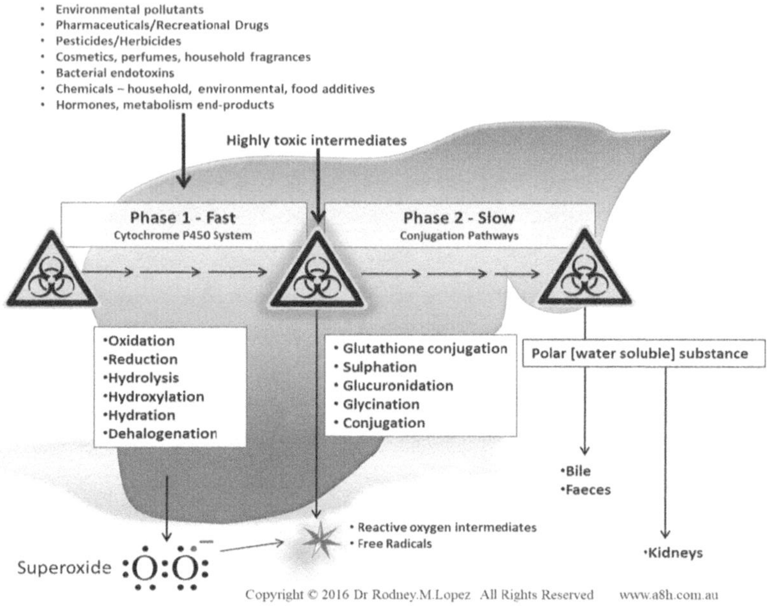

N-Acetylcysteine (NAC) is an inexpensive supplement (see Appendix 7) that can help your body provide the glutathione it needs for these important Phase-II reactions. As I have mentioned, you cannot change this ever-increasing toxic world but what you can do is make sure you prime these systems to function absolutely efficiently by ensuring all the elements are in place for them to work at their peak thus helping you get rid of toxicities you encounter in everyday life.

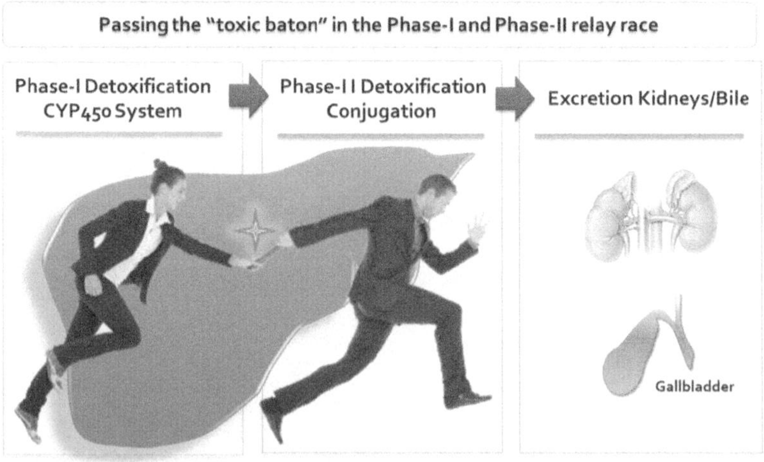

This system can be viewed as passing on the baton in a relay race. Compounds generated from Phase-I reactions are very toxic and need to be converted rapidly in the next phase i.e. Phase-II. If the baton is passed slowly or dropped, toxic damage can occur to the liver (fatty liver or cirrhosis), or damage to the body in general.

Appendix-7: N-Acetyl Cysteine or NAC

This is an interesting molecule found in every accident and emergency department. It is used in a life-saving way when someone presents with paracetamol (acetaminophen) overdose. Without NAC, the liver just 'implodes' and without a liver transplant, the patient dies. So NAC is not a 'plaything' it is an important compound used to save lives in emergency departments of hospitals and an important nutraceutical to protect your body against the ravages of a toxic world as discussed under biotransformation pathways (Appendix-6). Paracetamol poisoning severely depletes the body's glutathione supply, and glutathione is an extremely important innate antioxidant the body creates in vast amounts to offset metabolic oxidative stress caused by your cells simply producing energy from food or creating cellular components for survival.

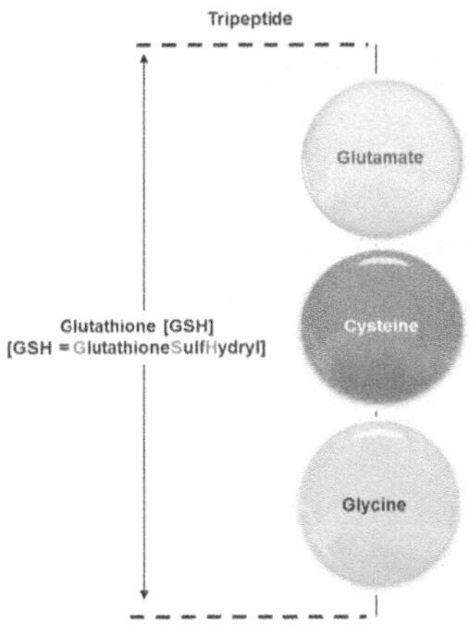

NAC replenishes glutathione reserves in your body effectively. Glutathione is your body's powerful antioxidant defence mechanism but has to be replenished constantly because trillions of cellular reactions that produce free radicals need to be quenched. Glutathione helps to regenerate Vitamin-C and E, boosting the antioxidant capacities of these vitamins. Even just 500 mg twice daily can help maximise immune system function and detoxification (biotransformation) systems helping to remove toxic compounds and heavy metals from the body. Glutathione is a tripeptide with cysteine being a component. NAC inhibits the master controller of inflammation NF-kB and can increase blood vessel vasodilation by supporting nitric oxide (NO) production.

N-Acetyl Cysteine (NAC) is a modification of the sulphur containing amino acid, cysteine. In the chapter on antioxidants, I painted a picture of how complex the antioxidant system is, and the countless trillions of reactions every second let alone the unfathomable number of cellular reactions in any given day producing free radicals and reactive oxygen species (ROS). Trying to offset these with oral antioxidants is futile and akin to the effect of throwing a bucketful of water into an ocean to increase its volume. However, a better strategy is to ensure you support the body's innate antioxidant system through a rigorous diet rich in phytochemicals and food diversity and then to provide the sulphur containing amino acid, cysteine in the form of NAC which is easy to take and only needs to be taken in small amounts to have a significant effect. It is very safe when taken in the recommended amounts but like any food or pharmaceutical, there is no guarantee that no reaction will occur. Side-effects are more common with intravenous delivery of NAC in medical settings. NAC acts like a mucolytic breaking down mucus in the sinuses and lungs and helps switch off the master controller of inflammation, NFkB. In terms of bowel cancer prevention, just 600 mg/day, resulted in a 40% reduction in polyp recurrence (De Leon and Roncucci 1997).Homocysteine a marker for heart disease was lowered by 45% with the use of NAC in a Swedish study (Wiklund, Fager et al. 1996). NAC has been shown to effectively protect against influenza with one study showing a 54% decrease in the number of people experiencing flu symptoms (De Flora, Grassi et al. 1997). Anyone with chronic obstructive pulmonary disease (COPD) and those with insulin resistance (prediabetes, PCOS or diabetes) should consider using NAC to offset the inflammation that can drive these diseases. Oxidative stress and inflammation is strongly associated with bowel cancer and NAC has been shown in preliminary studies to decrease the recurrence of bowel polyps by a staggering 40% (De Leon and Roncucci 1997).

NAC can help you recover from exercise and to help support Nitric Oxide (NO) formation in exercise. Just a small dose of 500 mg to 1 gram which is a tip of a teaspoon full is all you need once or twice daily to help with antioxidant and nitric oxide support and to help you recover after exercise.

Appendix-8: The Clean-15 & Dirty Dozen

The Environmental Working Group (EWG) has produced a shopper's guide to pesticides to help individuals and families steer clear of high pesticide ridden foods that add to our body's toxic load. This is based on 35,200 samples tested by the United States Department of Agriculture (USDA) and the Food and Drug Administration (FDA). In essence as a rough guide, any fruit and vegetable with a hard shell, seems to be protective of pesticides entering the edible inner portion of those foods. Any fruit or vegetable with soft shells, allow pesticides to enter those foods easily. Washing all fruit and vegetables is wise to remove any surface contaminants. Some key findings on the EWG's website were; more than 98 percent of strawberry samples, peaches, nectarines, and apples tested positive for at least one pesticide residue. The average potato had more pesticides by weight than any other produce. A single grape sample and a sweet bell pepper sample contained 15 pesticides. Single samples of strawberries showed 17 different pesticides. This guide tells you which ones you should consider buying in organic form (Dirty-Dozen)

The name 'Clean-15' and 'Dirty-Dozen' is catchy and is just represents the concept but in reality, there are many more products that could be added to each list.

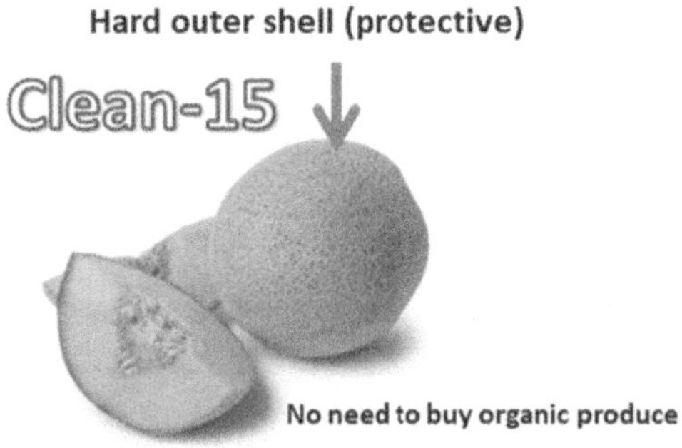

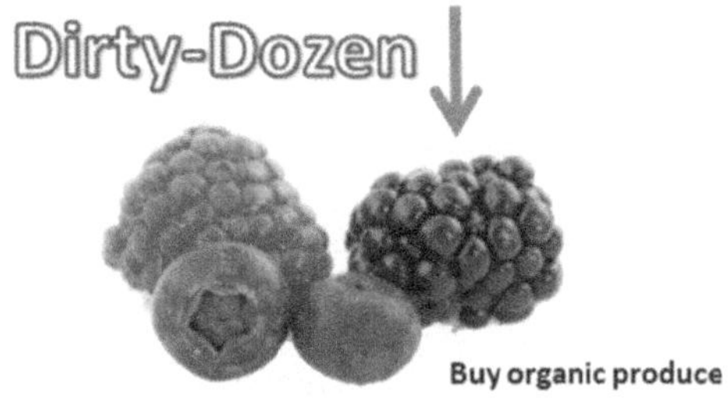

Clean -15	Dirty–Dozen (Buy organic forms)
Avocado	Apples
Asparagus	Berries
Rock Melon	Cherries
Watermelon	Cucumbers
Eggplant	Celery
Cabbage	Grapes
Pineapples	Nectarines
Mangoes	Peaches
Grapefruit	Spinach
Kiwifruit	Tomatoes and Cherry Tomatoes
Onions	Hot Peppers (Chillies)
Mushrooms	Kale/Collard Greens
Sweet Corn	
Sweet Peas	
Papaya	

Appendix-9: Acid-Base Balance

The graphic highlights how high acid loads can rob both muscles and bones of components to neutralise the acid presenting at the kidneys.

Meat, dairy and grains all produce high daily acid loads (DALs). Studies have been conflicting in the past but research can often be a blunt tool. Only now can we see how factors such as a low calcium intake can compound problems associated with a high acid load on the body. An important study showed a higher risk of osteoporosis of the femur in men with low calcium intakes and high renal acid loads (Mangano, Walsh, Kenny, Insogna, & Kerstetter, 2014). Such associations will be teased out as more and more research will look for factors that magnify acid load risk. Glutamine robbed from muscle and organs to offset acid loads will result in sarcopenia and organ shrinkage long-term and the loss of calcium carbonate and calcium citrate from bones to neutralise acid load will, in turn, lead to osteoporosis long-term.

The body cannot excrete urine with a pH lower than 5. A can of cola containing phosphoric acid with a pH of 3.0, results in a very high acid load. With the intake of just one can of cola, your body would have to dilute this 100 fold to ensure the urine has a pH of 5 resulting in 33 litres of urine needed to achieve this effect! (Barzel & Massey, 1998). This does not happen due to the buffering shown in the graphic below.

An abundance of organic anions from fruit and vegetables will go a long way to help buffer acid loads. Progressive muscle loss (sarcopenia) and osteoporosis are common problems in society and remember, this is a cumulative process over a lifetime. You just need to consider that 6 out of 10 people are overweight or obese and observe how people eat in terms of a vast intake of calories coming from meat, grains and dairy to see how food affects people long-term. What escapes may dietetic experts is this effect is small, incremental and occurs over a lifetime.

The graphic visually summarises what happens with high acid load foods being consumed.

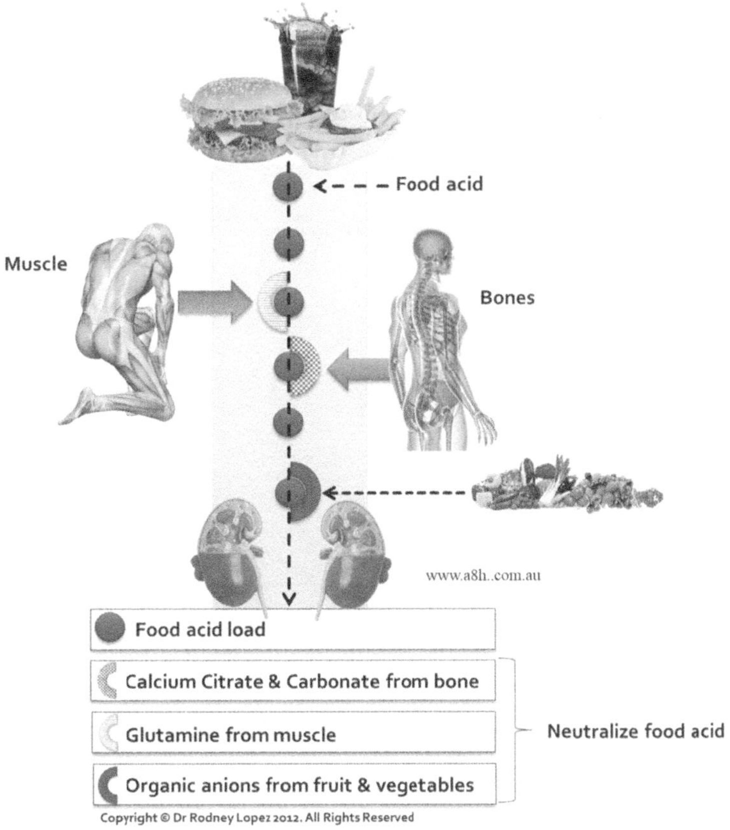

Appendix-10: The Activ8Health Whey Blend

Features of the Activ8Health Whey Blend

- ✓ High protein concentration
- ✓ Whey Protein Isolate (WPI)
- ✓ High bioavailability
- ✓ Organic
- ✓ Pesticide and Herbicide Free
- ✓ Solvent-free
- ✓ Grass Fed Cows
- ✓ New Zealand Product
- ✓ Low in lactose
- ✓ Low in carbohydrate
- ✓ Low in fat
- ✓ Added Pharmaceutical Grade Essential Amino Acids (EAAs) – 5 grams extra per serve
- ✓ Naturally high in BCAAs with additional BCAAs from the EAAs added
- ✓ Added L-Arginine; L-Glutamine and Citrulline as Nitric Oxide Boosters
- ✓ Vegetable Enzyme Matrix added
- ✓ Thaumatin Sweetened – a natural protein based sweetener with an excellent safety record

Many protein products contain various artificial sweeteners or flavours and have a protein that is not at the highest of grades and includes protein that does not come from a country such as New Zealand renowned for the purity and quality of their food products. What the cow eats will find its way into the milk being produced. Thus organic whey is ideal in an increasingly toxic world. As stated in this book, whey has many advantages and it would be good to refresh your memory on the benefits of whey. Whey Protein Isolate or WPI is very low in fat and it is the fat component that has the hormone component found in milk. So the hormones are discarded along with the fat. Like all proteins, it is best not to overdo it and use the recommended intakes for your weight in this book. WPI has the highest protein content whereas Whey Protein Concentrate has more lactose (carb) and is lower in protein than a WPI.

The Activ8Health Whey Blend is essentially 4 products in one:

- ✓ A premium, organic whey protein isolate (WPI)
- ✓ Added Essential Amino Acids (EAAs)
- ✓ Nitric Oxide Support (Arginine/Glutamine/Citrulline)
- ✓ Vegetable Enzyme Matrix in the mix for digestive support

NB: Brown Rice Protein for Vegetarians/Vegans is also available

Essential Amino Acids (EAAs) can be used as a low-calorie way of providing all the amino acids needed for protein synthesis. Remember, non-essential amino acids can be created by your body.

Appendix-11: Home-Based, Beginner's Routine

What is suggested is that you perform home-based exercises 2 – 3 times a week with rest between the exercises for repair and growth. It would be wise to perform gym based exercises either:

- ✓ **Total body workout** - once a week. Full-body routine just once a week only
- ✓ **Split Routine** - twice a week where you work say the upper body one day, allow 1 – 2 days of rest, repair and growth and then do the lower body on another day.

Gym-based exercise routines allow you to train at a greater intensity and provide a greater variety of aerobic and resistance training exercises.

The whole idea with a home- based routine is to perform a HIIT routine and then some resistance training with inexpensive equipment that requires minimal space to store.

Super-Slow Exercises: The resistance home-based exercises should be performed at a normal pace initially and then super-slow. This means performing the eccentric and concentric exercises at a very slow pace for example with a push-up you will go down slowly (eccentric movement), counting down to 10 seconds and then up 10 seconds or longer then down again for 10 seconds or longer. This forces the weakest muscle fibres from the Type-I's, then the lower intermediates through to the upper intermediates to the Type-IIX's to exhaust rapidly so that you make an inroad through these fibre types effectively. You can concentrate more on the eccentric move which will provide a greater muscle building effect. This allows complete muscle fibre activation from the Type-I's to the Type-IIX's but most likely not activating the Type-IIX's completely as the load may not be enough for this. This is where the gym exercises come in handy. Take the super-slow exercises to exhaustion with at least two (x2) eccentric movements completed. **Remember to always start your super-slow routine in the eccentric phase of the movement.**

The following exercises could be completed in 10 minutes. Get a functional assessment by an Exercise Physiologist first and check with your doctors if you have an injury or a medical condition before beginning any exercise routine.

Remember with Super-Slow exercises, start off at the beginning of the eccentric part of the exercise so that you finish off with x2 eccentric moves. See the chapter on exercise on Super-Slow moves and how to effectively perform these. They are an excellent finish to all resistance exercises.

See next page.

Exercise	Equipment
Exercise Bike – HIIT	You can find inexpensive exercise bikes in equipment stores or online as second hand units. Just 2 – 3, 30 second all-out efforts with 2 minutes in-between to catch your breath. This is a warm-up as well. 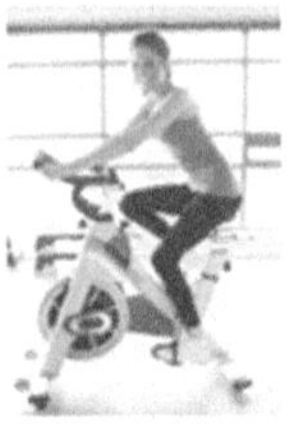
Push-Up Bars	This piece of equipment may cost around $10 in places like K-Mart. Start off with say 10 – 12 normal paced movements going down (eccentric) and then going up (concentric) Then do as many super slow reps as you can to exhaustion – i.e. you cannot do another move 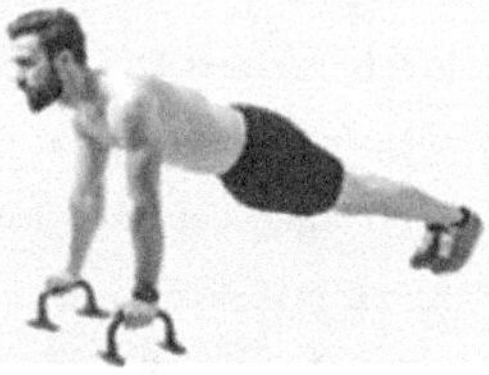
Resistance Bands	Another very inexpensive piece of equipment that you can easily take on holidays. These often come with a booklet so view these different exercises. I have shown 3 easily performed exercises that work multiple muscle groups. Perform at a normal pace for 10 – 12 reps, then super slow to exhaustion i.e. you cannot do another move 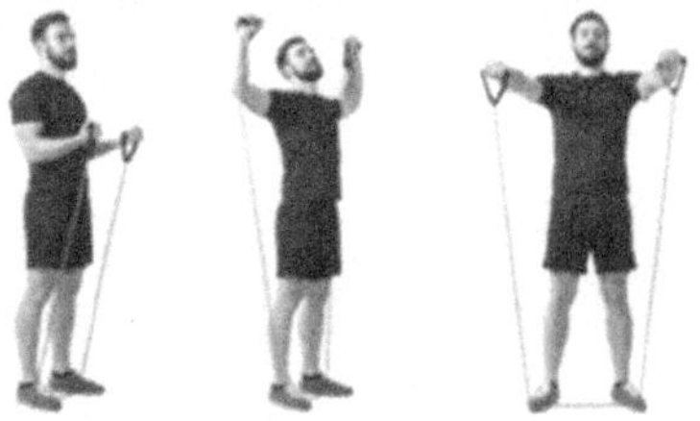
Kettlebells or Free Weights 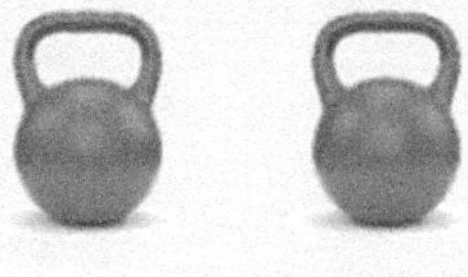	Using two light kettlebells whatever you think you can handle and then do squats as shown. Once again a normal pace for 10 – 12 reps then super slow till you can't do another rep. 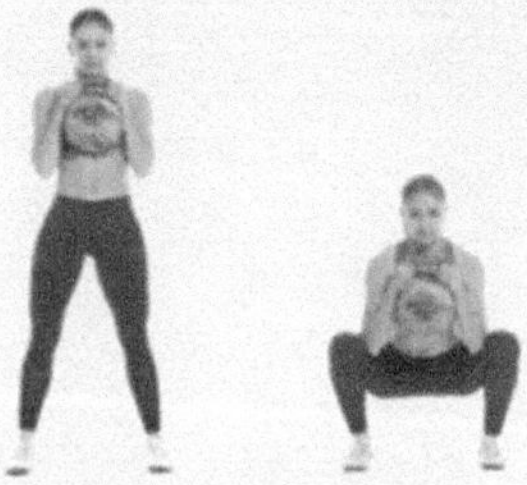

Appendix-12: Home-Based Exercise Intermediate to Advanced

These intermediate to advanced exercises can be added to the previous beginner's routine. Remember; by 'exhaustion' means that you just can't perform a particular exercise anymore. Exercising on uneven surfaces means you will need to call into play many more muscles just to stay stable. This makes it even more difficult if you do these exercises super-slow. Super slow exercises help you deplete muscle glycogen so stick to your Activ8Health Plan-A diet to mobilise your fat stores to replace the glycogen as I have discussed extensively in this book. These are inexpensive exercise tools that can be used in small dwellings.

You can certainly also have exercise balls, perform planks etc. but these suggested exercises are challenging and can provide a total body, glycogen depleting workout and all in 10 – 15 minutes. You do not need anything more in a home exercise setting. More strenuous, challenging and varied exercises can be done in the gym 1 – 2 times a week as mentioned in the beginner's section.

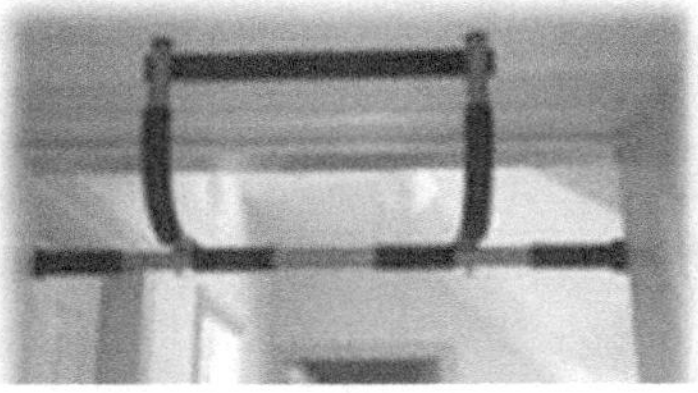

The exercises in the table can easily be done at home with simple inexpensive equipment like a door frame exercise bar for the hanging leg lifts, pull-ups or chin-ups as shown. Check the loads it can bear but many sporting stores keep these home gym products. The abdominal roller is a great exercise to use for the abdominal muscles as you can get an effective eccentric contraction (the movement away from you, stretching the abs) and doing this Super-Slow really works the abdominals and this one movement is worth a large number of concentric contractions (crunches).

Exercise	Equipment
Exercise Bike – HIIT	Perform 2 – 3, 30 second all-out efforts with 2 minutes in-between to catch your breath. This is a warm-up as well. 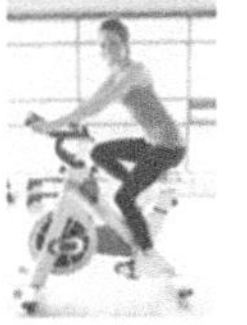
Door Gym 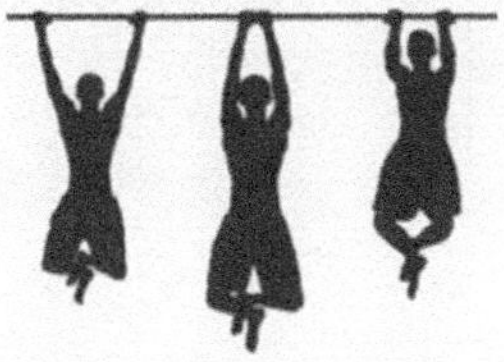	These devices are very inexpensive and yet very challenging. They simply sit in your door frame and can carry a lot of weight (check the limit if you are overweight). You can perform: 1. A chin up - Palms facing you 2. A pull-up - Palms facing away from you 3. Use narrow or wide grips 4. Leg raises while you are hanging 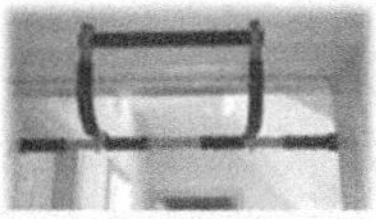 Perform exercises at a normal pace and then super slow until you cannot perform another rep.
Kettlebell Squat-Press	You can perform a squat. Going down is the eccentric phase. Do this at a normal pace and then super slow to exhaustion where you cannot perform another rep. You can also do a squat-press one-handed where you can raise the kettlebell over your head. 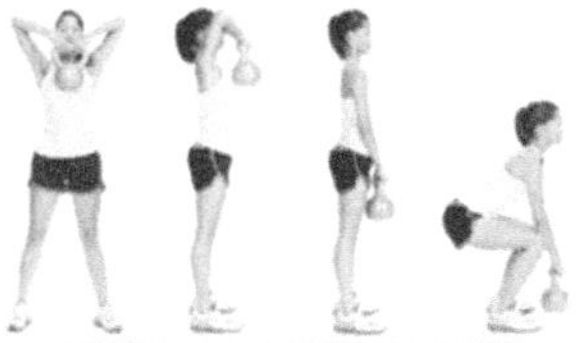
Squats & Presses on a Wobbleboard	Use a wobble board such as a Spri® Wobble Board Stand with one foot either side and then perform a squat-press on this uneven surface. Excellent for building not only strength but great balance as well. Once again, perform at a normal pace then super slow to exhaustion. This will be challenging on a platform that moves but this will call into play many muscles in the process. Don't do this exercise if you have problems with balance or weaknesses in lower-limb joints where that joint can give-way. 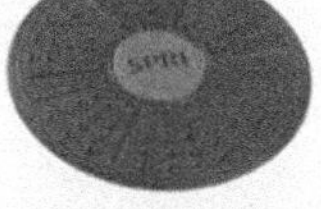
Abdominal Roller 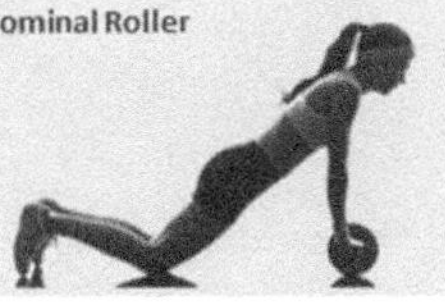	This may look easy but it is one of the few exercises that stretches the abdominal muscles i.e. creates an eccentric movement. Doing this at normal pace and then super slow will challenge you and help develop your core. 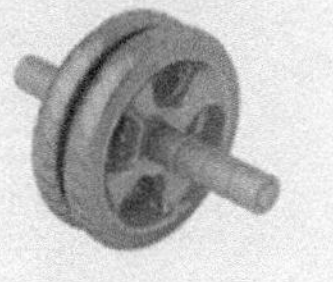

Appendix-13: The Activ8Health Plan-A Blended Meal

A blended meal is **not** a juiced meal – the fibre is preserved in the mix. There are many blenders on the market like a Vitamix® or a NutriBullet® and many other brands. The whole idea with a blended meal is to ensure you have a wide variety of vegetables and fruit that are not high in fructose and where the whole blended meal is low-glycemic-index (Low-GI) and low glycemic load (Low-GL). It is rich in complex carbohydrates from the vegetables and fruit and rich in fibre and phytochemicals. In my mind, a blended meal choice is a great one in the morning as it is very quick to make, quick to consume and you are ready for the day. There is absolutely no comparison in terms of nutritional value between a blended meal and something that comes out of a box. Anything that you pour out of a box is riddled with grain-based carbs that are highly processed with minimal nutritional value. Do not buy into the marketing hype. Nourish your body with a vegetable (mainly) and some fruit blend with protein or essential amino acids (EAAs) for an amazingly high phytochemical, fibre-rich blend to start your day. We are going to add a number of components shown that will make sense and we need a protein source and a whey protein is an excellent one but other forms of protein can be added or even Essential Amino Acids (EAAs) where the equivalent of 3 – 4 grams of L-Leucine in that amount added will provide the protein synthesis power of a full meal. **The Activ8Health Plan-A diets are designed to assist with fat loss or to maintain weight.** This Plan-A diet is not appropriate for those who are involved in elite sports or high intensity/load exercises or those engaged in physically demanding work on a daily basis as this may cause depletion of glycogen that cannot be replaced by fat stores fast enough. These individuals can hit-the-wall i.e. become extremely lethargic because of very low glycogen stores. An Activ8Health Plan-B with carbs will be more appropriate. Dietitians are available for a fee to discuss your needs at www.a8h.com.au

Food	Add to Blender Cup	Food Type Plan-A Blended Meal	Comment
Greens	1 – 2 cups	Rocket; Baby Spinach; Bok Choy; Kale; Collard Greens; Swiss Chard; Lettuce	Rich in magnesium, potassium, chlorophyll, Fibre, Carotenoids
Fruit	1/3 cup	Any seasonal fruit ; Exotic Fruits (Dragon fruit; Lychee; Prickly Pear; Durian)	Variety is key ; Experiment
Berries	1/4 cup	Blueberries; Blackberries; Raspberries; Cranberries, Strawberries	Organic if possible. Frozen is an excellent choice.
Citrus	See comment	Lemon, lime, mandarin, grapefruit, tangelo, orange, kumquat	Kumquats can be added whole as they are small and others in small pieces with the skin for the bioflavonoids and pectin.
Watery Items	To increase the fluid state of the blend	Watermelon; Cucumber; Tomatoes; Lemon; Lime ; Squash	The amount at your discretion. Will water down the mix as we want this to be fluid and not mush
Liquids	Determining how thick or thin the blend will be	Juices: Pomegranate (rich in punicalagins); Sour Cherry (anthocyanins); Prune (fibre/antioxidants); Cranberry (fibre; polyphenols)	¼ cup juice then topped up with unsweetened nut milks (low carb i.e. 5 grams or less) or Soda or Mineral water – add to the blender cup
Oil	1 teaspoon	Extra virgin olive oil; Avocado oil; Macadamia oil; Hemp seed oil; Walnut oil. Fresh frozen avocado can also be added (rich in monounsaturated fat)	Vitamins A/D/E/K are all fat soluble including the carotenoids. Blends mainly have Vitamin E/K/Carotenoids that need oils for optimal absorption. Rotate oils. Don't use the same thing every day
Lignans	1 tablespoon	Flaxseed meal; Black Sesame seeds	These are rich in lignans for glandular tissue health and rich in soluble/insoluble fibre, mucilage
Kelp	1 teaspoon	Organic: Wakame; Nori; Dulce; Kombu	Rich in iodine, trace elements. Vital you use organic forms
Prebiotics	See comments	Frozen Green Banana, Green Banana Powder, Hydrolyzed Guar Gum, Benefiber®, Inulin Powder or Teff Flour, Apple Fibre with Pectin NB: Inulin through various mechanisms including beneficial acidification of the bowel interior due to short chain fatty acids can increase the absorption of many minerals.	Purchase green bananas rich in resistant starch. Cut into 1/5's, coat with one of the oils above and freeze. Use 1 – 2 pieces in your blend. Inulin is a FODMAP and all prebiotics should be started at very low amounts one by one initially before combining them. Teff is a GF grain high in resistant starch (~40%)
Protein	See comments See Appendix 10	1. A good whey protein can be used in this blend and for exercise purposes. 2. EAAs can be used by anyone sensitive to various proteins as 3 – 4 grams of L-Leucine can provide the protein synthesis power of a full meal. Very low allergy potential. Very low in calories 3. Rice protein for vegans. Low allergy potential Check your recommended intake of protein in this book	The Activ8Health whey blend (See Appendix 10) has an excellent level of essential amino acids (EAAs) including the important BCAAs, grass-fed whey protein of the highest grade and enzymes for digestion. <u>Activ8Health EAAs are Vegan/Vegetarian friendly</u> (check www.a8h.com.au)

Appendix 14: Activ8Health Plan-A Solid Meal

There is no rule to say you cannot have some fruit on a plate when you eat a meal. Add phytochemical complexity by doing this. Do not forget to add vinaigrette (see below). If you need advice about food sensitivities or need a personalised diet, contact a Dietitian at the Activ8Health website – www.a8h.com.au

Food	Add to plate	Food Type Plan-A Solid Meal	Comment
Greens	1 – 2 cups	Rocket; Baby Spinach; Bok Choy; Kale; Collard Greens; Swiss Chard; Lettuce	Rich in magnesium, potassium, chlorophyll, Fibre, Carotenoids, Lutein & Zeaxanthin
Fruit	1/3 cup	Any seasonal fruit; Exotic Fruits (Dragon fruit; Lychee; Prickly Pear; Durian)	Variety is key; Experiment. Don't overdo it on fruit as we want to keep fructose levels down
Berries	1/4 cup	Blueberries; Blackberries; Raspberries; Cranberries, Strawberries	Organic if possible.
Vegetables	Large portions – 3 or more cups – multicoloured veggies	Capsicum, Cucumbers, Celery, Zucchini, Broccoli, Cauliflower, Brussels Sprouts, Raw Carrots, Bamboo Shoots, Radishes, Okra, Green Beans, Snow Peas, Tomatoes, Spaghetti Squash, Artichoke, Bean Sprouts	Low-carb veggies are a wonderful source of phytochemicals and fibre and don't have the energy dense problem of starchy carbs. Remember, vegetables are carbs but have a low GI and low GL
Oil	1 teaspoon (see vinaigrette below)	Extra virgin olive oil; Avocado oil; Macadamia oil; Hemp seed oil; Walnut oil. Fresh frozen avocado can also be added (rich in monounsaturated fat) – See Vinaigrette below	Vitamins A/D/E/K are all fat soluble including the carotenoids. Blends mainly have Vitamin E/K/Carotenoids that need oils for optimal absorption. Rotate oils. Don't use the same thing every day
Lignans	1 tablespoon	Flaxseeds; Sesame seeds esp. Black Sesame Seeds	These are rich in lignans for glandular tissue health and rich in soluble/insoluble fibre, mucilage
Kelp	1 teaspoon	Organic Wakame; Nori; Dulce; Kombu	Rich in iodine, trace elements. Vital you use organic forms of kelp.
Prebiotics	Small amounts initially and gradually increasing	Jerusalem artichokes, Leeks, Garlic, Onions	Jerusalem artichokes are very rich in inulin (long chains of fructose). Inulin may not be tolerated by someone who has irritable bowel syndrome (IBS). Always use small amounts initially.
Probiotic Foods	Small amounts	Kimchi, Sauerkraut, Fermented Cabbage, Natto, Miso	Low in calories and high in fibre. These foods are teeming with probiotics (microorganisms) that are beneficial for the gut microbiome. Avoid if you are histamine intolerant. Lactobacillus Plantarum may help degrade histamines (Capozzi, Russo et al. 2012).
Protein (Omnivores)	See comments	1. Main Animal Sources: Chicken breast, turkey, sardines, herring, mackerel, trout, salmon 2. Occasional. Grass-fed beef, venison, pork, lamb. Avoid if possible 3. EAAs 10-12 grams can provide the protein synthesis power of a whole meal. Very low in calories. Can be used in place of a solid meal as the need arises to decrease caloric intake	Organic preferable. Fish should be wild such as salmon or trout not farmed which are often labelled 'Atlantic Salmon'. Just two 100g servings of sardines will provide a weeks worth of Vit-B12. Try to avoid red meat as this is a health risk as discussed in the book. EAAs will lack the micronutrients of a whole meal. Activ8Health EAAs are Vegan/Vegetarian friendly
Protein (Vegetarians)		Tofu, tempeh, Quorn (mycoprotein), soy protein, nuts, seeds, NB: Legumes are high in carbs and so excluded in a Plan-A meal	Getting your protein from Quinoa or lentils or beans means you will be eating a lot of carbs with all the problems associated with this. Quorn comes in Vegan options (Schnitzel and Nuggets)
Herbs	Add to a Vinaigrette	Oregano, Parsley, Coriander (Cilantro), Thyme, Dill, Fennel	Add to a salad or to a vinaigrette. Rich in antioxidants and phytochemicals.
Vinaigrette	See comments	Add an oil (see above) to a vinegar and some spices and include tumeric and pepper.	This is a lost art and results in extremely important fat-soluble vitamins not being absorbed. The acetate in vinegar can attach to the GPR43 receptors of immune system cells to decrease inflammation (Macia, Tan et al. 2015).

Need advice to personalise your diet? Find an Accredited Practicing Dietitian (APD) to help you. Go to:

www.a8h.com.au

Appendix-15: Activ8Health Plan-B Blended Meal

Activ8Health Plan-B meals have carbohydrate in them and the reason for this is that some people do hard manual labour or exercise intensely and regularly or engage in resistance training with high loads. Glycogen can be depleted well within 2 hours of high intensity training and the body then cannibalises itself by drawing glucogenic amino acids from muscle, bone and organs. These glucogenic amino acids as the name suggests can undergo conversion to glucose in the liver in a process called gluconeogenesis. Constantly exercising in a glycogen depleted state may increase the risk of muscle loss, osteoporosis and organ shrinkage. The individual can 'hit-the-wall' and feel very lethargic and depleted with the risk of immune system dysfunction. Such individuals need to have carbohydrates in the system to replace the glycogen stores. Carbohydrate sources such as Poly-Joule® a maltodextrin polymer (glucose) and higher fructose containing foods **in this circumstance** may be helpful in re-establishing muscle glycogen (glucose) and liver glycogen (fructose) (Conlee, Lawler et al. 1987). The amount of maltodextrin will need to be determined based on energy expenditure and hence should be calculated by a Dietitian. The Activ8Health website (www.a8h.com.au) can be a portal to find a Dietitian that can assist you.

Remember nutritional resources need to match the intensity of exercise. The Activ8Health Plan-B diet is the smart way to increase glycogen stores.

Food	Add to Blender Cup	Food Type Plan-B Blended Diet	Comment
Greens	1 – 2 cups	Rocket; Baby Spinach; Bok Choy; Kale; Collard Greens; Swiss Chard; Lettuce	Rich in magnesium, potassium, chlorophyll, Fibre, Carotenoids, Lutein & Zeaxanthin
High Fructose Fruit	1/3 cup	Blueberries, lychee, persimmon, pomegranate, grapes, cherries, apple, pear, custard apple, mango, rock melon, loquat, rambutan	We try to avoid high fructose normally but in liver glycogen depleted individuals, fructose can help rapidly replete liver glycogen stores
Poly-Joule®	See comment	Maltodextrin Often used post-exercise due to minimal gut fluid shifts and rapid absorption.	This is a rapidly absorbed glucose polymer and thus unlikely to cause fluid shifts in the bowel. The amount needs to be individualized and determined by a Dietitian (www.a8h.com.au)
Citrus	See comment	Lemon, lime, mandarin, grapefruit, tangelo, orange, kumquat	Kumquats can be added whole as they are small and others in small pieces with the skin for the bioflavonoids and pectin.
Watery Items	To increase the fluid state of the blend	Watermelon; Cucumber; Tomatoes; Lemon; Lime ; Squash	The amount at your discretion. Will water down the mix as we want this to be fluid and not mush
Liquids	Determining how thick or thin the blend will be	Juices: Pomegranate (rich in punicalagins); Sour Cherry (anthocyanins); Prune (fibre/antioxidants); Cranberry (fibre; polyphenols)	¼ cup juice then topped up with unsweetened nut milks (low carb i.e. 5 grams or less) or Soda or Mineral water – add to the blender cup
Oil	1 teaspoon	Extra virgin olive oil; Avocado oil; Macadamia oil; Hemp seed oil; Walnut oil. Fresh frozen avocado can also be added (rich in monounsaturated fat)	Vitamins A/D/E/K are all fat soluble including the carotenoids. Blends mainly have Vitamin E/K/Carotenoids that need oils for optimal absorption. Rotate oils. Don't use the same thing every day
Lignans	1 tablespoon	Flaxseed meal; Sesame seeds	These are rich in lignans for glandular tissue health and rich in soluble/insoluble fibre, mucilage
Kelp	1 teaspoon	Organic Wakame; Nori; Dulce; Kombu	Rich in iodine, trace elements. Vital you use organic forms
Prebiotics	See comments	Frozen Green Banana, Green Banana Powder, Hydrolyzed Guar Gum, Benefiber®, Inulin Powder or Teff Flour, Apple Fibre with Pectin NB: Inulin through various mechanisms including beneficial acidification of the bowel interior due to short chain fatty acids can increase the absorption of many minerals.	Purchase green bananas rich in resistant starch. Cut into 1/5's, coat with one of the oils above and freeze. Use 1 – 2 pieces in your blend. Inulin is a FODMAP and all prebiotics should be started at very low amounts one by one initially before combining them. Teff is a GF grain high in resistant starch (~40%)
Protein Or EAA's	See comments See Appendix 10	1. A good whey protein can be used in this blend and for exercise purposes. 2. EAAs can be used by anyone sensitive to various proteins as 3 – 4 grams of L-Leucine can provide the protein synthesis power of a full meal. Very low allergy potential 3. Rice protein for vegans. Low allergy potential Check your recommended intake of protein in this book	The Activ8Health whey blend (See Appendix 10) has an excellent level of essential amino acids including the important BCAAs, grass-fed whey protein of the highest grade and enzymes. EAAs are low in calories Activ8Health EAAs are Vegan/Vegetarian friendly

Activ8Health Whey, EAAs, Creatine, Citrulline can be found at:

www.a8h.com.au

Appendix-16: The Activ8Health Plan-B Solid Meal

White potatoes, white rice, processed grains or white bread have little nutrition or fibre. A Plan-B diet concentrates on tubers or grains that have far more nutritional complexity. For example, black rice is rich in anthocyanins and Teff, a gluten-free Ethiopian grain found readily now in many stores, has around 40% resistant starch that is so important for the gut microbiome. Exercising intensely or performing hard labour does not mean you should consume empty calories just to get the glycogen stores back to normal at the cost of immediate and long-term health. This makes no sense. Both the Plan-A and Plan-B diets require nutrient density and nutrient diversity. Food rotation is encouraged. Ensuring constantly changing components in the same class of food e.g. greens could consist of Baby Spinach or Rocket (Arugula) or Bok Choy or Kale etc. so that you are constantly adding diversity and the same goes for fruit or protein sources as food diversity equals bowel organism diversity. See vegetarian choices in the Plan-A solid meal

Food	Add to Plate	Food Type Plan-B Solid Meal	Comment
Greens	2 – 3 cups	Rocket (Arugula); Baby Spinach; Bok Choy; Kale; Collard Greens ; Swiss Chard; Lettuce other green leaf veg varieties	Rich in magnesium, potassium, chlorophyll , Fibre, Carotenoids, Lutein & Zeaxanthin
Vegetables	Large portions – 3 or more cups – multicoloured veggies	Capsicum, Cucumbers, Celery, Zucchini, Broccoli, Cauliflower, Brussels Sprouts, Raw Carrots, Bamboo Shoots, Radishes, Okra, Green Beans, Snow Peas, Tomatoes, Spaghetti Squash, Artichoke, Bean Sprouts	Low-carb veggies are a wonderful source of phytochemicals and fibre and don't have the energy dense problem of starchy carbs. Remember, vegetables are carbs but have a low GI and low GL
Okra	½ cup	-	Rich in mucilage important for bowel health
Grains	Carbs See comment next column	Quinoa, Black Rice, Red Rice, Amaranth, Teff (All Gluten-Free) Needs based on intensity of exercise. Discuss with a Dietitian at www.a8h.com.au	Use grains that have nutritional qualities other than just carbs. Black and red rice for example is rich in anthocyanins and quinoa and amaranth are complete proteins.
Legumes	Carbs	Black Beans, Chickpeas, Lentils	High in carbs so use small amounts like a ¼ of a cup depending on your needs
Roots & Tubers	½ to 1 cup	Parsnip, Sweet Potato, Kumra, Yam, Celeriac, Rutabaga, Turnip, Beetroot	Lower in carbs than potato and higher in fibre and minerals.
High Fructose Fruit	1/3 cup	Blueberries, lychee, persimmon, pomegranate, grapes, cherries, apple, pear, custard apple, mango, rock melon, loquat, rambutan	We try to avoid high fructose normally but in liver depleted individuals, this can help rapidly replete liver glycogen
Citrus	See comment	Lemon, lime, mandarin, grapefruit, tangelo, orange, kumquat	Small pieces with the skin for the bioflavonoids and pectin.
Oil	1 teaspoon	Extra virgin olive oil; Avocado oil; Macadamia oil; Hemp seed oil; Walnut oil. Avocado can also be added to the meal (rich in monounsaturated fat) Add Vinaigrette below	Vitamins A/D/E/K are all fat soluble including the carotenoids. Blends mainly have Vitamin E/K/Carotenoids that need oils for optimal absorption. Rotate oils. Don't use the same thing every day
Lignans	1 tablespoon	Flaxseeds; Sesame seeds esp. Black Sesame Seeds – sprinkle on your salad or vegetables.	These are rich in lignans for glandular tissue health and rich in soluble/insoluble fibre, mucilage - can be added to the salad
Kelp	1 teaspoon	Organic Wakame; Nori; Dulce; Kombu	Rich in iodine, trace elements. Vital you use organic forms. Mix in with the salad or Vinaigrette
Prebiotics	See comments	Jerusalem artichokes , Leeks , Garlic , Onions	Jerusalem artichokes are very rich in inulin (long chains of fructose). Inulin may not be tolerated by someone who has irritable bowel syndrome (IBS). Always use small amounts initially.
Probiotic Foods	Small amounts	Kimchi, Sauerkraut, Fermented Cabbage, Natto, Miso	Low in calories and high in fibre. These foods are teeming with probiotics (microorganisms) that are beneficial for the gut microbiome. Avoid if you are histamine intolerant. Lactobacillus Plantarum may help degrade histamines (Capozzi, Russo et al. 2012).
Protein (Omnivores)	See comments	1. Main Animal Sources: Chicken breast, turkey, sardines, herring, mackerel, trout, salmon 2. Plant Based: Veggies, fruit, soy, Quorn, seeds, nuts 3. Occasional. Grass-fed beef, venison, pork, lamb. Avoid if possible 4. EAAs 10-12 grams can provide the protein synthesis power of a whole meal. Very low in calories. Can be used in place of a solid meal as the need arises to decrease caloric intake	Organic preferable. Fish should be wild such as salmon or trout not farmed which are often labelled 'Atlantic Salmon'. Just two 100g servings of sardines will provide a weeks worth of Vit-B12. Try to avoid red meat as this is a health risk as discussed in the book. EAAs will lack the micronutrients of a whole meal. Activ8Health EAAs are Vegan/Vegetarian friendly Search www.a8h.com.au
Herbs	Add to a Vinaigrette	Oregano, Parsley, Coriander (Cilantro), Thyme, Dill, Fennel	Add to a salad or to a vinaigrette. Rich in antioxidants and phytochemicals.
Vinaigrette	See comments	Add an oil (see above) to a vinegarand some spices and include tumeric and pepper and lemon/lime for the Vitamin-C. Pour onto your salad	This is a lost art and results in extremely important fat-soluble vitamins not being absorbed. The acetate in vinegar can attach to the GPR43 receptors of immune system cells to decrease inflammation (Macia, Tan et al. 2015).

Appendix-17: Designing a Personalised Diet

Why would you consider a personalised diet? We are moving headlong into a world of personalised medicine as we know that a one-size-fits-all approach does not work for everyone. So why would a personalised approach by a qualified Dietitian be of benefit? There are many points to consider:

1. **Personal dietary intake** – having your diet assessed through a special App and professional software package, interpreted expertly by an Accredited Practicing Dietitian can make a world of difference in finding hidden problems in someone's diet. Often people do not perceive major dietary flaws as a problem because they have eaten like this throughout their lives through familial influence, and it becomes an ingrained habit or they choose to eat particular foods out of taste and preference. Either way, it puts that individual at risk long-term. See Appendix 19 'Dietary Analysis Made Simple'
2. **Genetics** – everyone is unique with potentially 10 million single nucleotide polymorphisms (SNPs) in a human that can lead to changes in enzyme function and how a protein behaves and this can alter the metabolism of drugs or of phytochemicals found in food. Nutrigenomics can detect many SNPs (See Appendix 22) and knowing your particular genes means you can take action from a dietary sense to offset the mutations that exist in you. You can find an Activ8Health's independent practitioner trained in nutrigenomics to guide you.
3. **Individual Needs** – Everyone is different. You need to match an individual's lifestyle to their energy and nutrient needs. With increasing activity comes the need for increasing nutritional resources to match those needs. Remember the 'Triage Theory of Nutrition'? Not having a nutritional resource means this mechanism of robbing Peter to pay Paul, kicks in!
4. **Individual preferences in food & avoidance of important foods**
5. **Food allergies or sensitivities**
6. **Medications** – Many medications may result in nutrient deficiencies. For example, Metformin may result in a Vitamin-B12 deficiency or Statins may require CoQ10 because the pathway shared in cholesterol metabolism is interrupted by the statin. The list is extensive but needs to be taken into consideration
7. **Chronic Illnesses** – may have their own nutrient needs and this is complex from heart failure requiring a low salt intake to chronic kidney disease requiring a lower protein intake to diabetics on insulin or oral medications.
8. **Age** – we know that under 65's need a lower protein intake whereas those over 65 years of age will need a higher protein intake due to changes in hormones or diminishing IGF-1 levels which can decrease anabolic responses
9. **Gastrointestinal Disorders** – are common and range from Coeliac Disease to irritable bowel syndrome (IBS) with FODMAP sensitivities, Crohn's Disease or Ulcerative Colitis. All of these may cause dysbiosis where the gut microbiome is greatly affected and this may result in many nutrient deficiencies due directly to the disease itself or due to the individual avoiding many foods they perceive to be a problem, thus putting themselves at long-term risk

A personalized approach makes a lot of sense

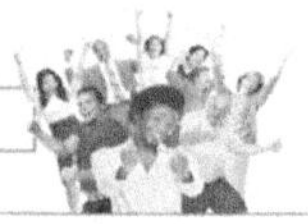

Let one of our highly qualified Accredited Practicing Dietitians guide your dietary needs. A full dietary analysis will be highly worthwhile and this is discussed in Appendix-19. Nutrigenomics discussed in Appendix-22 can help tailor your dietary needs to genetic mutations. Chronic disease may require either additional or even less of certain nutritional elements.

Please register at www.a8h.com.au first then look for the 'Personalized Diet' service, click the icon and then choose 'Broadcast Your Request'
Your request will go to all available independent practitioners that can provide this service.

Ask about body composition DEXA scans as a baseline before beginning any dietary programme. This will provide you with accurate measurements such as body fat percentage, whether you have deep visceral (abdominal) fat, if you bones are becoming thinner and how much lean muscle you have. Your nominated practitioner can advise you in this regard as well.

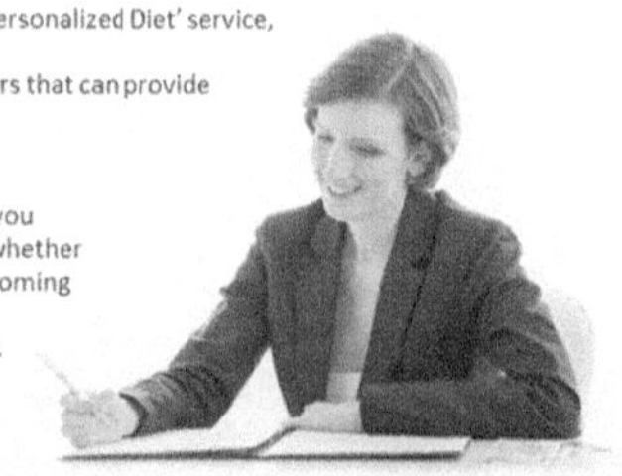

Appendix-18: Your Omega-3 and Omega-6 Levels and Lipid Subfractions

The omega-3 and omega-6 essential fatty acids were discussed in Appendix-2. So why measure these? As discussed, the Western diet is riddled with omega-6's putting an individual at great risk long-term from the myriad number of inflammatory driven chronic diseases. These dietary changes are often not even thought about in mainstream medicine and yet every aspect of this system has a profound impact on cellular function as omega-3's determine the fluidity of cell membranes or, as is the case with DHA a long-chain omega-3, it is concentrated in the brain and where the brain has the highest concentration of docosahexaenoic acid (DHA). This shows the importance of this vital compound in terms of brain structure and function. If you have an inflammatory condition, the last thing you want is a high omega-6 level in your body.

With regard to heart and vascular disease, Total Cholesterol is not the answer to determining risk. A considerable number of people who have had heart attacks have normal cholesterol levels and many with high cholesterol levels never have a heart attack. More and more research is being done on lipid subfractions such as small dense LDL (sdLDL), large buoyant LDL, VLDL, IDL. The test used by Activ8Health practitioner's measures:

1. **Total Cholesterol**
2. **Total LDL**
3. **HDL**
4. **VLDL**
5. **3 IDL fractions**
6. **7 LDL fractions**
7. **Oxidised-LDL and your Omega-6/Omega-3 ratio can also be measured to see how much of an inflammation risk you have with a high Omega-6 to Omega-3 ratio that can be measured along with the lipid subfractions.**

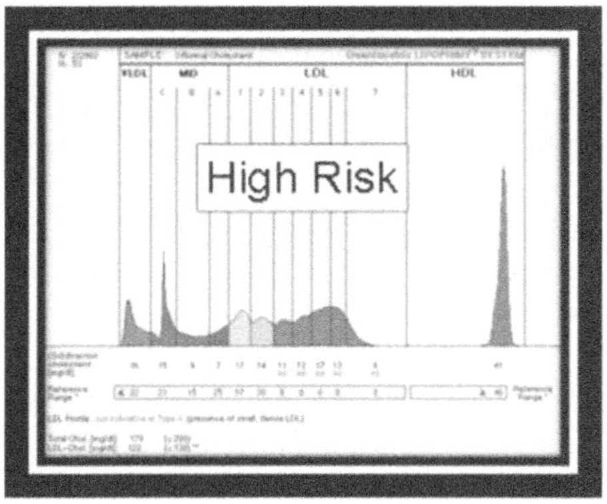

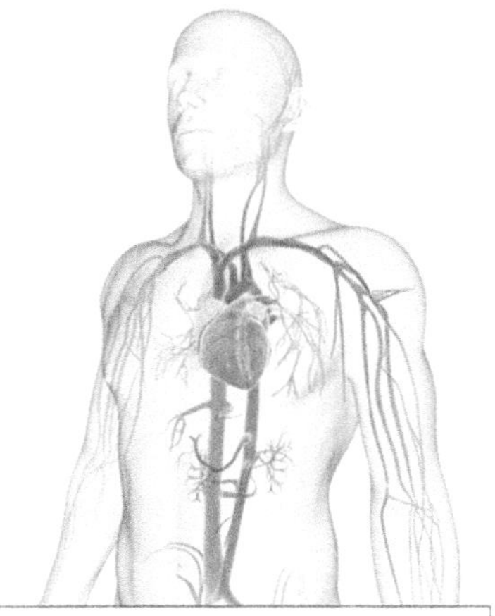

Simply look under 'Tests' or search for 'lipids' at www.a8h.com.au

Only registered clients at www.a8h.com.au can purchase products or order tests. It will be important to provide detailed clinical information enabling the practitioner to provide recommendations or products. Some countries may be excluded so please read the Terms & Conditions on the website. All practitioners work independently . The Activ8Health website is simply a portal for communication between you, a practitioner or supplier of products, services or tests. Always contact the relevant company or practitioner about products/services/tests if you have a query and not the website.

Appendix 19: Dietary Analysis made Easy

Analysing your diet – why is this important?

The term 'diet' simply means the sum total of all the foods and beverages that enter your mouth and are processed in your gastrointestinal tract. We have such a staggering variety of foods to choose from but how many people will know whether that combination of foods or fluids will contain all the macronutrients or micronutrients including all the trace elements you need for optimal health? We all know how a weak link in a chain will impair the whole system and this is no different to the nutrients your body needs to stay healthy. The 'Triage Theory' states that if there is a shortage of a nutrient, your body will rob Peter to pay Paul. In other words, your body will draw upon less important tissues like your bones, muscles and organ mass to shunt that much-needed nutrient to vital organs such as the heart or the brain. If this continues, the body weakens, your health deteriorates and your lifespan will decrease all because of a suboptimal nutrient intake and other factors that can exacerbate the situation. The trick in life is to ensure you provide your body with all the nutrients it needs to keep you living a vital life for as long as determined by your genes.

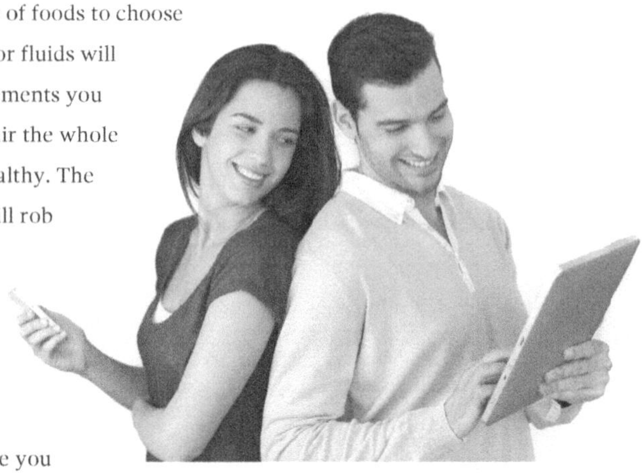

Just use an App on your Smartphone or Pad

A 3, 5 or 7-day diet diary using a Smartphone or iPad App can be kept which documents accurately your food and beverage intake. A file can then be emailed to the Dietitian for an in-depth analysis. This file can then be opened in a professional software package that has all the foods found in Australian supermarkets and food outlets. If your diet changes daily, then a 7-day database will be worthwhile but most people have a very similar intake on a day-to-day basis and herein underlies the problem for many a person – a lack of variety! One of our highly qualified independent Dietitians will be delighted to help you in this regard. Foods and quantities can also be documented manually and this can be analysed so this can be done for people in countries other than Australia. All reports and suggestions need to be filtered by your medical practitioner and/or specialist before you make any changes to your diet or exercise program.

Let one of our highly qualified Accredited Practicing Dietitians look over your results and guide you. They can view your analysis from the perspective of the principles discussed in this book and also take into consideration any sensitivities and preferences in food that you may have. You will be provided with a detailed report. Payments will be discussed for this reporting and there are also further payment packages available if you need additional personalized information, further analysis or advice.

Please register first then look for the 'Dietary Analysis' service, click the icon and then choose 'Broadcast Your Request'
Your request will go to all available practitioners that can provide this service.

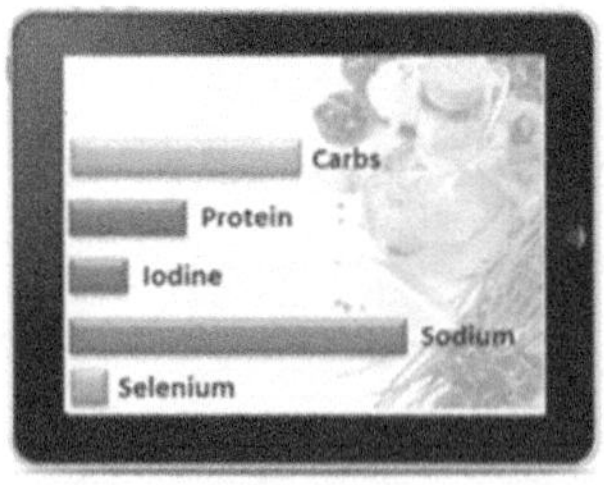

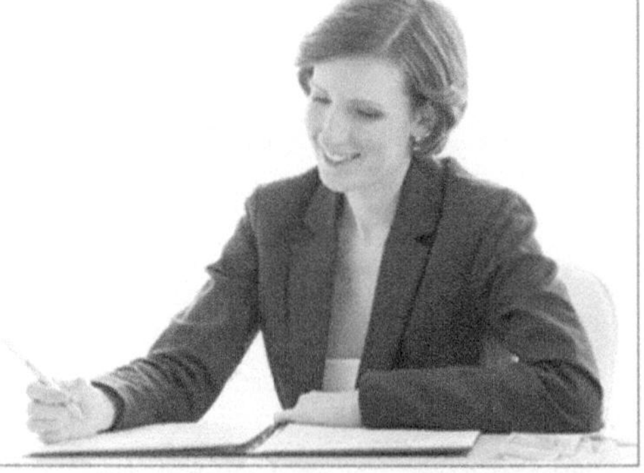

Appendix-20: Available Supplements

This is a short list of some important supplements. Many others may be found at www.a8h.com.au.

Type	Find at: www.a8h.com.au
Citrulline	As discussed in this book, Citrulline is an excellent donor of L-Arginine and Nitric Oxide (NO) synthesis so critical for cardiovascular health and as adjunctive treatment with a PDE5 inhibitor for erectile dysfunction and to use with Resveratrol and Nicotinaminde (NAD) to activate Sirtuins and FoxO
EAA's (Essential Amino Acids)	Excellent prior to exercising or post-exercise or to provide all the building blocks you need for protein synthesis without the calories. Search 'eaas'
Homocysteine Formulation	Try reducing protein intake to that recommended in this book. This will decrease methinoine and hence homocysteine. Supplementation may be needed if high homocysteine levels persist for perhaps genetic reasons. See Appendix-22 Nutrigenomic Testing
Iron chelates	Such as iron bisglycinate that is directly absorbed through the intestinal wall and does not interfere with absorption of other minerals. Lactoferrin helps with iron homeostasis, absorption and Vitamin-C that is a known helper for iron absorption.
Magnesium	Involved in 300 essential metabolic reactions. For everyone and in particular those suffering from irregular heart rhythms.
Multivitamin & Minerals	Activated B-Group vitamins and chelated minerals. Search for multivitamins. Recommended one every 2nd day
Nicotinamide (NAD^+)	NAD^+ is a master controller of the Sitruins and longevity pathways. Also evidence-based treatment of non-melanoma skin lesions
N-Acetyl Cysteine (NAC)	To improve antioxidant status and enhance biotransformation pathways. See Appendix-7 for more information.
Omega-3's	Critical for various reasons to maintain optimal health. Needs to be pharmaceutical grade, ultra low in contaminants and thus rigorously tested for heavy metals and other environmental toxins. Search for 'omega-3' or 'omegas'
Pregnancy Formulation	Needs to be high in iodine. Also having multiple forms of folic acid to help prevent neural tube defects. Ensuring micronutrient sufficiency is vital. Don't forget to include choline in your diet as discussed in this book. Look under 'pregnancy', 'natal' 'antenatal'
Probiotics	Need to be in large enough numbers, include a variety of beneficial probiotic bacteria and have a known adherence to gut mucosa and intestinal survival and colonization rate. Search under 'probiotics'
Protein	Whey, Brown Rice and Egg Protein forms are available for blending in the Plan-A and Plan-B Activ8Health diets and for exercise. Search for 'protein'
Resveratrol	Sirtuin and longevity pathway activation. A calorie restriction mimetic and can be used along with Nicotinamide and Citrulline. Search 'resveratrol'
Saccharomyces boulardii	To help maintain normal gut immunity and health. Search for 'saccharomyces' or 'probiotics'
Vitamin-A	For those with recurrent sinus, bladder, lung and gastrointestinal infections. Have a high intake of provitamin A carotenoids as well (red, organge fruit and vegetables). Look under 'vitamins'
Zinc	Over 300 enzymes depend upon zinc. Alternate with a Multivitamin

Appendix-21: Fructose concerns

There are many concerns with fructose and it all comes down to how fructose is metabolised. Of great concern is that fructose has no 'off switch' as fructokinase is not subjected to feedback inhibition by high fructose levels and so fructose is rapidly metabolised to Fructose-1-Phosphate (F1P) and onwards to increase triglyceride-rich, very low-density lipoproteins (VLDL) which are a cardiovascular risk.

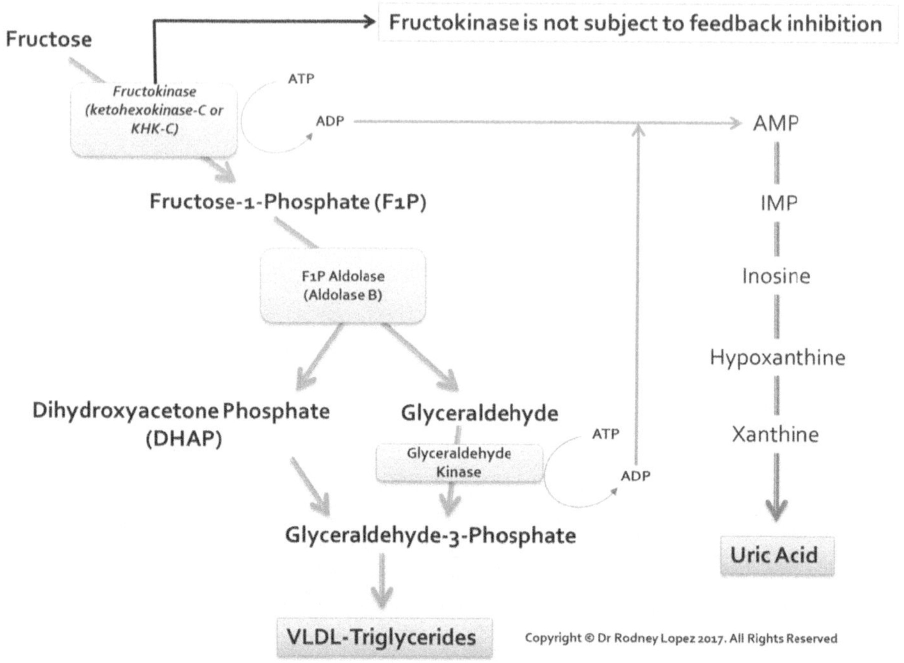

Fructokinase when it phosphorylates fructose to fructose-1-phosphate, it markedly depletes adenosine triphosphate (ATP) because there is no feedback inhibition of this enzyme and thus increases AMP levels (King 2017), which can then be converted to uric acid (UA). Uric acid causes gout and so high fructose consumption in these individuals is not a clever thing and uric acid is a very strong **independent** cardiovascular risk factor. Increasing AMP levels will result in increasing AMPK, which in turn will switch off critical protein synthesis pathways such as mTOR. We do not want to greatly inhibit mTOR by excessive intake of fructose which we also know, causes a high central (aortic) blood pressure (Pase, Grima et al. 2015). Imagine the elderly who have diminished protein synthesis drives and a risk for sarcopenia, decreasing mTOR in these individuals through high fructose intakes will be a disaster. What we want is to stop that uncontrolled bombardment of the mTOR pathway by high caloric and protein intakes. If you keep fruit consumption to low levels you automatically will be limiting fructose intake. Choosing fruit that contains lower fructose levels will mean you can have more of these. This is not rocket science and you do not have to read tables of fructose levels in foods. But beware that many processed products from sauces to condiments to protein powders may all be laced with fructose. All fruit can be fine as long as you limit their intake.

Excess Fructose: Fructose > Glucose	**High Fructose Load > 3g/Serving**	**Balanced Glucose/Fructose (Less likely to cause symptoms)**
Apple, pear, guava,, mango, nashi fruit, honeydew melon, pawpaw/papaya, quince, star fruit (carambola), Fructose powder Corn Syrup High fructose corn syrup Fruit concentrates	Dried fruit, fruit pastes such as tomato paste, chutney, sauces, fruit juices, fruits with a high sugar content (apple, pear, lychee, grapes, persimmon, cherries). Also coconut cream or milk, fruit bars, honey, agave syrup If wanting to have a low fructose load, have the equivalent of 1 serving of fruit at any time including blends, solid meals (1 medium sized piece of fruit or 2 small sized pieces of fruit such as an apricot)	**Berries:** Blueberry, blackberry, strawberry, raspberry, boysenberry, cranberry **Stone Fruit:** Peach, plum, nectarines, apricot (sorbitol in these may create symptoms in those with irritable bowel syndrome – IBS) **Citrus fruit:** Lemon, lime, mandarin, grapefruit, tangelo, orange, kumquat **Others:** Kiwi, passionfruit, pineapple, tamarillo, rhubarb, jackfruit, ripe banana **Low fructose vegetables:** Avocado, cucumber, Chinese cabbage, green pea, common lettuce, mushroom, parsnip, broccoli, celeriac, pumpkin (butternut), spinach, zucchini, snowpea, zucchini, endive, asparagus

Important: Fructose intolerance can cause irritable bowel symptoms (IBS) and this occurs when there is an imbalance in the concentration of fructose over glucose. However, keeping fructose levels at a low intake is wise due to the glycating effects and uric acid increasing effect of fructose and its association with insulin resistance.
Reference: (Shepherd and Gibson 2006); (Women's and Children's Health Network 2012)

Appendix-22; Genetic Testing - Nutrigenomics

Single nucleotide polymorphisms (SNPs) can now be tested for a relatively small sum of money. So why would you want this? Genes or gene variants, in particular, can determine the interaction between your genome and nutrient needs. Some genes such as the APOE4 provide a marker for Alzheimer's disease and cardiovascular disease and is associated with telomere shortening. Knowing you have this variant means you can ensure you decrease your risk through diet, exercise and supplementation. Paradoxical effects of dietary components with regard to disease states may also be found where polyunsaturated fatty acids like fish oil may actually increase the risk of cardiovascular disease. So a one-size-fits-all approach does not work. Nutrigenomics provides a far more targeted approach to dietary management and may be important in those with a high risk for chronic disease as indicated in say a family history or on blood testing. Once again, all reporting should be discussed with your medical team before implementing any dietary or exercise changes.

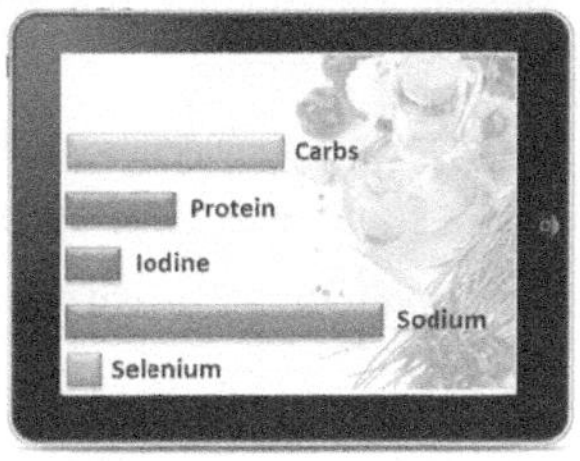	**Dietary Analysis** This provides a detailed analysis of exactly what your diet consists of and importantly the weaknesses, deficiencies, excesses
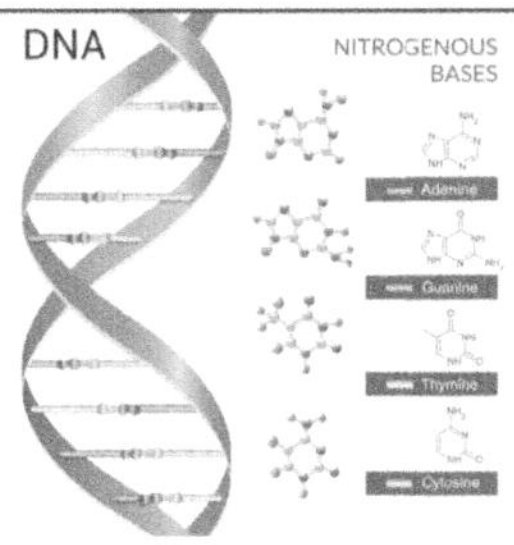	**Genetic Analysis** Can cross-check the genetic mutations you have with your dietary intake to see if there are any potential clashes. This enables personalization of diet to your genetic makeup.

Let one of our highly qualified Accredited Practicing Dietitians (APDs) look over your results and guide you. They can view your genomic analysis from the perspective of your dietary history and the principles discussed in this book. You will be provided with a detailed report by an expert molecular geneticist and this report will be viewed by one of our Accredited Practicing Dietitians who will then advise you in writing. Payments will be discussed for this reporting and there are also further payment packages available if you need further information and analysis or advice.

Please register first then look for the 'nutrigenomics' service, click the icon and then choose 'Broadcast Your Request' Your request will go to all available practitioners that can provide this service.

A full dietary analysis will be of tremendous help to the Dietitian so please consider this with a nutrigenomics assessment. This is all about personalizing the data to your needs as an individual.

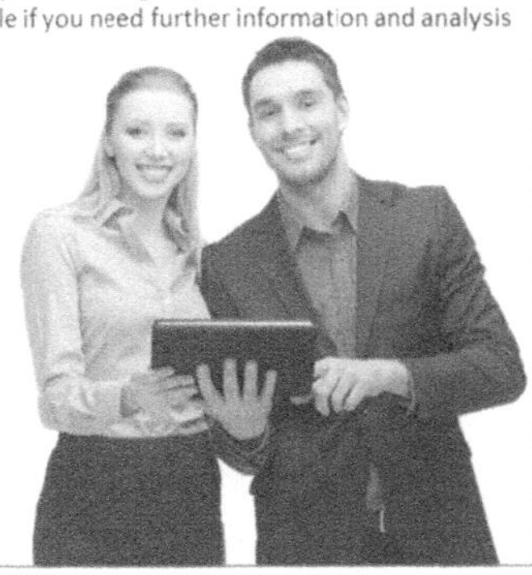

Over 100 SNPs can be analyzed and these provide insights into many molecular aspects that make you a unique individual. These include:

- ✓ Caffeine Metabolism
- ✓ Choline
- ✓ Coeliac Disease Risk (DQ2/DQ8)
- ✓ CoQ10 Metabolism
- ✓ Fat Gain Genes
- ✓ Inflammation
- ✓ Lactose Intolerance
- ✓ Lipid Metabolism
- ✓ Metabolic Syndrome and Diabetes
- ✓ Methylation, Folate and cofactors
- ✓ MTHFR
- ✓ Omega 3 and Omega 6
- ✓ Polyunsaturated Fat Risk (PUFAs)
- ✓ Sodium Sensitivity
- ✓ Sleep and Seasonal Variation
- ✓ Vitamins
- ✓ Oxidative Stress Genes
- ✓ Phase I Detoxification
- ✓ Phase II Detoxification
- ✓ Weight Management Genetic Issues
- ✓ Exercise Genes – what are you best doing in terms of exercise

Appendix-23: L-Citrulline, L-Arginine & Nitric Oxide (NO)

Nitric Oxide (NO) is critical for vasodilation (blood vessel muscles relaxing and thus increasing their diameter). NO can drop as you age and thus increase vascular resistance due to blood vessel stiffness thus increasing blood pressure and strain on the heart and worsening of vascular disease. Keeping Nitric Oxide levels high through the Citrulline to L-Arginine shuttle makes a great deal of sense. Nitric Oxide as you have learnt is connected to the SIRT1 sirtuin protein that helps keep your cells in molecular shape through repair and maintenance mechanisms. Those of you who are men and suffer from erectile dysfunction, then almost certainly, you have cardiovascular disease and endothelial dysfunction. If you are taking Cialis® or Viagra® then it is important to know that this won't work very well if there isn't enough Nitric Oxide (NO) to start the ball rolling. 30 – 40% of men do not respond to Cialis® or Viagra® (Pizzorno 2016), because there is not enough Nitric Oxide available for the critical first step in the erection cascade that begins with the activation of soluble guanylate cyclase (sGC) which then converts GTP to cGMP the molecule that results in smooth muscle relaxation - through PKG. Cialis® or Viagra® will keep cGMP levels high by blocking the enzyme that breaks this down i.e. the **Phosphodiesterase-5 Enzyme (PDE5 inhibitor)**. This helps maintain the erection. **So it all starts with Nitric Oxide!** As I have mentioned in the chapter on Sirtuins, the damaged endothelium which is the lining of all blood vessels including the damaged penile blood vessels causing erectile dysfunction (ED), will also have oxidised LDL (OxLDL) and this damaged LDL upregulates (increases) **arginase** an enzyme that rapidly converts L-Arginine to Ornithine and this, in turn, can increase the risk of collagen synthesis through Proline and Hydroxyproline production from Ornithine. This can be a significant problem for men with Peyronie's Disease (PD) a distortion of the penis on erection due to plaque formation. Citrulline can be highly beneficial when you are using a PDE5 inhibitor such as Cialis® or Viagra® or if you have a chronic illness such as hypertension, cardiovascular disease, Peyronie's disease of the penis or other scarring disease states which occur due to tissue remodelling. However, not all Citrulline supplements are created equal. It is important to have a pharmaceutical grade product that is not contaminated and one that is produced in a highly reputable manufacturing facility. **Look for 'Citrulline' at www.a8h.com.au**

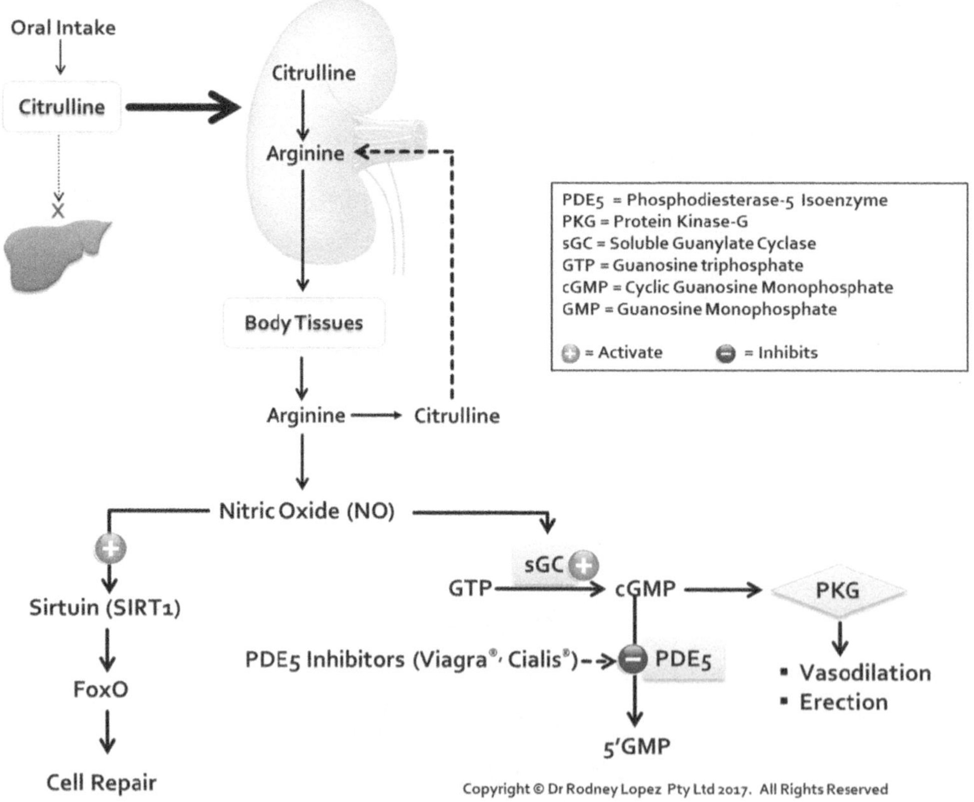

Appendix-24: Activ8Health Essential Amino Acids (EAAs)

There are 9 essential amino acids (EAAs) that cannot be manufactured in the human body. These by definition as being 'essential' need to be acquired in the diet. EAAs are a great way to stimulate protein synthesis without all the calories of whole protein. Included in this list of essential amino acids are the 3 Branched Chain Amino Acids (BCAAs) and thus you are getting all of these in the blend. The following table provides you with a list of the EAAs and highlights the 3 essential amino acids that are the BCAAs:

Essential Amino Acid (EAA)	Branched Chain Amino Acid (BCAA)
Histidine	
Isoleucine	Isoleucine a BCAA
Leucine	Leucine a BCAA
Lysine	
Methionine	
Phenylalanine	
Threonine	
Tryptophan	
Valine	Valine a BCAA

Only 6 grams of EAAs around exercise showed a doubling of protein synthesis. Some very important points regarding the consumption of EAA's are the following:

- EAAs stimulate actual protein synthesis
- They do not affect protein breakdown
- Non-Essential Amino Acids are not necessary
- Adding carbohydrate is absolutely not necessary and does not enhance protein synthesis
- Having more EAAs in a 2 hour period did not enhance protein synthesis at all. You need a drop in amino acid levels to reset protein synthesis (Børsheim, Tipton et al. 2002)

The research points to the incredible importance of EAAs in protein synthesis rather than carbohydrate or protein. One important paper states: *"Interestingly, addition of carbohydrate to protein affords no greater anabolic effects on protein turnover (neither increases in MPS nor depressions in MPB) after exercise, highlighting the central role of EAAs as the principal (and perhaps only!) macronutrients required to optimise anabolic responses in protein turnover to exercise" (Atherton and Smith 2012)* **MPS = Muscle Protein Synthesis; MPB = Muscle Protein Breakdown**

NB: The Activ8Health EAAs already have:
L-Citrulline + Glutamine + L-Arginine.

This tremendously supports Nitric Oxide (NO) formation but at the right dose. High doses increase oxidation (burning) of these compounds rather than being used for protein synthesis or nitric oxide (NO) formation. Reconstitute with water at the gym and have:
1/3 just before exercise, 1/3 during and 1/3 immediately after

It is known that insulin can be significantly elevated with EAAs and that adding carbohydrate is not necessary as the quote above states. Insulin's effects are anti-catabolic, not anabolic like the EAAs (Atherton and Smith 2012). **EAAs are what counts around exercise if you want muscle mass!**

Incredibly important points are --- all from (Atherton and Smith 2012)

1. Muscle Protein Synthesis (MPS) drive by nutrition alone will only last for 1.5 hours
2. Muscle Protein Synthesis (MPS) when combined with resistance training and EAAs can extend this anabolic protein synthesis point beyond 24 hours
3. Resistance training involving loads less than 70-90% 1RM, i.e. quite heavy loads maximise Muscle Protein Synthesis (MPS)
4. However, the important point is that much lower loads taken to exhaustion can equalise the Muscle Protein Synthesis (MPS) response to higher loads mentioned in point 3. This now ties in with the low loads mentioned in this book along with finishing a set with Super-Slow

Practitioner-only products can be viewed by someone who has **registered** on this website. No practitioner-only product can be purchased without the input of a qualified practitioner. It will be important to present detailed clinical information enabling the practitioner to provide recommendations or products. Some countries may be excluded so please read the Terms & Conditions on the website. All practitioners work independently . The Activ8Health website is simply a portal for communication between you, a practitioner or supplier of products, services or tests. Always contact the relevant company or person about products/services/tests if you have a exercises to exhaustion maximising eccentric contractions providing you with an amazing, evidence-based way of maximising Muscle Protein Synthesis (MPS) without excessive loads being used.

5. 6- 10 grams of EAA's is all you need to provide a maximum protein synthesis stimulus. EAAs are rapidly absorbed and thus this dose can be repeated in 2 hours. 1 teaspoon = 5 grams
6. If you want to add some whey, just a small amount of 5 – 10 grams along with the EAAs in a mixer and consume before, during and after as 1/3's described above

> As a guide using 0.1 g of EAAs per kg body weight has been shown to increase muscle protein balance (Williams 2005). So a 70 kg person will need 7 grams of EAAs in total.

Appendix-25: Creatine Monohydrate

This is a natural compound necessary for the transportation and storage of energy in every cell in the body. It is estimated that the body stores around 80 – 130 grams of Creatine but 1 – 2% of this is metabolised and thus need to be replaced every day.
It is important to note that significant and biologically relevant quantities can only be found in fish and meat and **<u>not in vegetables or dairy products.</u>**

<u>How does it work</u>

> Creatine monohydrate + Phosphate = Creatine Phosphate

The main supplier of energy in your cells and body is Adenosine Triphosphate (ATP). The end bond is the highest energy bond where significant amounts of energy are released when the terminal phosphate is removed. This enables you to run or lift heavy loads. When the terminal phosphate is cleaved, you are left with the remaining two phosphate bonds attached to the parent molecule and this is Adenosine Diphosphate (ADP).

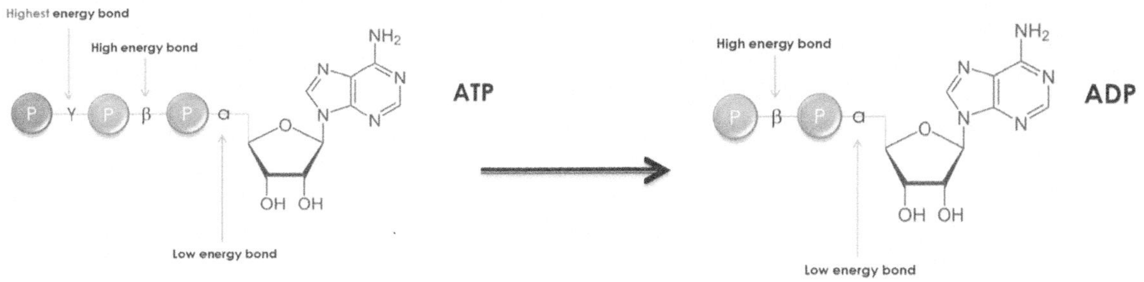

What phosphoCreatine does is supply the phosphate to ADP to regenerate ATP recharging the cell and improving stamina and strength.

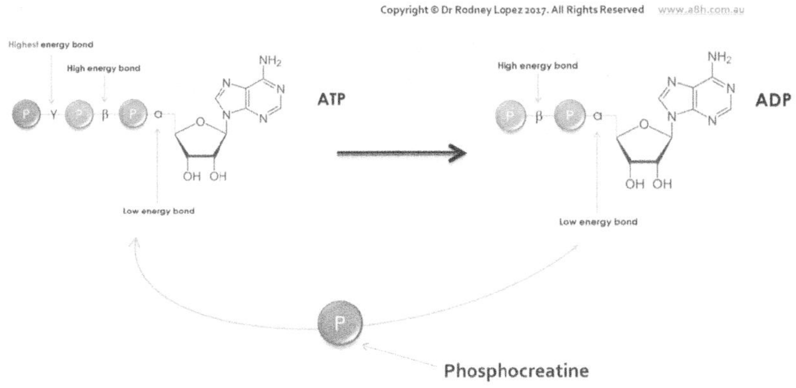

> Creatine is unstable in solution for any length of time so it is best taken in powder form to the gym at the recommended dose of 3 grams and then water added there and consumed relatively soon after it is in solution. Perhaps best to take Creatine in a separate mixer to your Whey/EAA/Citrulline blend to use 1/3 before/1/3 during/1/3 after exercise See Appendix-23 and 24 for tips to

<u>Age and decreased creation of phosphoCreatine</u>

Around 50% comes from your diet and the other 50% from your body's ability to create this compound. However, from the age of 30 years, your ability to regenerate phosphoCreatine diminishes and further deteriorates by around 8% every 10 years. Vegetarians and the elderly are at significant risk of phosphoCreatine deficiency. Just 3 grams per day is very safe and recommended especially for those who poorly recover after exercise and for seniors engaging in resistance training. Products like Creapure® are pharmaceutical grade and made in a dedicated factory with meticulous attention to detail to avoid contaminants like dicyandiamide and dihydro-1,3,5-triazine derivatives (http://www.efsa.europa.eu/de/efsajournal/pub/36.htm). Stick to the recommended dose. If a little bit is very good then a lot is not necessarily better. The kidney and liver toxicities of the past were due to the contaminants mentioned above and thus the purest product you can obtain like Creapure® is critical to ensure safety. Visit www.a8h.com.au and simply search for 'Creatine'.

Appendix-26: Exercise Supplementation Summarised

1. Take all supplements in powder form and mix at the gym
2. Have your 3g serve of Creatine Monohydrate (Creapure®) just prior to the exercise as Creatine is unstable in solution and needs to be consumed ASAP after being in solution
3. Add 1 – 2 scoops of EAAs (The Activ8Health EAA's are enriched with L-Citrulline + Glutamine + L-Arginine to support Nitric Oxide production). Thus if you purchase the Activ8Health form of EAAs you have this added support.
4. You can add a small amount of Activ8Health Whey if you like. Only a very small amount is needed, say 1 – 2 teaspoons (5 – 10 grams of whey). The Activ7Health Whey is enriched with L-Citrulline, EAAs, Glutamine and L-Arginine and so you do not want to add too much. The potential advantage of the whey as whole protein is that this will be broken down slowly providing amino acids more so after exercise stops but the whey is not absolutely necessary if you have around 10 grams of EAAs
5. Have 1/3 of this mix prior to exercise just after you have had your Creatine then sip the other 1/3 during your routine and the remaining 1/3 after exercise.

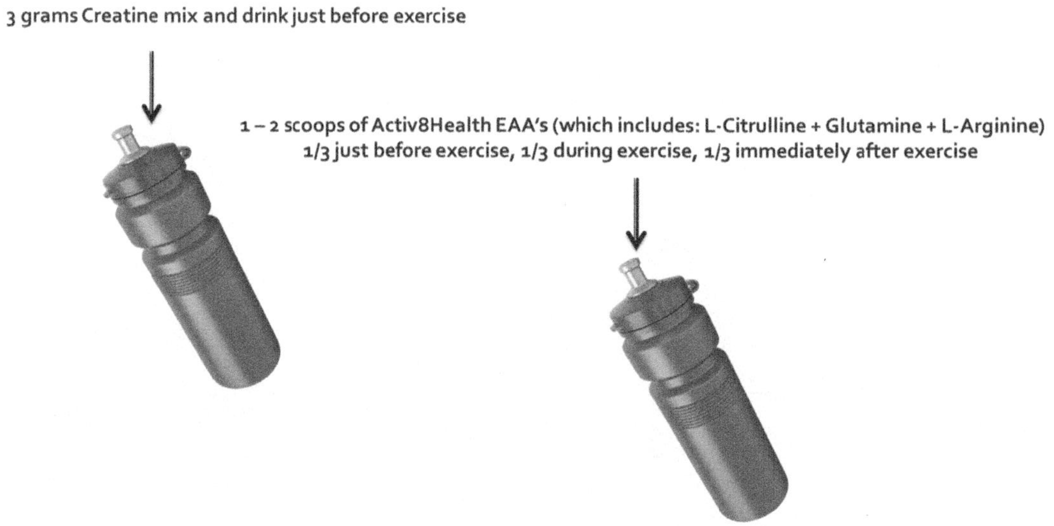

Note:

For those who think they need a massive hit of EAAs or Whey or any other protein around exercise, it is important to note that this has been researched. Researchers such as Levenhagen et al showed that it was amino acid availability rather than energy that was important with regard to protein synthesis around exercise (Levenhagen, CARR et al. 2002). The Levenhagen study only used 10 grams or less of protein and yet there was a significant increase in net protein synthesis.

As far as EAAs go, researchers like Atherton & Smith found that 10 grams of EAAs seem to be an optimal amount beyond which oxidation (burning) of the EAAs as fuel occurred (Atherton and Smith 2012). This is not what you want to do i.e. burn amino acids as energy as you want them to stimulate protein synthesis. Thus with the Activ8Health EAAs, you only need 1-2 scoops at the most and you will have a highly supportive mix for protein synthesis and at levels that prevent oxidation of the amino acids which is a waste of money because high doses are not necessary and this is evidence-based.

Appendix-27: Phytochemical Complexity

Ingredients: NanoGreens

- Greens blend
- Phytonutrient blend (Blueberry, Green Tea Extract, Grape Seed Extract, Cranberry, Raspberry, Tart Cherry, Pine Bark Extract, Broccoli, Tomato, Carrot, Spinach, Kale, Brussels Sprout, Bilberry, Elderberry, Pomegranate, Blackberry)
- Quercetin/Rutin
- Organic Rice Bran Soluble
- Raspberry Extract
- Organic Aloe Vera Powder Extract
- Fruit and Vegetable Blend (Apple, Carrot, Mango, Sweet Potato, Lemon, Parsley, Peach, Kale, Broccoli, Spinach*, Leek*, Beet , Cranberry* (Quinic Acid 6%)
- Organic Acerola Cherry Powder
- Green Tea Extract
- White Tea Extract
- Polygonum Cuspidatum
- Oat Bet Glucan

As I have indicated throughout the book, increasing phytochemical intake is of great importance to your health through the process of hormesis where these plant chemicals interact with genetic elements in your DNA to produce a multitude of effects on cell and protein repair mechanisms. Try to eat the 'rainbow' by adding a variety of multicoloured fruits and vegetables that you rotate constantly by eating salads, vegetables and fruits on a regular basis.

1 Serving NanoGreens® = Phytochemical 'Power' of 10 servings

Adding phytochemical complexity becomes even easier by the use of powders like NanoGreens which provide a huge phytochemical 'bang' in one serving of a phytochemical powder mix that can be added to the Plan-A and Plan-B blends described in this book or to water. There are 55 different components in the blend providing that enormous diversity of foods in an easily used form. However, the philosophy of the Activ8Health system is to ensure you do not have the same thing daily and so adding a phytochemical mix like this to your routine every 2nd day is all you would need.

The NanoGreens blend is 100 organic and vegan formulated.

It is designed to provide a high potency phytochemical 'hit' and also designed to taste good even in cold water.

Search www.a8h.com.au for these products.

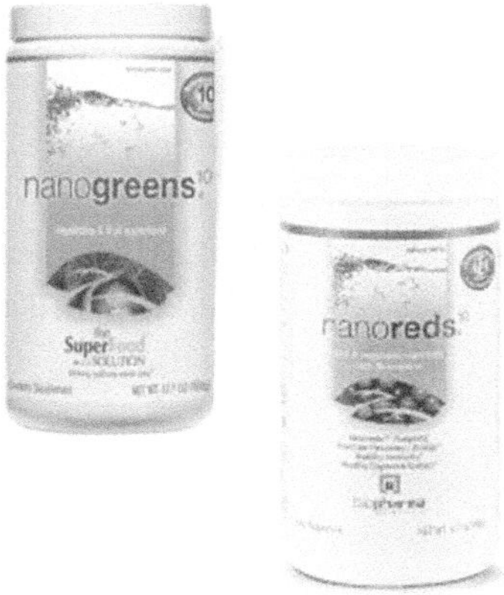

NanoGreens indredients continued

- Cinnamon Blend
- Milk Thistle
- Marigold Extract
- Dunaliella Salina
- Enzymes
- Lecithin
- Lycopene Extract-10%
- Organic Lemon Peel Powder
- Organic Quinoa Sprout
- Artichoke Extract
- Organic Atlantic Kelp Powder
- Stevia Leaf Crystals.

Appendix-28: Micronutrient content of various foods

You constantly hear the argument for including dairy or grains in your diet and the reason that is given time and again is to consume whole grains and milk due to the calcium content. To the "experts" calcium equals bone health and prevention of osteoporosis. This is very far from the truth as calcium is only a part of the equation and not the whole story. The table below pretty well destroys this myth of dairy (or grains) as being "supreme" choices for calcium when we compare cooked spinach with wheat, white flour and whole milk. Gram for gram, spinach has far more calcium than wheat and more calcium than milk! Whole wheat, wheat flour and milk have a huge disadvantage in terms of Vitamin-K1 (Phylloquinone) and as you can see the whopping dose of Vitamin-K1 of 927.2 mcg and this provides 7.7x the daily recommendation. Vitamin-K1 intake is vital to the production of Vitamin-K2 (Menaquinones). Vitamin-K1 is converted to a range of Menauinone compounds that are synthesized by intestinal microflora. Vitamin-K2 is a extremely important to enable diversion of calcium from blood vessels, heart valves and soft tissues towards bone. Individuals on Warfarin (Coumadin) anticoagulation suffer far more arterial calcification increasing the risk of arterial stiffness and heart failure.

The minerals in wheat and wheat flour are bound to phytates and hence are poorly bioavailable. So the nutritional panels on these grain-based products sound impressive but in terms of our health, it is pointless having a high level of any element if it cannot be absorbed effectively by the body. So, even with magnesium, wheat seems to have a higher level but the level in spinach will be far more efficiently absorbed.

For bone health you need far more than calcium. Spinach is rich in potassium, magnesium, calcium, amino acids and other trace elements that are vital for strong bones. Grains have a low Calcium to Phosphate (Ca/P) ratio and this can have a negative impact on bone growth and metabolism (Cordain 1999). Also of interest is the caloric value of the spinach in comparison to wheat or dairy.

Essential reading is a paper by Professor Loren Cordain, an excellent and in-depth article looking at the adequacies/inadequacies of cereal grains titled 'Cereal grains: humanity's double-edged sword' (Cordain 1999). Pushing grain consumption as being ideal sources of micronutrients is misleading. Higher consumption of grains will importantly displace vegetable and dairy consumption as sources of calcium. It is an absolute myth that you need to consume dairy to get enough calcium. You get an abundant amount of calcium gram for gram from spinach and other greens and you also get a range of phytochemicals such as Lutein and Zeaxanthin vital for eye health through dark green leafy vegetables. As you will notice in the table above, you do not get any Vitamin-A or K at all from grains like wheat. If someone is on a typical Western diet and you provide a food like whole grains in their diets then obviously you will get a positive health outcome. Adding anything remotely healthy to a pathetic diet will produce a positive health outcome and such outcomes no doubt help the grain industry sell its product. Positive health outcomes from grains are more likely due to the fibre content rather than micronutrient sufficiency because you can see two massive 'holes' where Vitamin-K and Vitamin-A both vital fat soluble vitamins are missing in whole grains.

Food	Quantity	Calcium	Magnesium	Potassium	Vitamin K (mcg)	Folate	Retinol	Calories (kcal)
Durum Wheat	**1 cup (192g)**	**65mg**	**276mg**	**828mg**	**0**	**83mcg**	**0**	**651 kcal**
White Wheat Flour	**192 grams**	**29mg**	**42 mg**	**205mg**	**0.6**	**50mcg**	**0**	**699 kcal**
Milk (3.7% Milkfat, whole)	**1 cup (192 grams)**	**228**	**25**	**290**	**0**	**10**	**60 mcg**	**123 kcal**
Spinach (cooked)	**192 grams**	**261mg**	**167mg**	**895mg**	**927.2 mcg**	**280mcg**	**Carotenoids**	**44 kcal**

Antioxidant Plates

All foods have a large number of nutrients but some are a rich source of a particular beneficial nutrient than others and these are the ones highlighted. There are a large number of trace elements vital to health. Many Nutritionists may not realise how vital say Nickel (Ni) is to the bowel microbiota and that methane production is Nickel-dependent due to the last step of methane production requiring a Ni-based enzyme (Zambelli and Ciurli 2013). Kelp is a rich source of many essential elements such as Co, Cr, Mo, Ni, Se, plus V, required by humans (de la Rocha, Sanchez-Muniz et al. 2009).

We need to ensure that we have our 14 essential minerals, 13 universally recognised vitamins, six macro-minerals (Sodium, Calcium, Magnesium, Potassium, Chloride and Phosphorus), fourteen trace minerals (Boron, Chromium, Cobalt, Copper, Iodine, Iron, Fluorine, Manganese, Molybdenum, Nickel, Selenium, Silica, Vanadium, Zinc) and two essentially fatty acids (Linoleic Acid and Alpha Linolenic Acid). We can also add Choline to this list, a vitamin-like compound. The Nutrient Reference Values for Australia and New Zealand states that "arsenic, boron, nickel, silicon and vanadium." do not have evidence for essentiality (https://www.nrv.gov.au/nutrients) but as shown above, a trace element such as Nickel is vital for the gut microbiota and this way of thinking of an individual as a human versus the holobiome i.e. human-microbiome hybrid may be the reason for these exclusions. Just because we (the human side) do not need something, it doesn't mean that our other half, the microbiota also doesn't need a micronutrient to survive.

This is a quaint, anachronistic way of thinking now. Boron is another example that in recent research has been found to lower prostatic PSA levels (LeBeau, Kostova et al. 2010), and protect against prostate cancer. Just 6 prunes can provide the boron necessary for this effect. Boron also supports bone health through various mechanisms. The trick is to ensure you are not deficient in all these recognised and important vitamins, minerals and trace elements.

In a report by the World Health Organization (WHO), an important point is made and that is to distinguish between:

1. **Basal Requirement** – the amount of an element required to prevent a detectable pathological effect on human health

2. **Normative Requirement** – the amount that provides a storage buffer against depletion caused by times of reduced intake or perhaps an
increased need for the nutrient resource due to illness or increased activity.

So you can see that just scraping through with calorie-rich, nutrient-poor foods eaten in Western societies is just not good enough. "Go and eat a balanced diet" is a simplistic statement made by so many 'experts' in nutrition when a struggling planet being depleted of resources like topsoil critical to keep us alive and where cultivars chosen for yield and not nutrient density are used and on top of this poor agricultural practices, transport, storage, cooking and individual genetic requirements all conspire to ensure our intakes are way below the normative requirement and that many are not even getting the basal requirements for a multitude of micronutrients.

Many other micronutrients high in compounds like Sulforaphane and Indole-3 Carbinol which are potent compounds are also important for health and these can influence biotransformation (detoxification) pathways and oestrogen metabolism. Rotate Broccoli with Kale, Cabbage, Cauliflower for these compounds.

Thus provide a large diversity of food to your body to enable it to not only survive but thrive. The following Antioxidant Plates (APs) are a suggestion and I am sure you will add other important foods to these plates.

Antioxidant Plate 1 (AP-1)

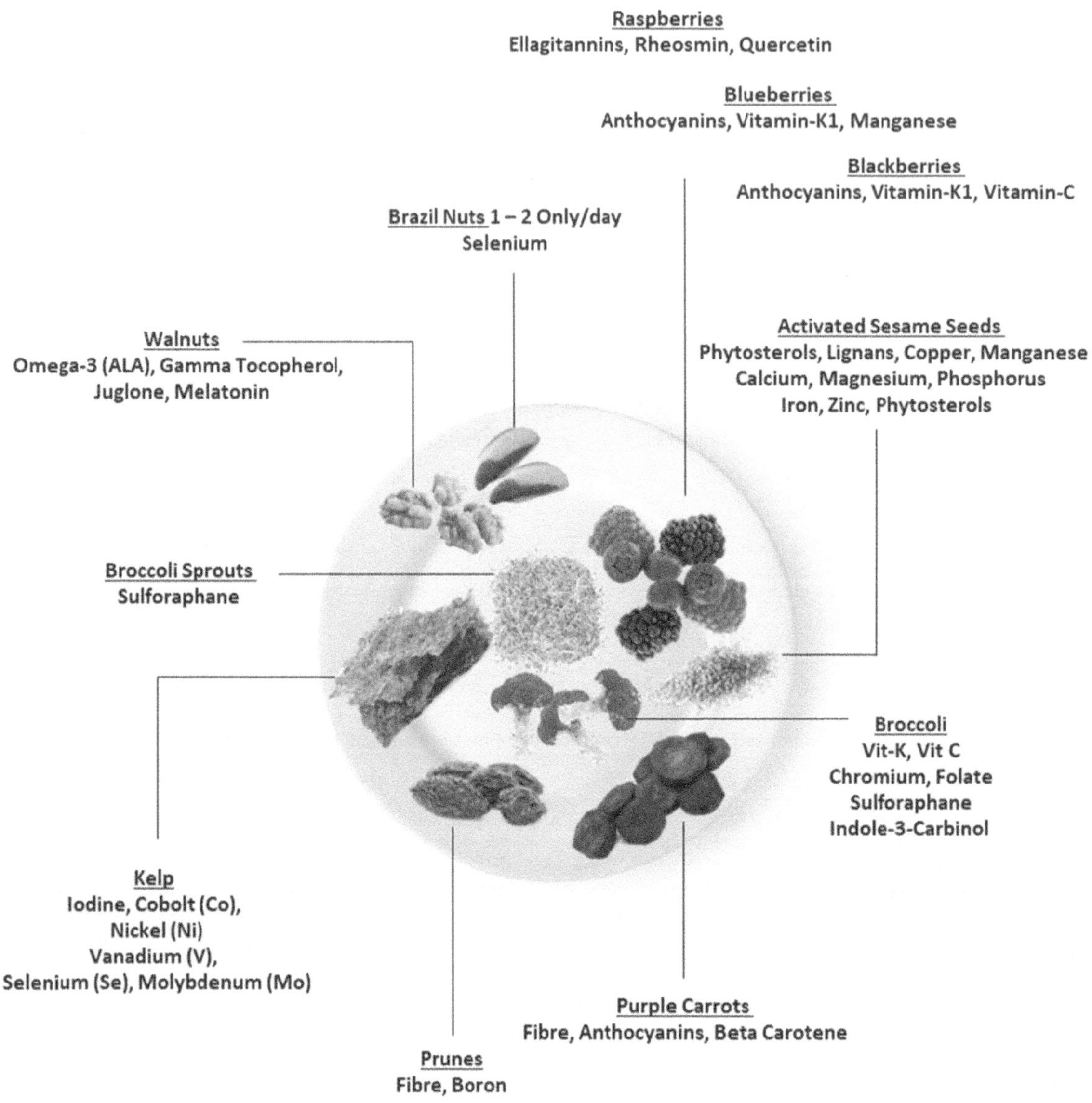

These plates provide a guideline on the various foods you need to consume to ensure you are meeting the recommended daily allowances of the various micronutrients and trace elements critical for optimal health. Do not have the same things every day, but alternate them in the spirit of rotating foods and to add variety to your diet. All foods have a large number of nutrients but some are a rich source of a few nutrients and these are highlighted. Nuts should be eaten raw and activated. Roasted nuts have their proteins denatured during the hot roasting process and this means the proteins in the nuts have been altered. This increases the risk of allergic responses to those proteins.

Antioxidant Plate 2 (AP-2)

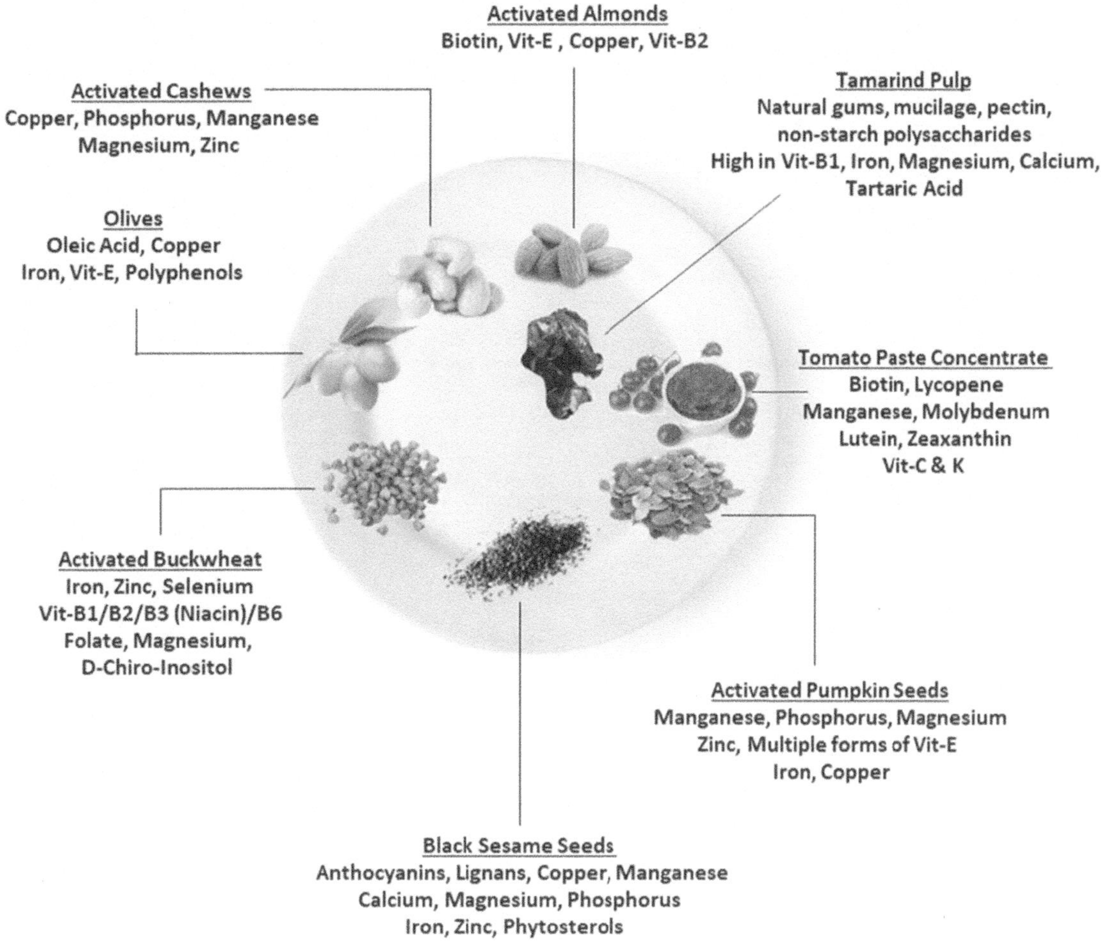

Nuts can be rotated. Have around 5 of each nut with perhaps two varieties on a plate at a time, include Hazelnuts, Macadamia, Pecans, Pistachios. Brazil nuts should be eaten most days because of the high Selenium content perhaps 5 days out of 7 in the spirit of including a washout period. Remember, Brazil nuts are very high in selenium if they actually come from the Amazon. Thus you risk selenium toxicity if you have too much. Limit these to 2 maximum per day. Peanuts which are legumes and not nuts, according to Professor Loren Cordain. Peanuts have a powerful lectin called PNA that can damage the bowel lining and peanuts can produce a lethal allergic reaction in susceptible individuals. PNA may increase the risk of cardiovascular disease. Until much more is found out about peanut safety in general, there is absolutely no need to include this in your diet.

Activation of nuts and seeds has been discussed in this book and the reasoning is sound in terms of releasing minerals. Soaking foods to improve nutrient value and digestibility is not new, but centuries old.

Getting into a habit of having these antioxidant plates will ensure you do not become depleted in essential micronutrients. Being sufficient in not only vitamins but the critical minerals and trace elements is key to your cells being able to function optimally and the key to a strong functional immune system.

Bibliography

Alberts, B., et al. (2013). Essential cell biology, Garland Science.

Angulo, P. and K. D. Lindor (2001). Treatment of non-alcoholic fatty liver: present and emerging therapies. Seminars in liver disease, Copyright© 2001 by Thieme Medical Publishers, Inc., 333 Seventh Avenue, New York, NY 10001, USA. Tel.:+ 1 (212) 584-4662.

Amar, J., Burcelin, R., Ruidavets, J. B., Cani, P. D., Fauvel, J., Alessi, M. C., . . . Ferriéres, J. (2008). Energy intake is associated with endotoxemia in apparently healthy men. *The American journal of clinical nutrition, 87*(5), 1219-1223.

Ames, B. N. (1999). "Micronutrient deficiencies: a major cause of DNA damage." Annals of the New York Academy of Sciences **889**(1): 87-106.

Ames, B. N. (2006). Low micronutrient intake may accelerate the degenerative diseases of aging through allocation of scarce micronutrients by triage. *Proceedings of the National Academy of Sciences, 103*(47), 17589-17594.

Änggård, E. (1990). "The endothelium–the body's largest endocrine gland?" Journal of Endocrinology **127**(3): 371-375.

ANH. (2012). Drugs as dangerous as war. Retrieved from http://anhinternational.org/2012/07/11/anh-exclusive-natural-health-products-ultra-safe-and-drugs-as-dangerous-as-war/

Arslan, N. (2014). "Obesity, fatty liver disease and intestinal microbiota." World Journal of Gastroenterology: WJG **20**(44): 16452.

Atherton, P. and K. Smith (2012). "Muscle protein synthesis in response to nutrition and exercise." The Journal of physiology **590**(5): 1049-1057.

Aune, D., De Stefani, E., Ronco, A. L., Boffetta, P., Deneo-Pellegrini, H., Acosta, G., & Mendilaharsu, M. (2009). Egg consumption and the risk of cancer: a multisite case-control study in Uruguay. *Asian Pac J Cancer Prev, 10*(5), 869-876.

Aune, D., et al. (2016). "Fruit and vegetable intake and the risk of cardiovascular disease, total cancer and all-cause mortality–a systematic review and dose-response meta-analysis of prospective studies." International Journal of Epidemiology.

Aymard, J.-P., et al. (1988). "Haematological adverse effects of histamine H2-receptor antagonists." Medical toxicology and adverse drug experience **3**(6): 430-448.

Bailey, R. L., West Jr, K. P., & Black, R. E. (2015). The epidemiology of global micronutrient deficiencies. *Annals of Nutrition and Metabolism, 66*(Suppl. 2), 22-33.

Barker, D. (1995). Intrauterine programming of adult disease. *Molecular medicine today, 1*(9), 418-423.

Barzel, U. S., & Massey, L. K. (1998). Excess dietary protein can adversely affect bone. *The Journal of nutrition, 128*(6), 1051-1053.

Batty, G., Kivimäki, M., Smith, G. D., Marmot, M., & Shipley, M. (2008). Post-challenge blood glucose concentration and stroke mortality rates in nondiabetic men in London: 38-year follow-up of the original Whitehall prospective cohort study. *Diabetologia, 51*(7), 1123-1126.

Benedict, F. G., et al. (1919). Human vitality and efficiency under prolonged restricted diet, Carnegie institution of Washington.

Berdanier, C. D., Berdanier, L. A., & Zempleni, J. (2008). *Advanced nutrition: macronutrients, micronutrients, and metabolism*: CRC Press.

Berg, J., et al. (2002). "Biochemistry Fifth Edition." WH Freeman and Company. New York **423**: 436-437.

Best, C., et al. (1949). "Liver damage produced by feeding alcohol or sugar and its prevention by choline." British Medical Journal **2**(4635): 1001.

Bianconi, E., et al. (2013). "An estimation of the number of cells in the human body." Annals of human biology **40**(6): 463-471.

Billis, A. (1986). "Latent carcinoma and atypical lesions of prostate An autopsy study." Urology **28**(4): 324-329.

Bhathal, P., et al. (1985). "Frequency of benign and malignant breast lesions in 207 consecutive autopsies in Australian women." British journal of cancer **51**(2): 271.

Bianconi, E., Piovesan, A., Facchin, F., Beraudi, A., Casadei, R., Frabetti, F., . . . Piva, F. (2013). An estimation of the number of cells in the human body. *Annals of human biology, 40*(6), 463-471.

Bjørnholt, J. V., Erikssen, G., Aaser, E., Sandvik, L., Nitter-Hauge, S., Jervell, J., . . . Thaulow, E. (1999). Fasting blood glucose: an underestimated risk factor for cardiovascular death. Results from a 22-year follow-up of healthy nondiabetic men. *Diabetes Care, 22*(1), 45-49.

Bonkowski, M. S. and D. A. Sinclair (2016). "Slowing ageing by design: the rise of NAD+ and sirtuin-activating compounds." Nature Reviews Molecular Cell Biology.

Børsheim, E., et al. (2002). "Essential amino acids and muscle protein recovery from resistance exercise." American Journal of Physiology-Endocrinology And Metabolism **283**(4): E648-E657.

Blackburn, E. H. (2017). The Telomere Effect, Orion Spring.

Blumenthal, C., Barlow, E., & Wrigley, C. (1993). Growth environment and wheat quality: the effect of heat stress on dough properties and gluten proteins. *Journal of Cereal Science, 18*(1), 3-21.

Brook, R. D. and S. Julius (2000). "Autonomic imbalance, hypertension, and cardiovascular risk." American journal of hypertension **13**(S4): 112S-122S.

Buchman, A. L., et al. (1992). "Lecithin increases plasma free choline and decreases hepatic steatosis in long-term total parenteral nutrition patients." Gastroenterology **102**(4): 1363-1370.

Burke, L., Cox, G., & Deakes, N. (2010). *The Complete Guide to Food for Sports Performance: Peak Nutrition for Your Sport*: Allen & Unwin Australia.

Butler, J. (2014). White Lies: A Viva. www.whitelies.org.uk

Calle, E. E. and R. Kaaks (2004). "Overweight, obesity and cancer: epidemiological evidence and proposed mechanisms." Nature Reviews Cancer **4**(8): 579-591.

Campbell, B., Kreider, R. B., Ziegenfuss, T., La Bounty, P., Roberts, M., Burke, D., . . . Antonio, J. (2007). International Society of Sports Nutrition position stand: protein and exercise. *Journal of the International Society of Sports Nutrition, 4*(1), 1.

Cani, P. D., Amar, J., Iglesias, M. A., Poggi, M., Knauf, C., Bastelica, D., . . . Chabo, C. (2007). Metabolic endotoxemia initiates obesity and insulin resistance. *Diabetes, 56*(7), 1761-1772.

Capozzi, V., et al. (2012). "Biogenic amines degradation by Lactobacillus plantarum: toward a potential application in wine."

Capra, S. (2006). Nutrient reference values for Australia and New Zealand: Including recommended dietary intakes.

Carding, S., et al. (2015). "Dysbiosis of the gut microbiota in disease." Microbial ecology in health and disease **26**.

Casey, D. (2012). "Elixir of immortality? Wine, resveratrol and sirtuins: an overview." Journal of wine research **23**(3): 247-252.

Ceriello, A. (2000). The post-prandial state and cardiovascular disease: relevance to diabetes mellitus. *Diabetes/metabolism research and reviews, 16*(2), 125-132.

Ceriello, A. (2003). The possible role of postprandial hyperglycaemia in the pathogenesis of diabetic complications. *Diabetologia, 46*.

Ceriello, A., et al. (2002). "Evidence for an independent and cumulative effect of postprandial hypertriglyceridemia and hyperglycemia on endothelial dysfunction and oxidative stress generation." Circulation **106**(10): 1211-1218.

Champagne, E. T. (1989). Low gastric hydrochloric acid secretion and mineral bioavailability. Mineral Absorption in the Monogastric GI Tract, Springer: 173-184.

Chang, C.-Y., et al. (2009). "Essential fatty acids and human brain." Acta Neurol Taiwan **18**(4): 231-241.

Chen, A. C., et al. (2015). "A phase 3 randomized trial of nicotinamide for skin-cancer chemoprevention." New England Journal of Medicine **373**(17): 1618-1626.

Cheetham, M. E., Boobis, L., Brooks, S., & Williams, C. (1986). Human muscle metabolism during sprint running. *Journal of Applied Physiology, 61*(1), 54-60.

Chen, A. C., et al. (2015). "A phase 3 randomized trial of nicotinamide for skin-cancer chemoprevention." New England Journal of Medicine **373**(17): 1618-1626.

Clarkson, P. M. and M. J. Hubal (2002). "Exercise-induced muscle damage in humans." American journal of physical medicine & rehabilitation **81**(11): S52-S69.

Cone, M. (2012). Low Doses of Hormonelike Chemicals May Have Big Effects. *Scientific American*.

Conlee, R., et al. (1987). "Effects of glucose or fructose feeding on glycogen repletion in muscle and liver after exercise or fasting." Annals of Nutrition and Metabolism **31**(2): 126-132.

Conlon, M. A. and A. R. Bird (2014). "The impact of diet and lifestyle on gut microbiota and human health." Nutrients **7**(1): 17-44.

Corbin, K. D. and S. H. Zeisel (2012). "Choline metabolism provides novel insights into non-alcoholic fatty liver disease and its progression." Current opinion in gastroenterology **28**(2): 159.

Cordain, L. (1999). Cereal grains: humanity's double-edged sword. *World Review of Nutrition and Dietetics, 84*, 19-19.

Cordain, L., et al. (2003). "Hyperinsulinemic diseases of civilisation: more than just Syndrome X." Comparative Biochemistry and Physiology, Part A **136**(1): 95-112.

Cordain, L. (2011). *The Paleo Answer: 7 Days to Lose Weight, Feel Great, Stay Young*: Wiley.

Costill, D. L., Wilmore, J. H., & Kenney, W. L. (2012). Physiology of sport and exercise. *Physiology Of Sport And Exercise-9780736094092-66, 78*.

Cremon, C., et al. (2010). "Intestinal dysbiosis in irritable bowel syndrome: etiological factor or epiphenomenon?" Expert review of molecular diagnostics **10**(4): 389-393.

Cronin, F. J., et al. (1987). "Developing a food guidance system to implement the dietary guidelines." Journal of Nutrition Education **19**(6): 281-302.

Cummings, J. H., & Bingham, S. A. (1998). Diet and the prevention of cancer. *British Medical Journal, 317*(7173), 1636.

Curis, E., et al. (2005). "Almost all about Citrulline in mammals." Amino Acids **29**(3): 177-205.

Cuthbertson, D. (2017). "Just 2 weeks of inactivity could lead to changes that increase risk of developing disease." Retrieved 22nd May 2017, from https://news.liverpool.ac.uk/2017/05/17/just-2-weeks-of-inactivity-could-lead-to-changes-that-increase-risk-of-developing-disease/.

D'Antona, G., Ragni, M., Cardile, A., Tedesco, L., Dossena, M., Bruttini, F., . . . Carruba, M. (2010). Branched-Chain Amino Acid Supplementation Promotes Survival and Supports Cardiac and Skeletal Muscle Mitochondrial Biogenesis in Middle-Aged Mice. *Cell Metabolism, 12*(4), 362-372.

Darden, E. (2014). The Body Fat Breakthrough: Tap the muscle-building power of negative training and lose up to 30 pounds in 30 days, Rodale.

Davis, D. R. (2009). "Declining fruit and vegetable nutrient composition: What is the evidence?" HortScience **44**(1): 15-19.

de la Rocha, S. R., et al. (2009). "Trace elements determination in edible seaweeds by an optimised and validated ICP-MS method." Journal of Food Composition and Analysis **22**(4): 330-336.

Dibaba, D., et al. (2015). "Magnesium intake and incidence of pancreatic cancer: the VITamins and Lifestyle study." British journal of cancer.

Davis, D. R., et al. (2004). "Changes in USDA food composition data for 43 garden crops, 1950 to 1999." Journal of the American College of Nutrition **23**(6): 669-682.

Dean, R. C. and T. F. Lue (2005). "Physiology of penile erection and pathophysiology of erectile dysfunction." The Urologic clinics of North America **32**(4): 379.

De Flora, S., et al. (1997). "Attenuation of influenza-like symptomatology and improvement of cell-mediated immunity with long-term N-acetylcysteine treatment." European Respiratory Journal **10**(7): 1535-1541.

Delanghe, J. R., et al. (2007). "Vitamin C deficiency and scurvy are not only a dietary problem but are codetermined by the haptoglobin polymorphism." Clinical chemistry **53**(8): 1397-1400.

De Leon, M. P. and L. Roncucci (1997). "Chemoprevention of colorectal tumors: role of lactulose and of other agents." Scandinavian journal of gastroenterology **32**(sup222): 72-75.

De Paepe, M., et al. (2014). "Bacteriophages: an underestimated role in human and animal health?" Frontiers in cellular and infection microbiology **4**: 39.

Doherty, T. J. (2003). "Invited review: aging and sarcopenia." Journal of Applied Physiology **95**(4): 1717.00347.2003.

Dollahite, J., Franklinms, D., & McNew, R. (1995). Problems encountered in meeting the Recommended Dietary Allowances for menus designed according to the Dietary Guidelines for Americans. *Journal of the American Dietetic Association, 95*(3), 341-347.

Downey, M., & Edmonds, B. (2007, 01). Triage theory offers a new look at aging.Natural Foods Merchandiser, 28, 56.

Dreyer, H. C., et al. (2006). "Resistance exercise increases AMPK activity and reduces 4E-BP1 phosphorylation and protein synthesis in human skeletal muscle." The Journal of physiology **576**(2): 613-624.

Durnin, J. (1981). Basal metabolic rate in man. *Joint FAO WHO UNU expert consultation on energy and protein requirements. Rome: World Health Organization.*

Eaton, S. (2006). "The ancestral human diet: what was it and should it be a paradigm for contemporary nutrition?" Proceedings of the Nutrition Society **65**(01): 1-6.

Ebbeling, C. B., Swain, J. F., Feldman, H. A., Wong, W. W., Hachey, D. L., Garcia-Lago, E., & Ludwig, D. S. (2012). Effects of dietary composition on energy expenditure during weight-loss maintenance. *JAMA: the journal of the American Medical Association, 307*(24), 2627-2634.

Enders, G. (2015). Gut: The inside story of our body's most underrated organ, Greystone Books Ltd.

Epe, B. (2012). "DNA damage spectra induced by photosensitization." Photochemical & Photobiological Sciences **11**(1): 98-106.

Erridge, C., Attina, T., Spickett, C. M., & Webb, D. J. (2007). A high-fat meal induces low-grade endotoxemia: evidence of a novel mechanism of postprandial inflammation. *The American journal of clinical nutrition, 86*(5), 1286-1292.

Evans, W. and W. Campbell (1993). "Sarcopenia and age-related changes in body composition and functional capacity." Journal of Nutrition **123**(2 Suppl): 465.

Felisberto, M. H. F., et al. (2015). "Use of Chia (Salvia hispanica L.) mucilage gel to reduce fat in pound cakes." LWT-Food Science and Technology **63**(2): 1049-1055.

Fischer, L. M., et al. (2010). "Dietary choline requirements of women: effects of oestrogen and genetic variation." The American journal of clinical nutrition **92**(5): 1113-1119.

Ford, E. S., et al. (2010). "Prediabetes and the risk for cardiovascular disease." Journal of the American College of Cardiology **55**(13): 1310-1317.

Foster-Powell, K., et al. (2002). "International table of glycemic index and glycemic load values: 2002." American Journal of Clinical Nutrition **76**(1): 5.

Fowler, S. P., et al. (2008). "Fueling the obesity epidemic? Artificially sweetened beverage use and long-term weight gain." Obesity **16**(8): 1894-1900.

Francis, G., Upton, F., Ballard, F., McNeil, K., & Wallace, J. (1988). Insulin-like growth factors 1 and 2 in bovine colostrum. Sequences and biological activities compared with those of a potent truncated form. *Biochemical Journal, 251*(1), 95-103.

Fraser, G., et al. (1992). "A possible protective effect of nut consumption on risk of coronary heart disease: the Adventist Health Study." Archives of Internal Medicine **152**(7): 1416.

Frei, B., et al. (2014). "Enough is enough." Annals of internal medicine **160**(11): 807.

Fuge, R. (1996). "Geochemistry of iodine in relation to iodine deficiency diseases." Geological Society London Special Publications **113**(1): 201.

Gallego, G., et al. (2010). "Iodine deficiency in Australia: is iodine supplementation for pregnant and lactating women warranted." Med J Aust **192**(8): 461-463.

Gerber, J. "A Review of Mineral Absorption with Special Consideration of Chelation as a Method to Improve Bioavailability of Mineral Supplements." Magnesium **21**: 27.

Graham, R. D. (2008). Micronutrient deficiencies in crops and their global significance. Micronutrient deficiencies in global crop production, Springer: 41-61.

Ganmaa, D., & Sato, A. (2005). The possible role of female sex hormones in milk from pregnant cows in the development of breast, ovarian and corpus uteri cancers. *Medical Hypotheses, 65*(6), 1028-1037.

Ghosh, H. S., et al. (2010). "SIRT1 negatively regulates the mammalian target of rapamycin." PLoS ONE **5**(2): e9199.

Gilbert, J.-A., Bendsen, N. T., Tremblay, A., & Astrup, A. (2011). Effect of proteins from different sources on body composition. *Nutrition, Metabolism and Cardiovascular Diseases, 21*, B16-B31.

Giovannucci, E., et al. (1998). "Multivitamin use, folate, and colon cancer in women in the Nurses' Health Study." Annals of internal medicine **129**(7): 517-524.

Godlee, F. (2017). Red meat: another inconvenient truth, British Medical Journal Publishing Group.

Gomes, A. P., et al. (2013). "Declining NAD+ induces a pseudohypoxic state disrupting nuclear-mitochondrial communication during aging." Cell **155**(7): 1624-1638.

Gosby, A., Conigrave, A., Raubenheimer, D., & Simpson, S. (2014). Protein leverage and energy intake. *Obesity reviews, 15*(3), 183-191.

Greer, E. L. and A. Brunet (2005). "FOXO transcription factors at the interface between longevity and tumor suppression." Oncogene **24**(50): 7410-7425.

Grilo, E. C., et al. (2014). "Alpha-tocopherol and gamma-tocopherol concentration in vegetable oils." Food Science and Technology (Campinas) **34**(2): 379-385.

Groff, J. L., & Gropper, S. A. S. (2000). *Advanced nutrition and human metabolism*: West/Wadsworth Belmont, CA.

Grønholdt, M.-L. M., et al. (1996). "Echolucent carotid artery plaques are associated with elevated levels of fasting and postprandial triglyceride-rich lipoproteins." Stroke **27**(12): 2166-2172.

Grune, T., et al. (2010). "■-Carotene is an important vitamin A source for humans." The Journal of nutrition **140**(12): 2268S-2285S.

Guallar, E., et al. (2013). "Enough is enough: stop wasting money on vitamin and mineral supplements." Annals of internal medicine **159**(12): 850-851.

Guarente, L. (2008). "Mitochondria—a nexus for aging, calorie restriction, and sirtuins?" Cell **132**(2): 171-176.

Hackethal, V. (2017). "Dramatic Rise in Colorectal Cancer in Younger Adults." 2017, from http://www.medscape.com/viewarticle/876409.

Hall, J. E. (2015). *Guyton and Hall textbook of medical physiology*: Elsevier Health Sciences.

Heaney, R. P. and D. K. Layman (2008). "Amount and type of protein influences bone health." The American journal of clinical nutrition **87**(5): 1567S-1570S.

Heilmeyer, L. M. (2012). Signal transduction and protein phosphorylation, Springer Science & Business Media.

Henry-Vitrac, C., et al. (2010). "Contribution of chlorogenic acids to the inhibition of human hepatic glucose-6-phosphatase activity in vitro by Svetol, a standardized decaffeinated green coffee extract." Journal of Agricultural and Food Chemistry **58**(7): 4141-4144.

Hirakawa, Y., Ninomiya, T., Mukai, N., Doi, Y., Hata, J., Fukuhara, M., . . . Kiyohara, Y. (2012). Association Between Glucose Tolerance Level and Cancer Death in a General Japanese Population The Hisayama Study. *American journal of epidemiology, 176*(10), 856-864.

Hariri, N., & Thibault, L. (2010). High-fat diet-induced obesity in animal models. *Nutrition research reviews, 23*(02), 270-299.

Hoffman, J. R. and M. J. Falvo (2004). "Protein-Which is best." Journal of Sports Science and Medicine **3**(3): 118-130.

Högström, G., et al. (2015). "Aerobic fitness in late adolescence and the risk of early death: a prospective cohort study of 1.3 million Swedish men." International Journal of Epidemiology: dyv321.

Holt, S., Miller, J., & Petocz, P. (1997). An insulin index of foods: the insulin demand generated by 1000-kJ portions of common foods. *The American journal of clinical nutrition, 66*(5), 1264-1276.

Hoyt, G., Hickey, M., & Cordain, L. (2005). Dissociation of the glycemicand insulinaemic responses to whole and skimmed milk. *British Journal of Nutrition, 93*(2), 175.

Hultman, E. (1967). "Muscle glycogen in man determined in needle biopsy specimens method and normal values." Scandinavian journal of clinical and laboratory investigation **19**(3): 209-217.

Hunter, J. E., Zhang, J., & Kris-Etherton, P. M. (2010). Cardiovascular disease risk of dietary stearic acid compared with trans, other saturated, and unsaturated fatty acids: a systematic review. *The American journal of clinical nutrition, 91*(1), 46-63.

Institute-Science-In-Society. (2014). Phosphorus Starvation Threatens the World. Retrieved from http://www.i-sis.org.uk/Phosphorus_Starvation_Threatens_the_World.php

Imai, S.-i. and L. Guarente (2014). "NAD+ and sirtuins in aging and disease." Trends in cell biology **24**(8): 464-471.

Ishii, T., et al. (1998). "Resistance training improves insulin sensitivity in NIDDM subjects without altering maximal oxygen uptake." Diabetes Care **21**(8): 1353-1355.

Ito, T. and R. T. Jensen (2010). "Association of long-term proton pump inhibitor therapy with bone fractures and effects on absorption of calcium, vitamin B12, iron, and magnesium." Current gastroenterology reports **12**(6): 448-457.

Jakubowicz, D., Froy, O., Ahrén, B., Boaz, M., Landau, Z., Bar-Dayan, Y., . . . Wainstein, J. (2014). Incretin, insulinotropic and glucose-lowering effects of whey protein preload in type 2 diabetes: a randomised clinical trial. *Diabetologia, 57*(9), 1807-1811.

Jessani, S., Gangopadhyay, K., Patel, J., Lip, G., & Millane, T. (2007). Should oral glucose tolerance testing be mandatory following acute myocardial infarction? *International Journal of Clinical Practice, 61*(4), 680-683.

Jiang, Q., et al. (2001). "γ-Tocopherol, the major form of vitamin E in the US diet, deserves more attention." The American journal of clinical nutrition **74**(6): 714-722.

Jiang, Q., et al. (2008). "Long-chain carboxychromanols, metabolites of vitamin E, are potent inhibitors of cyclooxygenases." Proceedings of the National Academy of Sciences **105**(51): 20464-20469.

Karjalainen, R., et al. (2008). A review on bioactive compounds in black currants (Ribes nigrum L.) and their potential health-promoting properties. I International Symposium on Biotechnology of Fruit Species: BIOTECHFRUIT2008 839.

Kenyon, C., Chang, J., Gensch, E., Rudner, A., & Tabtiang, R. (1993). A C. elegans mutant that lives twice as long as wild type. *Nature, 366*(6454), 461-464.

Keys, A., et al. (1950). "The biology of human starvation.(2 vols)."

Kim, C., et al. (2017). "Neurogenic Effects of Ghrelin on the Hippocampus." International journal of molecular sciences **18**(3): 588.

King, M. (2017). "Fructose Metabolism." 2017, from http://themedicalbiochemistrypage.org/fructose.php.

Koeth, R. A., Wang, Z., Levison, B. S., Buffa, J. A., Org, E., Sheehy, B. T., . . . Li, L. (2013). Intestinal microbiota metabolism of l-carnitine, a nutrient in red meat, promotes atherosclerosis. *Nature Medicine.*

Krebs-Smith, S. M., et al. (1996). "Fruit and vegetable intakes of children and adolescents in the United States." Archives of Pediatrics & Adolescent Medicine **150**(1): 81-86.

Kushi, L. H., et al. (1996). "Dietary antioxidant vitamins and death from coronary heart disease in postmenopausal women." New England Journal of Medicine **334**(18): 1156-1162.

Kragh-Hansen, U. (1981). "Molecular aspects of ligand binding to serum albumin." Pharmacological Reviews **33**(1): 17-53.

Kumar, V., Abbas, A. K., & Aster, J. C. (2012). *Robbins basic pathology*: Elsevier Health Sciences.

Kumar, V., Sinha, A. K., Makkar, H. P., & Becker, K. (2010). Dietary roles of phytate and phytase in human nutrition: A review. *Food Chemistry, 120*(4), 945-959.

Kuo, C., et al. (2010). "Gout and risk of non-alcoholic fatty liver disease." Scandinavian journal of rheumatology **39**(6): 466-471.

Lai, S.-W. and K.-F. Liao (2013). "Body mass index and non-alcoholic fatty liver disease." Journal of gastroenterology **48**(4): 549-549.

Lal, R. (2011). Human Body: A virtual zoo of bacteria, Springer.

Laplante, M. and D. M. Sabatini (2012). "mTOR signaling in growth control and disease." Cell **149**(2): 274-293.

Lazarou, J., Pomeranz, B. H., & Corey, P. N. (1998). Incidence of adverse drug reactions in hospitalized patients: a meta-analysis of prospective studies. *JAMA, 279*(15), 1200-1205.

Leaf, A. (1999). "Dietary Prevention of Coronary Heart Disease : The Lyon Diet Heart Study." Circulation **99**(6): 733-735.

LeBeau, A. M., et al. (2010). "Prostate-specific antigen: an overlooked candidate for the targeted treatment and selective imaging of prostate cancer." Biological chemistry **391**(4): 333-343.

Lee, G. E., et al. (2008). "Association between BMI and metabolic syndrome and adenomatous colonic polyps in Korean men." Obesity **16**(6): 1434-1439.

Lee, J. M., Lee, H., Kang, S., & Park, W. J. (2016). Fatty Acid Desaturases, Polyunsaturated Fatty Acid Regulation, and Biotechnological Advances. *Nutrients, 8*(1), 23.

LEVENHAGEN, D. K., C. CARR, M. G. CARLSON, D. J. MARON, M. J. BOREL, and P. J. FLAKOLL. Postexercise protein intake enhances whole-body and leg protein accretion in humans. Med. Sci. Sports Exerc., Vol. 34, No. 5, pp. 828-837, 2002.

Levi, B., & Werman, M. J. (1998). Long-term fructose consumption accelerates glycation and several age-related variables in male rats. *The Journal of nutrition, 128*(9), 1442-1449.

Levine, J. A. (2004). Non-exercise activity thermogenesis (NEAT). *Nutrition Reviews, 62*(suppl 2), S82-S97.

Levine, M. E., Suarez, J. A., Brandhorst, S., Balasubramanian, P., Cheng, C.-W., Madia, F., . . . Wan, J. (2014). Low protein intake is associated with a major reduction in IGF-1, cancer, and overall mortality in the 65 and younger but not older population. *Cell Metabolism, 19*(3), 407-417.

Li, M., et al. (2001). "Re[redacted]emergence of iodine deficiency in Australia." Asia Pacific journal of clinical nutrition **10**(3): 200-203.

Li, Q., et al. (2010). "Analysis of glucose levels and the risk for coronary heart disease in elderly patients in Guangzhou Haizhu district." Nan fang yi ke da xue xue bao= Journal of Southern Medical University **30**(6): 1275-1278.

Li, M., Verdijk, L. B., Sakamoto, K., Ely, B., van Loon, L. J., & Musi, N. (2012). Reduced AMPK-ACC and mTOR signaling in muscle from older men, and effect of resistance exercise. *Mechanisms of Ageing and Development, 133*(11), 655-664.

Lin, Y., et al. (2000). "Variability of the conversion of ß-carotene to vitamin A in women measured by using a double-tracer study design." The American journal of clinical nutrition **71**(6): 1545-1554.

Lipovetzky, N., et al. (2004). "Heavy meals as a trigger for a first event of the acute coronary syndrome: a case-crossover study." Isr Med Assoc J **6**(12): 728-731.

Loprinzi, P. D., et al. (2015). "Movement-based behaviors and leukocyte telomere length among US adults." Med Sci Sports Exerc **47**(11): 2347-2352.

Lu, W., Chen, H., Niu, Y., Wu, H., Xia, D., & Wu, Y. (2016). Dairy products intake and cancer mortality risk: a meta-analysis of 11 population-based cohort studies. *Nutrition Journal, 15*(1), 91.

Lyons, D., et al. (1997). "Impaired nitric oxide-mediated vasodilatation and total body nitric oxide production in healthy old age." Clinical Science **93**(6): 519-525.

Macia, L., et al. (2015). "Metabolite-sensing receptors GPR43 and GPR109A facilitate dietary fibre-induced gut homeostasis through regulation of the inflammasome." Nature communications **6**.

MacIntosh, B. R., et al. (2006). Skeletal muscle: form and function, Human Kinetics 1.

Macrina, A. L., et al. (2012). "Oestrone and oestrone sulfate concentrations in milk and milk fractions." Journal of the Academy of Nutrition and Dietetics **112**(7): 1088-1093.

Maedler, K., Oberholzer, J., Bucher, P., Spinas, G. A., & Donath, M. Y. (2003). Monounsaturated fatty acids prevent the deleterious effects of palmitate and high glucose on human pancreatic [redacted]-cell turnover and function. *Diabetes, 52*(3), 726-733.

Mangano, K. M., Walsh, S. J., Kenny, A. M., Insogna, K. L., & Kerstetter, J. E. (2014). Dietary acid load is associated with lower bone mineral density in men with low intake of dietary calcium. *Journal of Bone and Mineral Research, 29*(2), 500-506.

Mansoor, M., et al. (1999). "Plasma total homocysteine response to oral doses of folic acid and pyridoxine hydrochloride (vitamin B6) in healthy individuals. Oral doses of vitamin B6 reduce concentrations of serum folate." Scandinavian journal of clinical and laboratory investigation **59**(2): 139-146.

Margioris, A. N. (2009). Fatty acids and postprandial inflammation. *Current Opinion in Clinical Nutrition & Metabolic Care, 12*(2), 129.

Marsh, K. A., Munn, E. A., & Baines, S. K. (2012). Protein and vegetarian diets. *Med J Aust, 1*(Suppl 2), 7-10.

Martin, C. K., Heilbronn, L. K., Jonge, L., DeLany, J. P., Volaufova, J., Anton, S. D., . . . Ravussin, E. (2007). Effect of calorie restriction on resting metabolic rate and spontaneous physical activity. *Obesity, 15*(12), 2964-2973.

Martin, B. C., et al. (1992). "Role of glucose and insulin resistance in development of type 2 diabetes mellitus: results of a 25-year follow-up study." The Lancet **340**(8825): 925-929.

Maslowski, K., et al. (2009). "Regulation of inflammatory responses by gut microbiota and chemoattractant receptor GPR43." Nature **461**(7268): 1282-1286.

Mason, S. (1962). "Some aspects of gastric function in the newborn." Archives of disease in childhood **37**(194): 387-391.

McCann, J. C. and B. N. Ames (2009). "Vitamin K, an example of triage theory: is micronutrient inadequacy linked to diseases of aging?" The American journal of clinical nutrition **90**(4): 889-907.

McCrady-Spitzer, S. K., & Levine, J. A. (2012). Nonexercise activity thermogenesis: a way forward to treat the worldwide obesity epidemic. *Surgery for Obesity and Related Diseases, 8*(5), 501-506.

McCullough, F., Northrop-Clewes, C., & Thurnham, D. (1999). The effect of vitamin A on epithelial integrity. *Proceedings of the Nutrition Society, 58*(02), 289-293.

McGill, H. C., et al. (2008). "Preventing heart disease in the 21st century." Circulation **117**(9): 1216-1227.

McMillen, M. (2016). "Colorectal Cancers on the Rise in Younger Adults." 2017, from http://www.medscape.com/viewarticle/872749.

McPherson, J. D., Shilton, B. H., & Walton, D. J. (1988). Role of fructose in glycation and cross-linking of proteins. *Biochemistry, 27*(6), 1901-1907.

Melnik, B. C., John, S. M., & Schmitz, G. (2011). Over-stimulation of insulin/IGF-1 signaling by western diet may promote diseases of civilisation: lessons learnt from laron syndrome. *Nutrition & Metabolism, 8*(1), 41.

Merck Manual. Professional Version. http://www.merckmanuals.com/professional

Merksamer, P. I., et al. (2013). "The sirtuins, oxidative stress and aging: an emerging link." Aging (Albany NY) **5**(3): 144-150.

Messier, S. P., Gutekunst, D. J., Davis, C., & DeVita, P. (2005). Weight loss reduces knee joint loads in overweight and obese older adults with knee osteoarthritis. *Arthritis & Rheumatism, 52*(7), 2026-2032.

Milo, R., & Phillips, R. (2015). *Cell biology by the numbers*: Garland Science.

Minehira, K., Bettschart, V., Vidal, H., Vega, N., Vetta, V., Rey, V., . . . Tappy, L. (2003). Effect of carbohydrate overfeeding on whole body and adipose tissue metabolism in humans. *Obesity research, 11*(9), 1096-1103.

Mirmiran, P., Esfandiari, S., Bahadoran, Z., Tohidi, M., & Azizi, F. (2016). Dietary insulin load and insulin index are associated with the risk of insulin resistance: a prospective approach in tehran lipid and glucose study. *Journal of Diabetes & Metabolic Disorders, 15*(1), 23.

Mirsky, S. (2007). The World Is Fat: Obesity Now Outweighs Hunger WorldWide. Scientific American.

Misra, R., et al. (2001). "An unusual photohaemolytic property of riboflavin." Food and chemical toxicology **39**(1): 11-18.

Moore, D., Robinson, M., Fry, J., Tang, J., Glover, E., Wilkinson, S., . . . Phillips, S. (2009). Ingested protein dose response of muscle and albumin protein synthesis after resistance exercise in young men. *Am J Clin Nutr, 89*, 161 - 168.

Moyer, M. W. (2013). The myth of antioxidants. *Scientific American, 308*(2), 62-67.

Müller, M. J., et al. (2010). "Is there evidence for a set point that regulates human body-weight." F1000 Med Rep **2**(59.10): 3410.

Munn, A., et al. (2013). "Energy, water and space use by free-living red kangaroos Macropus rufus and domestic sheep Ovis aries in an Australian rangeland." Journal of Comparative Physiology B **183**(6): 843-858.

Muti, P., Quattrin, T., Grant, B. J., Krogh, V., Micheli, A., Schünemann, H. J., . . . Trevisan, M. (2002). Fasting Glucose Is a Risk Factor For Breast Cancer A Prospective Study. *Cancer Epidemiology Biomarkers & Prevention, 11*(11), 1361-1368.

Health, N. Y. (2016). "Chronic Disease and Conditions ". Retrieved 05/10/2016, 2016, from https://www.health.ny.gov/diseases/chronic/.

Neis, E. P., Dejong, C. H., & Rensen, S. S. (2015). The role of microbial amino acid metabolism in host metabolism. *Nutrients, 7*(4), 2930-2946.

Neuhouser, M. L., et al. (2003). "Fruits and vegetables are associated with lower lung cancer risk only in the placebo arm of the [redacted]-carotene and retinol efficacy trial (CARET)." Cancer Epidemiology Biomarkers & Prevention **12**(4): 350-358.

Newgard, C. B. (2012). "Interplay between lipids and branched-chain amino acids in development of insulin resistance." Cell Metabolism **15**(5): 606-614.

Nguyen, D., et al. (2013). "Impaired mitochondrial fatty acid oxidation and insulin resistance in aging: novel protective role of glutathione." Aging Cell **12**(3): 415-425.

NLM (2017). "What are Single Nucleotide Polymorphisms (SNPs)?". 2017.

Nordio, M., & Pajalich, R. (2013). Combined treatment with Myo-inositol and selenium ensures euthyroidism in subclinical hypothyroidism patients with autoimmune thyroiditis. *Journal of thyroid research, 2013.*

Norton, L. and G. J. WILsoN (2009). "Optimal protein intake to maximise muscle protein synthesis." AgroFood industry hi-tech **20**: 54-57.

O'Donovan, G., et al. "Association of "Weekend Warrior" and Other Leisure Time Physical Activity Patterns With Risks for All-Cause, Cardiovascular Disease, and Cancer Mortality." JAMA Internal Medicine.

O'Hara, A. M., & Shanahan, F. (2006). The gut flora as a forgotten organ. *EMBO reports, 7*(7), 688-693.

O'Keefe, J. H., Gheewala, N. M., & O'Keefe, J. O. (2008). Dietary Strategies for Improving Post-Prandial Glucose, Lipids, Inflammation, and Cardiovascular Health. *J Am Coll Cardiol, 51*(3), 249-255. doi:10.1016/j.jacc.2007.10.016

O'Keefe, J. H. and D. S. Bell (2007). "Postprandial hyperglycemia/hyperlipidemia (postprandial dysmetabolism) is a cardiovascular risk factor." The American Journal of Cardiology **100**(5): 899-904.

O'Sullivan, T. A., Bremner, A. P., O'Neill, S., & Lyons-Wall, P. (2010). Glycemicload is associated with insulin resistance in older Australian women. *European Journal of Clinical Nutrition, 64*(1), 80-87.

Oldstone, M. (1998). Molecular mimicry and immune-mediated diseases. *The FASEB Journal, 12*(13), 1255.

Outwater, J., Nicholson, A., & Barnard, N. (1997). Dairy products and breast cancer: the IGF-I, oestrogen, and bGH hypothesis. *Medical Hypotheses, 48*(6), 453-461.

Ozner, M. D. (2008). The Great American Heart Hoax: Lifesaving Advice Your Doctor Should Tell You about Heart Disease Prevention (But Probably Never Will!), BenBella Books.

Pamplona, R. and G. Barja (2006). "Mitochondrial oxidative stress, aging and caloric restriction: the protein and methionine connection." Biochimica Et Biophysica Acta (BBA)-Bioenergetics **1757**(5): 496-508.

Park, E. J., Thomson, A. B., & Clandinin, M. T. (2010). Protection of intestinal occludin tight junction protein by dietary gangliosides in lipopolysaccharide-induced acute inflammation. *Journal of pediatric gastroenterology and nutrition, 50*(3), 321-328.

Pase, M. P., et al. (2015). "Habitual intake of fruit juice predicts central blood pressure." Appetite **84**: 68-72.

Pepino, M. Y., et al. (2013). "Sucralose affects glycemic and hormonal responses to an oral glucose load." Diabetes Care **36**(9): 2530-2535.

Pingali, P. (2007). Westernization of Asian diets and the transformation of food systems: Implications for research and policy. *Food policy, 32*(3), 281-298.

Pirmohamed, M., James, S., Meakin, S., Green, C., Scott, A. K., Walley, T. J., . . . Breckenridge, A. M. (2004). Adverse drug reactions as cause of admission to hospital: prospective analysis of 18 820 patients. *Bmj, 329*(7456), 15-19.

Pizzorno, L. (2016). "Managing Erectile Dysfunction—When Viagra Doesn't." Longevity Medicine Review. from http://www.lmreview.com/articles/print/l-Citrulline-restoring-erectile-function-viagra-doesnt/.

Pojer, E., et al. (2013). "The case for anthocyanin consumption to promote human health: a review." Comprehensive Reviews in Food Science and Food Safety **12**(5): 483-508.

Pontzer, H., et al. (2016) "Constrained Total Energy Expenditure and Metabolic Adaptation to Physical Activity in Adult Humans." Current Biology.

Popkin, B. M., et al. (2012). "Global nutrition transition and the pandemic of obesity in developing countries." Nutrition Reviews **70**(1): 3-21.

Qiao, Y.-L., et al. (2009). "Total and cancer mortality after supplementation with vitamins and minerals: follow-up of the Linxian General Population Nutrition Intervention Trial." Journal of the National Cancer Institute.

Rand, W. M., Pellett, P. L., & Young, V. R. (2003). Meta-analysis of nitrogen balance studies for estimating protein requirements in healthy adults. *The American journal of clinical nutrition, 77*(1), 109-127.

Rea, P. A. and A. Y. Tien (2017). "Metformin: Out of Backwaters and into the Mainstream." American Scientist **105**(2): 102.

Redlich, G., Zanger, U. M., Riedmaier, S., Bache, N., Giessing, A. B., Eisenacher, M., . . . Marcus, K. (2008). Distinction between human cytochrome P450 (CYP) isoforms and identification of new phosphorylation sites by mass spectrometry. *Journal of proteome research, 7*(11), 4678-4688.

Richman, E. L., Kenfield, S. A., Stampfer, M. J., Giovannucci, E. L., & Chan, J. M. (2011). Egg, red meat, and poultry intake and risk of lethal prostate cancer in the prostate-specific antigen-era: incidence and survival. *Cancer Prevention Research.*

Rimm, E. B., et al. (1998). "Folate and vitamin B6 from diet and supplements in relation to risk of coronary heart disease among women." JAMA **279**(5): 359-364.

Risbridger, G. P., Bianco, J. J., Ellem, S. J., & McPherson, S. J. (2003). Oestrogens and prostate cancer. *Endocrine-Related Cancer, 10*(2), 187-191.

Ross, R. G., et al. (2013). "Perinatal choline effects on neonatal pathophysiology related to later schizophrenia risk." American Journal of PsyChiatry **170**(3): 290-298.

Round, J. L., & Mazmanian, S. K. (2009). The gut microbiota shapes intestinal immune responses during health and disease. *Nature Reviews Immunology, 9*(5), 313-323.

Salway, J. (2006). Medical biochemistry at a glance, Wiley-Blackwell.

Salway, J., & Granner, D. (2004). *Metabolism at a Glance*: Blackwell Pub.

Sanders, L. (2010). Every patient tells a story: medical mysteries and the art of diagnosis, Harmony Books.

Sandhu, M. S., et al. (2002). "Insulin, insulin-like growth factor-I (IGF-I), IGF binding proteins, their biologic interactions, and colorectal cancer." Journal of the National Cancer Institute **94**(13): 972-980.

Sarris, J., et al. (2015). "Nutritional medicine as mainstream in psychiatry." The Lancet Psychiatry **2**(3): 271-274.

Scientific American Reports. (2006). Eating to Live. Special Edition. Scientific American.

Scrimshaw, et al. (1968). Interactions of nutrition and infection, World Health Organization.

Selvin, E., et al. (2010). "Glycated hemoglobin, diabetes, and cardiovascular risk in nondiabetic adults." N Engl J Med **2010** (362): 800-811.

Shaw, J., & Tanamas, S. (2012). Diabetes: the silent pandemic and its impact on Australia. *Melbourne: Baker IDI Heart and Diabetes Institute.*

Shepherd, S. J. and P. R. Gibson (2006). "Fructose malabsorption and symptoms of irritable bowel syndrome: guidelines for effective dietary management." Journal of the American Dietetic Association **106**(10): 1631-1639.

Shi, J., et al. (2005). Asian functional foods, CRC press.

Simopoulos, A. P., & Sidossis, L. (2000). What is so special about the traditional diet of Greece. *Mediterranean Diets. World Rev Nutr Diet, 87*, 24-42.

Singh, M. (2005). "Essential fatty acids, DHA and human brain." Indian Journal of Pediatrics **72**(3): 239-242.

Soldatos, G., & Cooper, M. E. (2006). Advanced glycation end products and vascular structure and function. *Current hypertension reports, 8*(6), 472-478.

Song, B., & Thomas, D. M. (2007). Dynamics of starvation in humans. *Journal of mathematical biology, 54*(1), 27-43.

Spector, T. (2015). *The Diet Myth: The Real Science Behind What We Eat*: Hachette UK.

Spence, J. D. (2002). "Importance of diet in vascular prevention: vastly underestimated." Circulation **106**(18): e133-e133.

Steiber, A., Kerner, J., & Hoppel, C. L. (2004). Carnitine: a nutritional, biosynthetic, and functional perspective. *Molecular Aspects of Medicine, 25*(5), 455-473.

Stipp, D. (2012). A new path to longevity. *Scientific American, 306*(1), 32-39.

St-Onge, M.-P., et al. (2017). "Meal timing and frequency: implications for cardiovascular disease prevention: a scientific statement from the American Heart Association." Circulation **135**(9): e96-e121.

Strasser, S. I. and V. Pattullo (2017). "Managing the rising burden of chronic liver disease: non-alcoholic fatty liver disease and alcoholic liver disease."

Strong, K., Mathers, C., Leeder, S., & Beaglehole, R. (2005). Preventing chronic diseases: how many lives can we save? *TheLancet, 366*(9496), 1578-1582.

Sturniolo, G., et al. (1991). "Inhibition of gastric acid secretion reduces zinc absorption in man." Journal of the American College of Nutrition **10**(4): 372-375.

Suharno D, West CE, Muhilal, Karyadi D, Hautvast JG. Supplementation with vitamin A and iron for nutritional anaemia in pregnant women in West Java, Indonesia. Lancet. 1993;342(8883):1325-1328.

Sulakvelidze, A., et al. (2001). "Bacteriophage therapy." Antimicrobial agents and chemotherapy **45**(3): 649-659.

Tabá, G., Herder, C., Rathmann, W., Brunner, E., & Kivimäk, M. (2012). Prediabetes: A High-Risk State for Developing Diabetes. *Lancet, 379*(9833), 2279-2290.

Temme, E., Mensink, R. P., & Hornstra, G. (1997). Effects of medium chain fatty acids (MCFA), myristic acid, and oleic acid on serum lipoproteins in healthy subjects. *Journal of lipid research, 38*(9), 1746-1754.

TGA (2010). Australian Public Assessment Report for Omega-3-acid ethyl esters 90. Department of Health & Ageing. Therapeutic Goods Administration.

Thaiss, C. A., et al. (2016). "Persistent microbiome alterations modulate the rate of post-dieting weight regain." Nature 540(7634): 544-551.

Time. (2012). What If the World's Soil Runs Out? *Time.* Retrieved from http://world.time.com/2012/12/14/what-if-the-worlds-soil-runs-out/

Tidball, J. G. (2005). "Inflammatory processes in muscle injury and repair." American Journal of Physiology-Regulatory, Integrative and Comparative Physiology **288**(2): R345-R353.

Thorburn, A. N., McKenzie, C. I., Shen, S., Stanley, D., Macia, L., Mason, L. J., . . . Robert, R. (2015). Evidence that asthma is a developmental origin disease influenced by maternal diet and bacterial metabolites. *Nature communications, 6.*

Thyroid Foundation Ltd, T. A. "Iodine Deficiency & Nutrition ". 2017, from https://www.thyroidfoundation.org.au/page/13/iodine-nutrition-iodine-deficiency.

Tofler, G. H. and J. E. Muller (2006). "Triggering of acute cardiovascular disease and potential preventive strategies." Circulation **114**(17): 1863-1872.

Trialists'Collaboration, A. (2002). "Collaborative meta-analysis of randomised trials of antiplatelet therapy for prevention of death, myocardial infarction, and stroke in high risk patients." Bmj **324**(7329): 71-86.

Twigg, S. M., Kamp, M. C., Davis, T. M., Neylon, E. K., & Flack, J. R. (2007). prediabetes: a position statement from the australian diabetes society and australian diabetes educators association. *Medical Journal of Australia, 186*(9), 461.

van Baak, M. A. (2008). "Meal-induced activation of the sympathetic nervous system and its cardiovascular and thermogenic effects in man." Physiology & Behavior **94**(2): 178-186.

Vander Heiden, M. G., et al. (2009). "Understanding the Warburg effect: the metabolic requirements of cell proliferation." Science **324**(5930): 1029-1033.

Vighi, G., et al. (2008). "Allergy and the gastrointestinal system." Clinical & Experimental Immunology **153**(s1): 3-6.

Vigneri, P. G., et al. (2015). "The insulin/IGF system in colorectal cancer development and resistance to therapy." Frontiers in oncology **5**: 230.

Villamena, F. A. (2013). *Molecular basis of oxidative stress: chemistry, mechanisms, and disease pathogenesis*: John Wiley & Sons.

Vuksan, V., et al. (2010). "Reduction in postprandial glucose excursion and prolongation of satiety: possible explanation of the long-term effects of whole grain Salba (Salvia Hispanica L.)." European Journal of Clinical Nutrition **64**(4): 436-438.

Wang, X. and P. J. Quinn (2010). Endotoxins: structure, function and recognition, Springer Science & Business Media.

Wester, K., et al. (2008). "Incidence of fatal adverse drug reactions: a population based study." British journal of clinical pharmacology **65**(4): 573-579.

Westerterp-Plantenga, M., Luscombe-Marsh, N., Lejeune, M., Diepvens, K., Nieuwenhuizen, A., Engelen, M., . . . Westerterp, K. (2006). Dietary protein, metabolism, and body weightregulation: dose–response effects. *International Journal of Obesity, 30*, S16-S23.

WHO, E. C. (2008). "Waist circumference and waist-hip ratio." Report of a WHO Expert Consultation Geneva: World Health Organization: 8-11.

Wiklund, O., et al. (1996). "N-acetylcysteine treatment lowers plasma homocysteine but not serum lipoprotein (a) levels." Atherosclerosis **119**(1): 99-106.

Willems, J. L. and N. H. Low (2012). "Major carbohydrate, polyol, and oligosaccharide profiles of agave syrup. Application of this data to authenticity analysis." Journal of Agricultural and Food Chemistry **60**(35): 8745-8754.

Willett, W. (2006). "Multivitamins: Should you buy this insurance?". from http://www.health.harvard.edu/newsletter_article/multivitamins-should-you-buy-this-insurance.

Williams, M. (2005). "Dietary supplements and sports performance: amino acids." Journal of the International Society of Sports Nutrition **2**(2): 63.

Wilmore, J., Costill, D., & Kenney, W. (2008). *Physiology of sport and exercise*: Human Kinetics Publishers.

Wilson, J. D. (1980). The pathogenesis of benign prostatic hyperplasia. *The American journal of medicine, 68*(5), 745-756.

Wolk, A. (2016). "Potential health hazards of eating red meat." Journal of internal medicine.

Women's and Children's Health Network (2012). Low fructose diet for children. Pamphlet. Department of Health, South Australian Government.

Wright, M. E., et al. (2007). "Supplemental and dietary vitamin E intakes and risk of prostate cancer in a large prospective study." Cancer Epidemiology and Prevention Biomarkers **16**(6): 1128-1135.

Xu, Q., et al. (2009). "Multivitamin use and telomere length in women." The American journal of clinical nutrition: ajcn. 26986.

Yeum, K. J., & Russell, R. M. (2002). Carotenoid bioavailability and bioconversion. *Annual review of nutrition, 22*(1), 483-504.

Yoon, M.-S. (2016). The Emerging Role of Branched-Chain Amino Acids in Insulin Resistance and Metabolism. *Nutrients,* 8(7), 405.

Zaletel, K., & Gaberscek, S. (2011). Hashimoto's thyroiditis: from genes to the disease. *Current genomics, 12*(8), 576-588.

Zambelli, B. and S. Ciurli (2013). Nickel and human health. Interrelations between Essential Metal Ions and Human Diseases, Springer: 321-357.

Zambito, D. A. (2007). Oestrogens in bovine milk: Effects of milk synthesis, The Pennsylvania State University.

Zeisel, S. H. (2004). "Nutritional importance of choline for brain development." Journal of the American College of Nutrition **23**(suppl 6): 621S-626S.

Zeevi, D., et al. (2015). "Personalised nutrition by prediction of glycemic responses." Cell **163**(5): 1079-1094.

Zeisel, S. H. and K.-A. Da Costa (2009). "Choline: an essential nutrient for public health." Nutrition Reviews **67**(11): 615-623.

Zipes, D. P. and H. J. Wellens (1998). "Sudden cardiac death." Circulation **98**(21): 2334-2351.

Zhang, C., et al. (2015). "Dietary modulation of gut microbiota contributes to alleviation of both genetic and simple obesity in children." EBioMedicine **2**(8): 968-984.

Zhang, Z., et al. (2001). Boron is associated with decreased risk of human prostate cancer. FASEB JOURNAL, FEDERATION AMER SOC EXP BIOL 9650 ROCKVILLE PIKE, BETHESDA, MD 20814-3998 USA.

Zota, A. R., et al. (2016). "Recent fast food consumption and bisphenol A and phthalates exposures among the US population in NHANES, 2003-2010." Environmental Health Perspectives.

Index

ABOUT THE AUTHOR

Dr Rodney Lopez MBBS (Sydney University), GradCertNutriMed (RMIT)

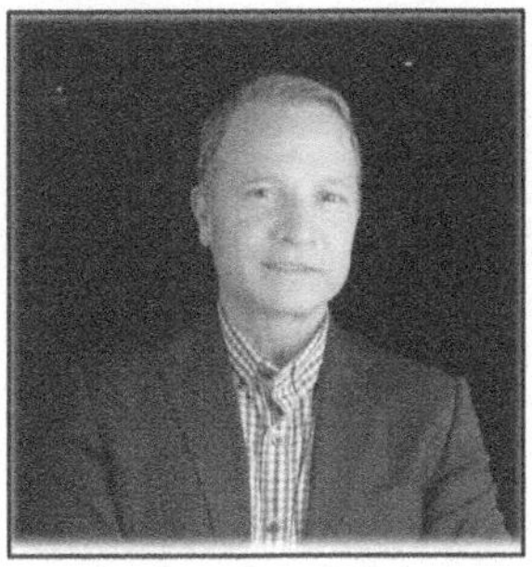

I graduated from the Faculty of Medicine at Sydney University, Australia in 1983. I was a fully qualified laboratory technician prior to medical studies and worked at the Institute of Clinical Pathology and Medical Research (ICPMR) before undertaking medical studies. I also worked in the Biochemistry laboratory at Westmead Hospital, Sydney as an undergraduate. My interest in preventative health care propelled me to study clinical nutrition and functional medicine with postgraduate qualifications from RMIT University, Melbourne in 2009. I continue to work full-time in general practice and constantly hone my skills and knowledge in medical practice and I avidly consume new and cutting-edge knowledge in clinical nutrition and preventative healthcare. The age of clinical nutrition as adjunctive treatment for a myriad number of diseases is now emerging as a powerful force in medicine. I hope you enjoy this book which is the culmination of many years of study.

Made in United States
Cleveland, OH
05 November 2026

47656818R00172